Gems of Ophthalm
GLAUCOM,

Gems of Ophthalmology
GLAUCOMA

Editors

HV Nema MS
Former Professor and Head
Department of Ophthalmology
Institute of Medical Sciences
Banaras Hindu University
Varanasi, Uttar Pradesh, India

Nitin Nema MS DNB
Professor
Department of Ophthalmology
Sri Aurobindo Institute of Medical Sciences
Indore, Madhya Pradesh, India

JAYPEE *The Health Sciences Publisher*
New Delhi | London | Panama

Jaypee Brothers Medical Publishers (P) Ltd

Headquarters
Jaypee Brothers Medical Publishers (P) Ltd.
4838/24, Ansari Road, Daryaganj
New Delhi 110 002, India
Phone: +91-11-43574357
Fax: +91-11-43574314
E-mail: jaypee@jaypeebrothers.com

Overseas Offices

JP Medical Ltd.
83 Victoria Street, London
SW1H 0HW (UK)
Phone: +44-20 3170 8910
Fax: +44(0)20 3008 6180
E-mail: info@jpmedpub.com

Jaypee-Highlights Medical Publishers Inc.
City of Knowledge, Bld. 235, 2nd Floor, Clayton
Panama City, Panama
Phone: +1 507-301-0496
Fax: +1 507-301-0499
E-mail: cservice@jphmedical.com

Jaypee Brothers Medical Publishers (P) Ltd.
17/1-B, Babar Road, Block-B, Shyamoli
Mohammadpur, Dhaka-1207
Bangladesh
Mobile: +08801912003485
E-mail: jaypeedhaka@gmail.com

Jaypee Brothers Medical Publishers (P) Ltd.
Bhotahity, Kathmandu, Nepal
Phone: +977-9741283608
E-mail: kathmandu@jaypeebrothers.com

Website: www.jaypeebrothers.com
Website: www.jaypeedigital.com

Inquiries for bulk sales may be solicited at: jaypee@jaypeebrothers.com

Gems of Ophthalmology—Glaucoma

First Edition: 2018

ISBN: 978-93-5270-249-7

Printed at: Sanat Printers

Contributors

Mermoud A MD
Professor
Department of Glaucoma
Hospital Ophtalmique
Jules-Gonin University of Lausanne
Lausanne, Switzerland

Murali A MS DNB FAICO
Head
Department of Glaucoma
MN Eye Hospital, Chennai
Director
Swamy Eye Clinic
Chennai, Tamil Nadu, India

Narayanaswamy A MS
Research Associate
Singapore Eye Hospital
Singapore

Parivadhini A MS
Consultant
Glaucoma Service
Department of Glaucoma
Sankara Nethralaya
Chennai, Tamil Nadu, India

Aparna AC MS
Consultant
Department of Glaucoma
MN Eye Hospital
Chennai, Tamil Nadu, India

Mandal AK MD
Director
Jasti V Ramanamma Children's
Eye Care Centre
LV Prasad Eye Institute
Hyderabad, Telangana, India

Rajendra K Bansal MD
Associate Clinical Professor
Department of Ophthalmology
Edward S Harkness Eye Institute
Columbia University Medical Center
NYC, New York, USA

Marshall DH MD FRCSC
Department of Ophthalmology and
Visual Sciences
University of Wisconsin System
Madison, Wisconsin, USA

Chandra Sekhar G MS FRCS
Director
LV Prasad Eye Institute
Hyderabad, Telangana, India

Puthuran GV MS
Consultant
Department of Glaucoma
Aravind Eye Hospital
Madurai, Tamil Nadu, India

Savleen Kaur MS
Senior Research Associate
Glaucoma Service
Advanced Eye Centre
Postgraduate Institute of Medical Education
and Research
Chandigarh, India

Kiran Chandra Kedarisetti MBBS
Junior Resident
Advanced Eye Centre
Postgraduate Institute of Medical Education
and Research
Chandigarh, India

Deshpande KV MS
Consultant
Mahatme Eye Bank and Eye Hospital
Mumbai, Maharashtra, India

Vijaya L MS
Senior Consultant
Glaucoma Service
Department of Glaucoma
Sankara Nethralaya
Chennai, Tamil Nadu, India

Moorthy LP MS
Senior Glaucoma Fellow
Zeiss Centre of Excellence in Glaucoma
Aravind Eye Hospital
Tirunelveli, Tamil Nadu, India

Gandhi M MS
Senior Consultant
Glaucoma and Anterior Segment
Dr Shroff Charity Eye Hospital
New Delhi, India

Malleswari M MS
Consultant
Glaucoma Service
Aravind Eye Hospital and
Postgraduate Institute
Madurai, Tamil Nadu, India

Nivean M MS FMRF
Consultant
Department of Vitreoretina
MN Eye Hospital
Chennai, Tamil Nadu, India

Palani M DO DNB FAICO (UK)
Consultant
Department of Glaucoma
MN Eye Hospital
Chennai, Tamil Nadu, India

Arjit Mitra MS
Consultant
Glaucoma Service
Aravind Eye Hospital
Tirunelveli, Tamil Nadu, India

Madhivanan N MS FMRF
Consultant
Department of Vitreoretina
MN Eye Hospital
Chennai, Tamil Nadu, India

Rangaraj NR MS DO
Director
Premier Eyecare and Surgical Center
Chennai, Tamil Nadu, India

Choudhari NS MS
Consultant
Department of Glaucoma
LV Prasad Eye Institute
Hyderabad, Telangana, India

Albis-Donado O MD
Ophthalmologist-Glaucoma
Associate Professor
Instituto Mexicano de Oftalmologia lap
Queretaro, Mexico

Ichhpujani P MD
Assistant Professor
Glaucoma and Neuro-ophthalmology
Government Medical College and Hospital
Chandigarh, India

Netland PA MD PhD
Siegel Professor of Ophthalmology
Hamilton Eye Institute
The University Tennessee
Health Science Center
Memphis, Tennessee, USA

Ki Ho Park MD
Assistant Professor
Department of Ophthalmology
Seoul National University
College of Medicine
Seoul, South Korea

Maris PJG Jr MD
Edward S Harkness Eye Institute
Columbia University Medical Center
NYC, New York, USA

Bhagat PR MS
Associate Professor
Glaucoma Clinic
M&J Western Regional Institute of
Ophthalmology
Civil Hospital and BJ Medical College
Ahmedabad, Gujarat, India

David R MS DNB
Associate Consultant
Department of Glaucoma
Sankara Nethralaya
Chennai, Tamil Nadu, India

Krishnadas R MS
Chief Medical Officer and Consultant
Glaucoma Service
Aravind Eye Hospital and
Postgraduate Institute
Madurai, Tamil Nadu, India

Sindhushree R MS FICO FAICO (Glaucoma)
Consultant
Aravind Eye Hospital
Tirunelveli, Tamil Nadu, India

R Ramakrishnan MS
Professor and Chief Medical Officer
Aravind Eye Hospital
Tirunelveli, Tamil Nadu, India

George RJ MS
Senior Consultant
Department of Glaucoma
Sankara Nethralaya
Chennai, Tamil Nadu, India

Bhartiya S MD
Consultant
Glaucoma Service
Fortis Memorial Research Institute
Gurugram, Haryana, India

Kaushik S MS
Professor
Glaucoma Service
Advanced Eye Centre
Postgraduate Institute of Medical Education
and Research
Chandigarh, India

Rajagopal S DO DNB
Consultant
Department of Retina
MN Eye Hospital
Chennai, Tamil Nadu, India

Chandravanshi SL MS
Associate Professor
Department of Ophthalmology
SS Medical College
Rewa, Madhya Pradesh, India

Pandav SS MS
Professor
Glaucoma Service
Advanced Eye Centre
Postgraduate Institute of Medical Education
and Research
Chandigarh, India

Dada T MD
Professor
Dr Rajendra Prasad Centre for
Ophthalmic Sciences
All India Institute of Medical Sciences
New Delhi, India

Shaarawy T MD
Professor
Department of Glaucoma
Hospital Ophtalmique
Jules-Gonin University of Lausanne
Lausanne, Switzerland

James C Tsai MD
Associate Professor of Ophthalmology
Director, Glaucoma Division
Edward S Harkness Eye Institute
Columbia University Medical Center
NYC, New York, USA

Perkins TW MD
Professor
Department of Ophthalmology and
Visual Sciences
University of Wisconsin System
Madison, Wisconsin, USA

Gothwal VK Opt M Appl Sc
Optometrist
LV Prasad Eye Institute
Hyderabad, Telangana, India

Preface

Glaucoma is a progressive optic neuropathy marked by damage to optic nerve head associated with visual field defects. It is the second important cause of blindness worldwide. According to one estimate there are more than 67 million people affected by glaucoma of which about 10% are blind. The blindness caused by glaucoma is irreversible. The glaucoma blindness may be silent or painful and stormy. It is estimated that by 2020, glaucoma may affect 80 million people globally. It is predicted that majority of people will be affected by primary open angle glaucoma (POAG) but primary angle closure glaucoma (PACG) will be more common in Asians. The disease is likely to cause bilateral blindness in more than 11 million individuals. Projection of glaucoma for the year 2040 is also reported; it is estimated that the number of people affected by glaucoma worldwide is likely to increase to 111.8 million.

Early detection and proper treatment of glaucoma can prevent blindness. Many tests are available for the diagnosis of glaucoma even in the early stage. Besides diagnosis, tests help in monitoring the treatment. The state-of-the-art glaucoma detection technology includes intraocular pressure recording, visual field testing, pachymetry, gonioscopy, digital fundus photography of optic nerve, retinal nerve fiber layer analysis by optical coherence tomography (OCT), anterior segment OCT and ultrasound biomicroscopy. As soon as glaucoma is detected, the treatment must be instituted immediately. Treatment includes topical or systemic medication or both, laser therapy and conventional filtration surgery.

The book on Glaucoma presents a detail account of routine glaucoma investigations, such as gonioscopy, optic nerve and visual fields examinations as well as advanced imaging technology. Different types of secondary glaucoma, uveitic, pigmentary, pseudoexfoliative, traumatic, neovascular, phacomorphic, etc. have been described in detail. The developmental glaucoma and management of glaucoma with coexisting cataract are also covered in the book. Treatment modalities, such as medical, laser and surgery of developmental and adult glaucoma have been described adequately.

The book is multi-authored, therefore, repetition could not be avoided. Readers can take the advantage of knowing the views of different authors. However, special effort has been put to avoid ambiguity.

The editors assure the readers that the major part of the work presented in this book comes from the Recent Advances in Ophthalmology series, edited by Dr HV Nema and Dr Nitin Nema. In each chapter, author/s have provided references to published work of their own group as well as relevant references from other experts for the benefit of those readers who want to read the topic in detail.

Hopefully, the book will help postgraduates, residents and general ophthalmologists to understand glaucoma in a better way and enable them to treat glaucoma at an early stage to prevent blindness.

HV Nema MS
Nitin Nema MS DNB

Acknowledgments

We wish to record our grateful thanks to all authors for their spontaneity, cooperation and hard work. Some of them have revised their chapters. Our special thanks go to Drs R Ramakrishnan, Murali Ariga, Malarchelvi Palani, Sushma Kaushik and Shibal Bhartiya for contributing their chapters on a short notice.

Credit goes to Mr Jitendar P Vij (Group Chairman), Jaypee Brothers Medical Publishers (P) Ltd who has agreed to start a new series—Gems of Ophthalmology. *Glaucoma* is the third book of this series.

Ms Charu Bali Siddhu and Ms Kritika Dua, Development Editors deserve our appreciation for her continued interest in refining chapters and eliminating plagiarism.

Contents

1

Gonioscopy

George RJ, Parivadhini A, Narayanaswamy A, Vijaya L

Gonioscopy, the visualization and assessment of the anterior chamber angle, is an essential procedure in the diagnosis and management of glaucoma. Gonioscopy serves two purposes:
1. To identify the eyes at risk for angle closure.
2. To detect any abnormalities in the angle.

Both of these can help in differentiating one type of glaucoma from another and provide guidance for appropriate therapy. The term *gonioscopy* was coined by Trantas in 1907. Subsequently, Goldmann introduced the gonioprism, and Barkan mastered the art of gonioscopy and highlighted its role in the management of glaucoma. All cases of glaucoma should undergo a routine and periodic gonioscopic evaluation for complete ophthalmic examination. The procedure is fairly easy to perform, but experience is needed for an accurate assessment and interpretation.

OPTICAL PRINCIPLES

The anatomy of the eye is such that the angle recess is not visualized by routine instrumentation due to total internal reflection of rays emerging from the angle recess. The gonioscope was evolved to overcome this optical problem of critical angle at the air–cornea interface (41°) (Fig. 1.1).

TYPES OF GONIOSCOPY

Direct Gonioscopy—Lenses

Direct gonioscopy is performed with the aid of concave contact lenses (e.g. Koeppe) placed over an anesthetized cornea with the patient in supine

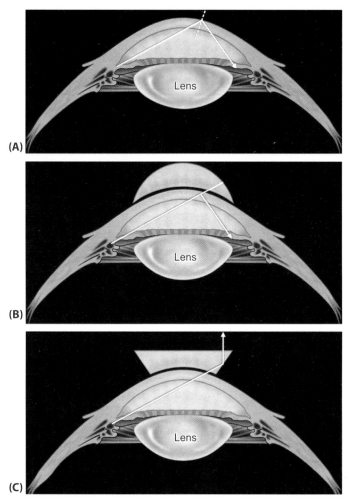

Figs. 1.1A to C: Optical principles of gonioscopy: (A) Incident light from angle exceeds critical angle resulting in total internal reflection and preventing visibility of the recess. (B and C) The gonio lens optically eliminates the cornea as shown in the schematic diagrams and allows visibility of the angle.

position and the space between the lens and cornea filled with normal saline or methyl cellulose as a coupling agent. Viewing is achieved directly using a handheld biomicroscope and an illuminator. Alternatively, the operating microscope can be used to evaluate the angle of the anterior chamber by making appropriate adjustments. Koeppe's lenses (Fig. 1.2A) are available in diameters of 16 and 18 mm, allowing easy use in pediatric patients. This technique can be practiced both in the outpatient clinic as well as in the operation theater. A major advantage of this method is that it allows simultaneous comparison of different quadrants of the angle. Apart from the diagnostic value, lenses like the Swan Jacob (Fig. 1.2B) and Barkan and Thorpe, Mori upright gonio lens aid in surgical intervention (Fig. 1.2C).

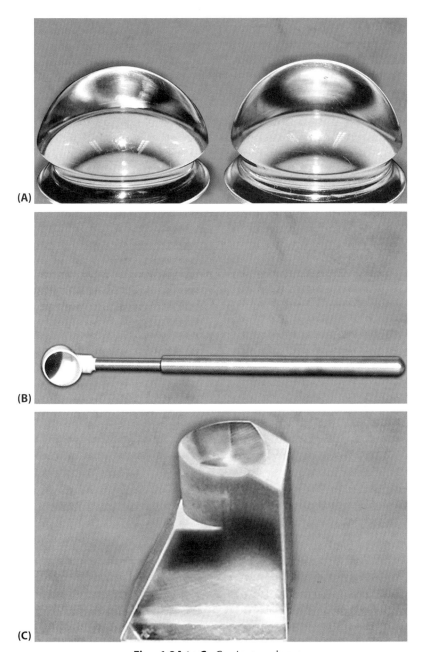

Figs. 1.2A to C: Gonioscopy lenses.

Indirect Gonioscopy Mirrors

Indirect gonioscopy employs reflecting prisms (e.g., Goldmann lens) mounted in a contact lens and angulated at appropriate degrees to evaluate the angle structures using the slit-lamp (Table 1.1). The most popular lenses are the Goldmann type (Fig. 1.3A), Sussman (Fig. 1.3B), Posner (Fig. 1.3C) and Zeiss four-mirrors (Fig. 1.4).

Table 1.1: Contact lenses used for gonioscopy.

Type	Lenses	Features
Direct		
	1. Koeppe	Diagnostic lens—50 diopters concave lens available in two sizes for infants (16 mm) and adults (18 mm)
	2. Barkan	Surgical lens—available in various sizes and has blunted edges, allowing access for goniotomy
	3. Thorpe	Surgical and diagnostic lens
	4. Swan-Jacob	Surgical lens for goniotomy
	5. Mori	Surgical lens for goniosurgery
	6. Layden	Diagnostic lens for evaluating neonatal angle
Indirect		
	1. Goldmann single mirror and three mirrors	Diagnostic and therapeutic lenses, provide excellent images with good magnification and globe stability
	2. Zeiss and Posner four mirrors	Ideal diagnostic lenses, patient-friendly and very valuable in evaluating narrow angles and to perform identation gonioscopy
	3. Sussman four mirrors	Handheld four mirrors similar advantages as the Zeiss lenses
	4. Ritch trabeculoplasty lens	Four-mirrored lens with pairs inclined at 59° and 62°. One of each set has a convex lens over it providing magnification—both diagnostic and therapeutic

Note: Goldmann lenses (Fig. 1.3A), are of two types: (i) Single mirrored—has a mirror angulated at 62°, (ii) Three-mirrored lens—has mirrors at 59° (tongue-shaped, used to evaluate the angle), 67° (midsized, used to view midperipheral fundus) and 73° (long, used to view peripheral fundus and ciliary body). The central well has a diameter of 12 mm and radius of curvature of 7.38 mm. A newer modified version with 8.4 mm radius of curvature eliminates the need of using a coupling solution. The three mirrors also aid in retinal evaluation and laser therapy.

Zeiss lens (has under holder), Sussman (handheld) four-mirrors (Fig. 1.3B) or Posner (has a screw-in handle) (Fig. 1.3C) has mirrors angulated at 64° spaced at 90° intervals and are among the most popular gonioscopy lenses. The Zeiss four-mirrors (Fig. 1.4) eliminates the need for rotation to evaluate the angle and its radius of curvature is 7.8 mm, closer to the corneal curvature, thereby eliminating the need for a viscous coupling agent. The diameter of the lens is 9.0 mm, which aids in dynamic or compression gonioscopy, an important technique in evaluating narrow angles and angle-closure glaucomas.

Manipulative gonioscopy can be performed by Goldmann two mirror lenses in which the patient is asked to look in the direction of angle to be visualized with pressure on the cornea. Indentation gonioscopy can be performed with Zeiss, Posner and Sussman lenses wherein indentation of the

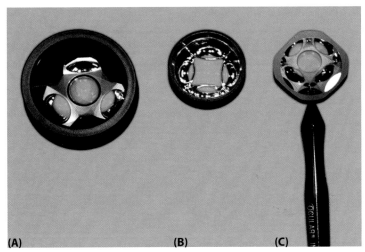

Figs. 1.3A to C: (A) Goldmann lens. (B) Sussman lens. (C) Posner four-mirror lens.

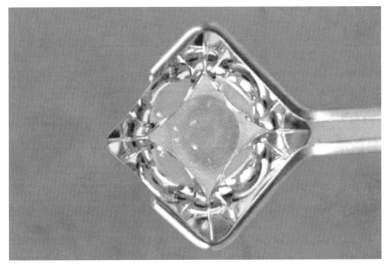

Fig. 1.4: Zeiss four-mirror lens.

central cornea displaces the aqueous into peripheral angle-closure, pushes the iris backward and widens the chamber angle.

PROTOCOL FOR A ROUTINE GONOSCOPY

- Explain the procedure to the patient
- Reassure the patient and ensure cooperation
- Corneal surface is examined to rule out any contraindication for gonioscopy (abrasion, infection, significant corneal edema or opacity).
- Adequate anesthesia is ensured using either 0.5% topical proparacaine or 4.0% lignocaine.

- The patient and examiner should be in a comfortable posture with adequate support to examiner's forearm and elbow to make sure of good control and minimal pressure over the eye throughout the procedure.
- The lens is held in the examiner's left hand for evaluating the right eye and vice versa.
- The three-mirror gonioscope is filled with viscous solutions and inserted as shown in Figure 1.5. The four-mirror Zeiss lens is applied directly.
- The patient is asked to maintain a straight gaze once the lens is in situ.
- Low, but adequate illumination (darkroom) and small beams (1 mm) are focused on the mirror, with viewing and illumination maintained in the same axis. The illumination arm is moved paraxial when needed to evaluate the nasal and temporal recesses. Magnification and illumination can be increased when needed to evaluate finer details like new vessels and foreign bodies.
- One quadrant can be evaluated at a time with the three-mirror by sequential rotation while with the four-mirror all four quadrants can be evaluated without rotation and with minimum adjustments of the slit-lamp. Always remember the opposite quadrant (e.g., with mirror at 7 o'clock, the 1 o'clock angle) is being evaluated and the image is reversed but not crossed.
- Other dynamic maneuvers like compression and over-the-hill evaluation are subsequently done. Over-the-hill maneuver involves asking the patient to look in the direction of the mirror, which in turn gives access to viewing angle recess over the convex iris. Compression techniques will be dealt with subsequently.

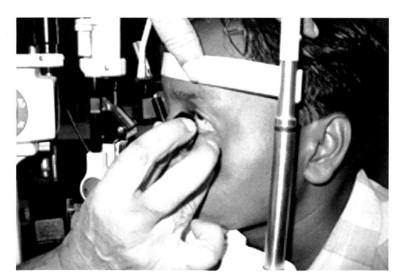

Fig. 1.5: The inferior rim of four-mirrors gonioscope is inserted in the lower fornix with patient in upgaze as shown and swiftly tilted on to the cornea preventing loss of any coupling fluid.

- Disinfection of lenses is necessary prior and after every use because of the potential of transmitting infection. Lenses can be swiped dry with bacillocid (2% glutearaldehyde) or alternatively lenses can be rinsed with soap solution and water and allowed to dry.

GONIOSCOPIC ANATOMY AND INTERPRETATION

Repeated and routine normal gonioscopic studies are essential in adding to one's experience in evaluating a pathological angle. A methodical evaluation of each structure from iris plane to Schwalbe's line should curtail errors in interpretation (Fig. 1.6).

To start with, from the peripheral iris plane one can follow upward to the insertion of iris root. The contour of iris has several variations. The normal adult eye has a slightly convex contour. The same may be exaggerated in hyperopic eyes, where in the anterior segment it is crowded. A flat iris configuration is commonly associated with myopia and aphakia. A flat iris configuration with a peripheral convex roll or hump of iris that lies in close relation to the trabecular meshwork and can be seen in phakic normal eyes, which often mimics a narrow angle and is referred to as *plateau iris configuration*. Contours could also be concave and are associated with high myopes and pigment dispersion syndrome. The insertion of iris root may vary from posterior, anterior or high insertions, thereby determining the visibility of the ciliary body band and the contour and depth of angle recess. The ciliary body band is composed of the anterior end of ciliary muscle and is seen as a slate gray or dark brown uniform band when insertion of iris root is posterior, anterior and high insertions preclude its view. An unusually wide ciliary body band may be seen in myopes and aphakes and may be confused with angle recession, but comparative gonioscopy and other signs of trauma help to distinguish between the normal and the pathological.

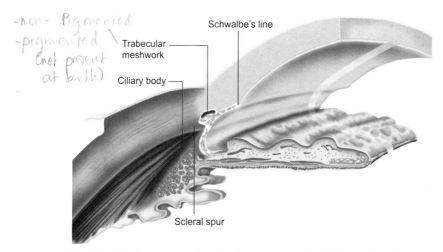

(handwritten annotation: -non- Pigmented / -pigmented (not present at birth))

Schwalbe's line

Trabecular meshwork

Ciliary body

Scleral spur

Fig. 1.6: Gonioscopic landmarks of a normal angle of the anterior chamber.

The next anterior transition is the scleral spur, the most prominent and most important landmark, identification of which is vital in terms of orientation of the angle. The scleral spur is the posterior lip of the scleral sulcus and is attached to the ciliary body band posteriorly and to the corneoscleral portion of trabecular meshwork anteriorly. It is visible as a glistening opaque white line between the ciliary body band and trabecular meshwork; however, identification at times may be difficult when the trabeculum is nonpigmented. The scleral spur may be obscured in the presence of dense pigmentation of angle structures like in posttraumatic or postsurgical situations. Iris processes, which are fine uveal strands arising from anterior iris surface and running up to the corneoscleral meshwork may also prevent a good view especially when they are prominent, as seen in congenital glaucomas. The spur is not visible in the presence of peripheral anterior synechiae (PAS) or appositional angle closure on routine gonioscopy.

The trabecular meshwork has a posterior functional, more pigmented portion and a less functional nonpigmented anterior portion. The corneoscleral part of the meshwork extends from the scleral spur to the Schwalbe's line. The pigmentation of the meshwork varies with the kind of eyes, age and other pathological conditions. Brown eyes and adult eyes tend to have a deeper pigmentation compared to blue eyes and younger individuals. A nonpigmented trabecular meshwork may often present a tricky situation as far as accurate assessment is concerned, since its color and texture seems to merge with the scleral spur. However, a careful evaluation reveals it to be a more translucent and less white structure. The *parallelopiped effect* is a useful adjunct that can be used in situations wherein the landmarks are indistinguishable. This effect causes a narrow-slit beam of light that is reflected from the anterior and posterior corneal surfaces to collapse at the Schwalbe's line. Once this point is identified the other landmarks can be assessed based on the distance from the line.

The Schlemm's canal is usually not visible, but can be seen through a less pigmented posterior trabeculum when reflux blood fills up either due to raised episcleral venous pressure, or rarely as a normal phenomenon. Excess pressure over the globe especially with a three-mirror gonioscope can also cause artifactual filling up of the Schlemm's canal with blood.

Schwalbe's line, as described before, represents the peripheral termination of the Descemet's membrane. Usually optically identified by the parallelopiped method, it also at times appears as a prominent white ridge known as *posterior embryotoxon*, a misnomer. This ridge is better appreciated when the patient looks in the direction of the mirror and is more prominent in the temporal quadrants. The line may occasionally be pigmented and is referred to as *Sampaolesi line* as seen in pseudoexfoliation and pigment dispersion syndrome.

Pediatric Eye

The pediatric eye has definite but subtle variations in its anatomy. The iris contour in a newborn is usually flat and its insertion is posterior to scleral spur with the anterior extension of ciliary body band visible. This contour does eventually become convex as the angle recess develops in 6–12 months. The trabecular meshwork is nonpigmented and appears thick and translucent. Congenital glaucomas present with anterior insertions of the iris directly on to the trabeculum and at times the anterior iris stroma sweeps upward in a concave fashion to insert onto the trabecular meshwork.

GRADING AND RECORDING OF GONIOSCOPIC FINDINGS

Though multiple individual variations in assessment and grading gonioscopic details are being followed, it is important to follow a certain protocol of documentation, which aids in follow up of the disease process. Among the systems described (Table 1.2), the Spaeth's system is thought to be complete as it covers details with regard to angle width, iris insertion and configuration. Any gonioscopic data should contain (a) width of angle recess, (b) iris contour and insertion of iris root, (c) degree of pigmentation, (d) presence

Table 1.2: Classification systems for gonioscopy.

System	System basis	Angle structures and classification	
Scheie (1957)	Extent of angle structures visualized	All structures visible	Wide open
		Angle recess not seen	Grade I narrow
		Ciliary body band not seen	Grade II narrow
		Posterior trabeculum obscured	Grade III narrow
		Only Schwalbe's line visible	Grade IV narrow
Shaffer (1960)	Angular width of recess	Wide open (30°–45°)	Grades III–IV, closure impossible
		Moderately narrow (20°)	Grade II, closure possible
		Extremely narrow (10°)	Grade I, closure probable
		Partly or totally closed	Grade 0, closure present
Spaeth (1971)	Insertion of iris root	Anterior to Schwalbe's line	A
		Behind (posterior) to Schwalbe's line	B
		Centred at scleral spur	C
		Deep into ciliary body band	D
		Extremely deep	E
	Angular approach to the recess	Slit	
		10°	
		20°	
		30°	
		40°	
	Configuration of peripheral iris	Regular (slightly convex)	r
		Queer (posterior bowing)	q
		Steep	s
	TM pigment	0 (none) to 4 (maximal)	

of abnormal structures in each quadrant. Figure 1.7 shows a wide-open angle (Shaffer's grade IV or Spaeth's D40r) with regular iris contour and deep recess. All the landmarks—iris root, ciliary body band, scleral spur and trabecular meshwork—are visible. When insertion of iris occurs at scleral spur, the peripheral iris appears slightly convex, the angle of the anterior chamber still remains open (Shaffer's grade III or Spaeth's C30r, Fig. 1.8).

Classification of Primary Angle-closure

* *Primary angle-closure suspect (PACS):* An eye in which appositional contact between the peripheral iris and posterior trabecular meshwork is

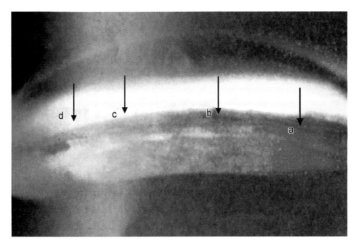

Figs. 1.7: Gonio-photograph of a grade IV Shaffer's angle (corresponds to Spaeth—D40r): (a) Iris root, (b) Ciliary body band, (c) Scleral spur, (d) Trabecular meshwork. Iris contour is regular with a deep recess.

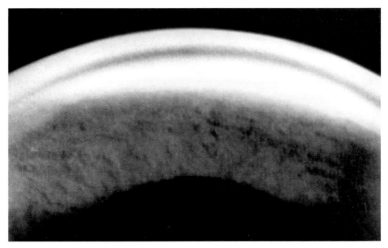

Fig. 1.8: Gonio-photograph of a grade III Shaffer's angle (corresponds to Spaeth—C30r). Landmarks are visible up to scleral spur with a mild iris convexity.

possible (if posterior trabecular meshwork is not visualized for >270°), is considered PACS.

- *Primary angle closure (PAC):* An eye with an occludable drainage angle and features indicating that trabecular obstruction by the peripheral iris has occurred, such as PAS, elevated intraocular pressure, iris whorling (distortion of the radially orientated iris fibers), 'glaucomfleken' lens opacities, or excessive pigment deposition on the trabecular surface. The optic disk does not have glaucomatous damage.
- *Primary angle-closure glaucoma (PACG):* PACG is defined when primary glaucoma is present with the evidence of angle closure.

COMPRESSION GONIOSCOPY

Compression or indentation gonioscopy is a simple and invaluable technique that one needs to know to assess narrow angles (Fig. 1.9) and chronic angle-closure situations. It helps distinguish appositional angle-closure from synechial angle-closure. The technique employs exerting external pressure over the cornea using the Zeiss, Posner or Sussman four mirror lenses, thereby forcing the lens iris diaphragm posteriorly and allowing visualizing the hidden angle recess (Fig. 1.10).

The technique involves a routine assessment of all quadrants, following which, if one subsequently decides the angle is narrow, each quadrant is re-evaluated using a narrow slit-beam (to prevent miosis causing artifactual opening of the angle recess), pressure is applied directed toward the center of the eye. It results in deepening of the anterior chamber in the area of recess caused by bowing back of peripheral iris along with stretching of the limbal scleral ring and straightening of the angle recess; following this one can see structures that were not visible earlier, or confirm the presence of PAS. Corneal folds often distort the view but this can be minimized with appropriate

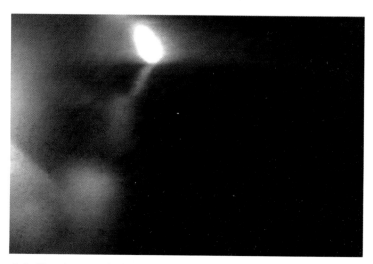

Fig. 1.9: The photograph shows a narrow angle visible up to the Schwalbe's line.

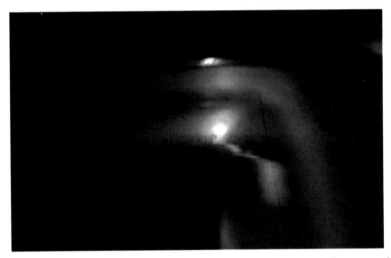

Fig. 1.10: The same angle on compression widens to reveal landmarks up to scleral spur.

technique in application of pressure. The physiological principles involved in compression gonioscopy have been depicted in Figure 1.11A to C. Compression may not be effective when intraocular pressures are beyond 40 mm Hg as this limits the expansion of the limbal scleral ring.

COMMON GONIOSCOPIC FINDINGS AND THEIR VARIATIONS

Peripheral Anterior Synechiae

The PAS (Fig. 1.12) is a pathological term referring to the adhesions of peripheral iris to the anterior angle structures, most often the functional trabecular meshwork, or rarely, extending to the Schwalbe's line. Typically, associated with PACG, uveitic and other secondary angle-closure glaucomas. PAS may often be confused with iris processes which are normal fine lacy cords of uveal tissue extending from the peripheral iris to the trabecular meshwork. PAS, on the other hand, are broad adhesions commonly localized to quadrants with areas in between widening with indentation technique of gonioscopy (Table 1.3). An angle that is closed 360° may often present a dilemma but one can follow the slit-beam from the posterior surface of the cornea which normally does not meet the beam on the iris directly in an angle that is open but instead lies alongside the other. A direct continuation of the beam without a break is suggestive of a closed angle. Clinical correlation and experience will often help overcome this hurdle.

Blood Vessels

Normally all vessels in the angle are restricted to the ciliary body band and iris root and do not extend to the scleral spur or trabecular meshwork.

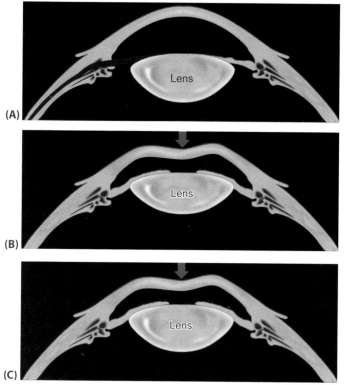

Figs. 1.11A to C: Compression gonioscopy: (A) The narrow angle appears closed on a routine gonioscopy. (B) Compression fails to allow visibility of angle structures due to peripheral anterior synechiae (PAS). (C) Compression widens the recess and allows a view of all structures in the absence of PAS.

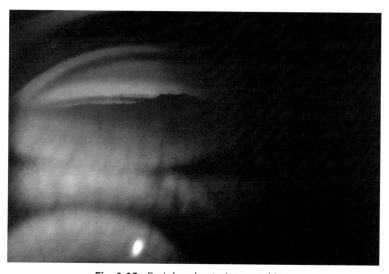

Fig. 1.12: Peripheral anterior synechiae.

Table 1.3: Differences between iris processes and peripheral anterior synechiae.

Iris processes	Peripheral anterior synechiae
Delicate and lacy	Broad and irregular
Follows concavity of angle recess	Bridges the angle recess
Does not obscure underlying structures	Obscures under lying structures
Does not inhibit posterior movement of the iris on indentation	Inhibits posterior movement
	Drag normal iris vessels with them
	Pigmentation of the cornea anterior to the synecheiae may be present

Anomalous vessels are not rare. They, however, can readily be distinguished from neovascularization (Fig. 1.13), which are vessels usually arising from the peripheral iris surface and branching out in an arborizing and lacy pattern onto the corneoscleral portion of trabecular meshwork. Varying amounts of PAS may also be associated depending on the stage of disease process.

Pigmentation

The trabecular meshwork has a varying amount of pigmentation varying from 0 to 4, which is a subjective grading that correlates to none (0), faint (1), average (2), heavy (3) and very heavy (4). Pigmentation increases with age under normal physiological conditions. Excessive pigmentation is usually pathological and is associated with pseudoexfoliation syndrome, pigment dispersion syndrome, traumatic and uveitic glaucomas. Patchy trabecular meshwork pigmentation can be seen corresponding to areas of gonioscopically identifiable previous closure (Fig. 1.14).

Other Abnormal Findings

A variety of surprises may be hidden in the angle recess. Angle recession may be seen as irregular widening of ciliary body band (Fig. 1.15). Iridodialysis, CD cleft (Fig. 1.16), KPs (Fig. 1.17), trabeculectomy stoma (Fig. 1.18) can also be observed. Blood in Schlemm's canal (Fig. 1.19) appears as a uniform linear reddish hue just anterior to pigmented trabecular meshwork and is associated with raised episcleral venous pressure. It can also be observed under normal conditions and as an artifact when excess external pressure is exerted during gonioscopy. Pseudoexfoliative material (Fig. 1.20), microscopic hyphema and hypopyon can be visualized. Foreign bodies, iris cyst (Fig. 1.21) and emulsified silicone oil globules (Fig. 1.22) are among the other things that can be picked up by a careful gonioscopy.

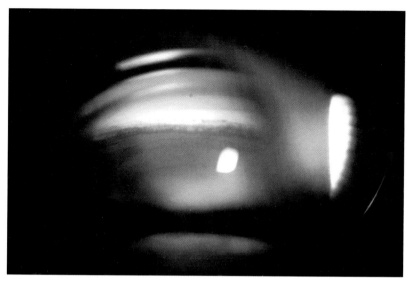

Fig. 1.13: Neovascularization of the angle.

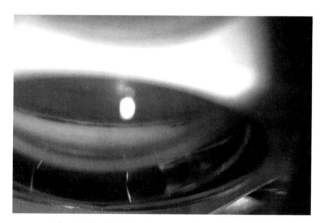

Fig. 1.14: Patchy pigmentation of the angle.

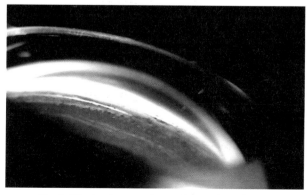

Fig. 1.15: Angle recession with a wide CB band.

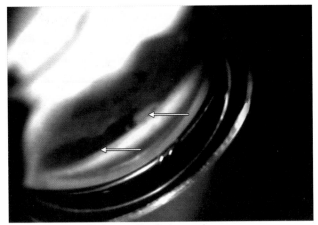

Best seen with a 3 mirror gonioscope

Fig. 1.16: Iridodialysis with a CD cleft.

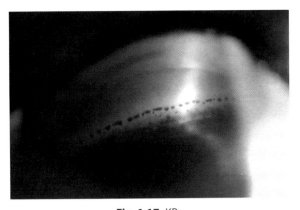

Fig. 1.17 KPs.

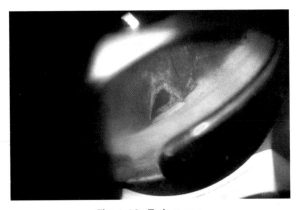

Fig. 1.18: Trab stoma.

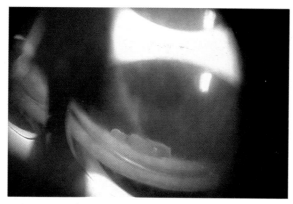

Fig. 1.19: Foreign bodies in the angle and blood in Schlemm canal.

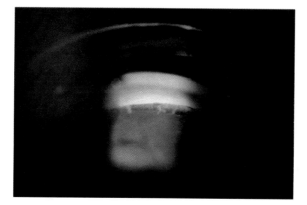

Fig. 1.20: PXF material in the inferior angle.

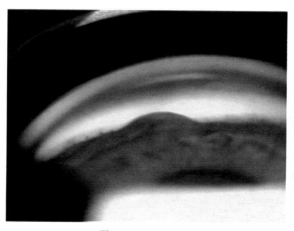

Fig. 1.21: Iris cyst.

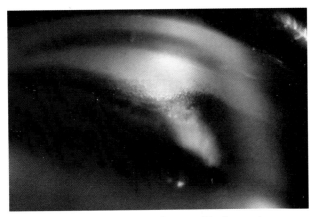

Fig. 1.22: Emulsified silicone oil in the angle.

CONCLUSION

In conclusion, the diagnostic basis of any glaucoma should be in correlation to the gonioscopic findings whenever possible. The management and prognosis of the disease depends on a complete diagnosis that includes a routine and periodic gonioscopic evaluation. Gonioscopy widens our scientific understanding of the disease process and guides us to manage the disease more effectively.

BIBLIOGRAPHY

1. Alward WL. A history of gonioscopy. Optom Vis Sci. 2011;88(1):29-35.
2. Foster PJ, Gazzard GA, Heath TG, et al. Pattern of trabecular surface pigment deposition in angle closure. Arch Ophthalmol. 2006;124(7);1062.
3. Foster PJ, Buhrmann R, Quigley HA, et al. The definition and classification of glaucoma in prevalence surveys. Br J Ophthalmol. 2002;86(2):238-42.
4. Friedman DS, He M. Anterior chamber angle assessment techniques. Diagnostic and surgical techniques. Surv Ophthalmol. 2008;53(3):250-73.
5. Grant WM, Schumen JS. The angle of the anterior chamber In: Epstein DL, Allingham RR, Schuman JS (Eds.). Chandler and Grant's Glaucoma, 4th edition. Baltimore, MD: Williams and Wilkins; 1996.
6. Kanski JJ, James AM, John FS. Glaucoma—A Colour Manual of Diagnosis and Treatment, 2nd edition. London: Butterworth-Heinemann; 1996.
7. Neil TC, Diane CL. Atlas of Glaucoma. London: Martin Dunitz; 1998. p. 39.
8. Savage JA. Gonioscopy in the management of glaucoma. In Focal Points Clinical Modules for Ophthalmologists. San Francisco, CA: AAO; 2006.
9. Stamper RL, Liebermann MF, Drake MV. Becker-Shaffer's Diagnosis and Therapy of the Glaucomas, 8th edition. Mosby: Elsevier; 2009.
10. Thomas R, Thomas S, Chandrashekar G. Gonioscopy. Indian J Ophthalmol. 1998;46(4):255-61.

Optic Disk Assessment in Glaucoma

Choudhari NS, Chandra Sekhar G

INTRODUCTION

Glaucoma is the second leading cause of blindness worldwide. The estimated number of people with open-angle and angle-closure glaucoma for 2020 using prevalence models is 79.6 million.[1] At least 50% of patients do not know that they have glaucoma since the disease is usually asymptomatic.[2] Rapid advances have been made in recent times in imaging technologies such as confocal scanning laser ophthalmoscopy, scanning laser polarimetry and optical coherence topography for the detection of glaucomatous damage. However, these technologies have only moderate ability to pick up glaucoma at an early stage.[3-5] New psychophysical tests such as short wavelength automated perimetry, frequency doubling perimetry and motion automated perimetry are targeted at specific visual functions and have been shown to be more sensitive and specific than standard automated perimetry for identifying early glaucomatous damage.[6-8] However, these techniques may not be available to all clinicians and have the limitations of any subjective test. Several studies have shown that abnormalities in the appearance of the optic disk may precede visual field defects.[9,10] Conventional stereoscopic clinical evaluation and imaging of the optic disk with fundus photographs is still the most frequently used and sensitive means of diagnosing glaucoma.[11] With some training, it is possible to clinically evaluate optic nerve head and retinal nerve fiber layer stereoscopically and detect early glaucomatous damage. The aim of this chapter is to highlight the techniques of clinical evaluation of the optic disk, describe the morphological changes of the optic nerve in glaucoma, and discuss the differential diagnosis.

METHODS OF OPTIC DISK EXAMINATION

Traditionally, the direct ophthalmoscope has been used for the evaluation of the optic nerve head. Though it has the advantage of providing a magnified view of the optic nerve head, it however, lacks stereopsis and permits color based instead of contour-based judgment of the neuroretinal rim (NRR). Therefore, the use of the direct ophthalmoscope is to be strongly discouraged.

A variety of contact and non-contact lenses are available that allow stereoscopic view of the fundus on the slit-lamp. Contact lenses such as Goldmann lenses are relatively uncomfortable for the patient, take longer time and the coupling fluid can cause transient blurring and difficulty in obtaining good quality fundus photographs. Non-contact lenses include +60 D, +78 D, +90 D and Volk superfield lenses. These provide excellent stereoscopic and magnified view of the optic disk.

It is important to draw the appearance of the optic nerve head based on these methods (Figs. 2.1A to E and 2.2). Though drawing of the optic disk suffers from the disadvantage of being subjective in nature, this does offer a quick and inexpensive method of monitoring the optic nerve head in patients with glaucoma over time. It also serves as a check against incomplete examination of the optic disk. Moreover, photographs may not be possible in all cases such as patients with rigid miotic pupils and those with significant media opacities. However, wherever possible, photographs are an indispensable adjunct to clinical evaluation.

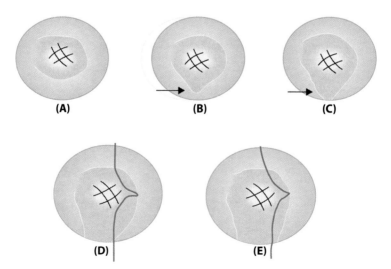

Figs. 2.1A to E: (A) Optic disk drawing. Conventionally, the outline of the cup is not drawn on the temporal side. Therefore, all these drawings are of right disk. (B) The arrows indicates inferior excavation and (C) inferior notch. (D and E) Note relation of vessel to the notch.

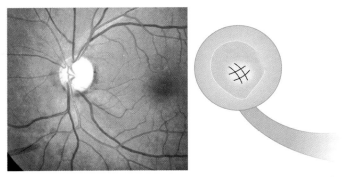

Fig. 2.2: Optic disk documentation: Note the inferior excavation and the inferior nerve fiber layer defect outlined by the two lines in the optic disk drawing.

FEATURES OF GLAUCOMATOUS DISK DAMAGE

Cup–Disk Ratio

Early studies by Armaly et al. have reported that the vertical and horizontal cup–disk diameters ratio are useful for the quantification of glaucomatous optic neuropathy and for early detection of glaucoma.[12] The ratio has limited value in the identification of glaucomatous damage, because of the wide variability in the size of the optic cup in the normal population.

Disk margin is defined by inner edge of white scleral ring (outer arrows), and the optic cup is the level at which NRR steeps (inner arrows) (Fig. 2.3). A large cup–disk ratio can be normal if the optic disk is large[13] and a small

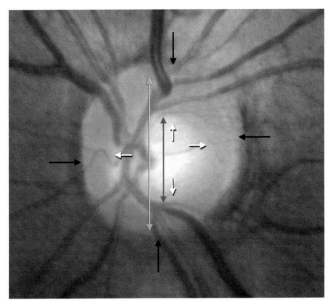

Fig. 2.3: Disk margin (black arrows) and cup margin (white arrows). Maximum vertical diameter of the cup (blue arrow) and the disk (green arrow).

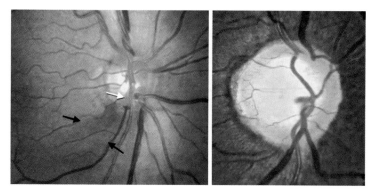

Fig. 2.4: Cup–disk ratio in relation to optic disk size. The optic disk on left is small with small cup and still has inferior excavation (white arrow) with nerve fiber layer defect (black arrow). In contrast, the optic disk right has a large physiological cup.

cup–disk ratio may be glaucomatous if the optic disk is small (Fig. 2.4).[14] The problem with estimating cup–disk ratio as a measure of glaucomatous damage is that it is difficult to decide if the cup is physiological in a large disk or pathological in a small- or normal-sized disk. In a study by Garway-Heath et al., vertical cup–disk diameter ratio *corrected for the optic disk size* was the best parameter to separate between normal subjects and patients of ocular hypertension with retinal nerve fiber layer defect.[15] Therefore, in the clinical description of the optic nerve head, it is important to state the vertical cup–disk diameter ratio in combination with the estimated disk size. The disk diameter can be measured by adjusting the slit-lamp beam height to the edges of the disk while viewing the disk with a 60 D lens (Fig. 2.5).[16] The measurement by this method is roughly equal to the measurement obtained by the planimetry of disk photographs by Litmann's correction. Measurements

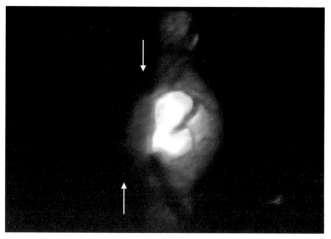

Fig. 2.5: During slit-lamp biomicroscopy, adjust the height of the slit-lamp beam to the vertical disk diameter, read the height of the beam and then multiply it by the correction factor of hand-held lens to obtain vertical optic disk diameter.

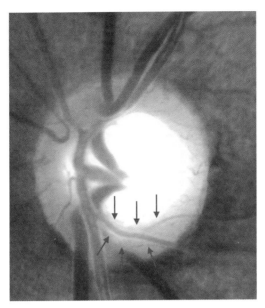

Fig. 2.6: Margin of color cup (red arrows) versus contour cup (blue arrows). The former may miss the inferior excavation.

can also be made with other lenses by multiplying the measured value with the appropriate magnification factor, Goldmann contact lens X1.26 and Volk superfield lens X1.5.[16]

It is important to differentiate contour cupping from color cupping. The margin of the cup should be determined by the bend of the small vessels across the disk rim and not by the central area of disk pallor (Fig. 2.6).

Asymmetry of Optic Disk Cupping

Asymmetry of cupping is seldom seen in normal eyes and until proven otherwise, it must be taken as an indication of early glaucomatous damage. However, while assessing asymmetry, it is important to rule out asymmetry of the disk size, which can be physiological or be the result of anisometropia. Intereye asymmetry in the size of the optic disk may result in difference in the cup–disk ratio between two eyes, in the absence of glaucoma (Fig. 2.7).

Neuroretinal Rim Evaluation

A focal or diffuse loss of the NRR is typical in glaucoma. Focal damage usually involves a particular area of the rim. If the rim is completely lost in a focal area, it is called complete notch (Fig. 2.8) whereas localized thinning of the rim is called incomplete notch or excavation (Figs. 2.2 and 2.9). Diffuse damage results in symmetrical enlargement of the cup. The ISNT rule states that normally the inferior rim is the thickest followed by the superior, the nasal and then the temporal (Fig. 2.10).[17] During optic nerve head evaluation, one

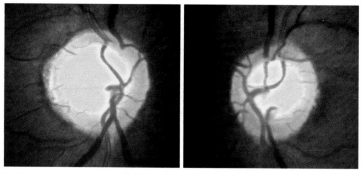

Fig. 2.7: Asymmetry on optic disk cupping is explainable by asymmetry in the size of the disk. Both optic disks are healthy.

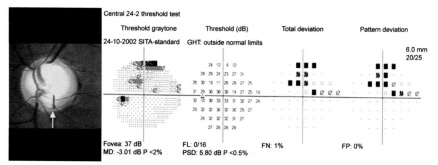

Fig. 2.8: Inferior optic disk notch (yellow arrows) and the visual field defect. The visual field defect corresponds with the glaucomatous changes in the optic disk. Blue arrows indicates bayoneting sign.

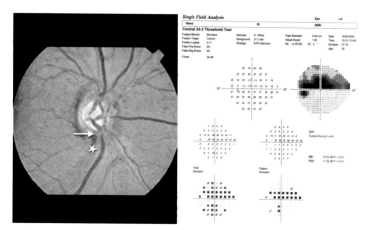

Fig. 2.9: The optic disk photograph shows early inferior excavation (arrow) with corresponding superior arcuate field defect. Note optic disk hemorrhage (star).

must look carefully for any areas of thinning of the NRR or for notching. If the cup is especially deep in the notch, it is known as a pseudo-pit. Notching and pseudo-pits are usually seen at the superior or inferior poles. The width of the notch tends to correspond to the extent of the visual field defect (Fig. 2.8).

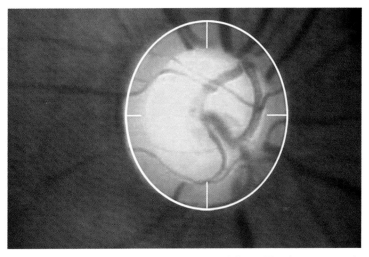

Fig. 2.10: ISNT rule: The inferior rim is the thickest followed by the superior, the nasal and then the temporal.

Optic rim pallor indicates vascular insult to the nerve. Although it is seen in a few subtypes of glaucoma, it may point toward a non-glaucomatous etiology of optic damage.

Vascular Changes

Splinter hemorrhages on the optic disk are a common finding in glaucoma patients (Figs. 2.9 and 2.11). Various studies have shown that disk hemorrhages in association with localized nerve fiber layer defects and notches of the NRR are more common among patients with normal tension glaucoma.[18,19] A possible explanation for the difference in frequency has been

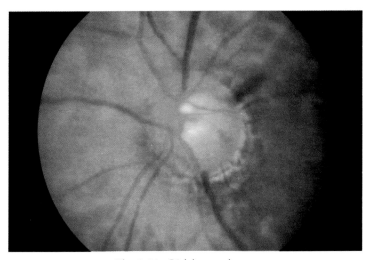

Fig. 2.11: Disk hemorrhage.

suggested by Jonas et al. They stated that the amount of blood leaking out of a vessel into the surrounding tissue depends on the intraocular pressure (IOP) when the bleeding occurs.[19] High transmural pressure gradient in normal pressure glaucoma leads to larger disk hemorrhages. Also, since the absorption rate of disk hemorrhages depends on the size of the disk bleed, the hemorrhages in patients of normal pressure glaucoma may take a longer time to disappear and thus have a higher chance to be detected than the disk hemorrhages in patients of high pressure glaucoma.[20]

Hemorrhages in glaucoma usually appear as splinter-shaped or flame-shaped hemorrhages on the disk surface (Fig. 2.9).[21] They usually precede NRR changes and visual field defects. The visual field defects corresponding to the location of the hemorrhage may be expected to appear weeks to year later.[22] The presence of disk hemorrhage(s) is considered an indication for further IOP lowering in the management of glaucoma.

Configuration of Vessels

The retinal vessels on the optic nerve head can provide clues about the topography of the disk. Nasalization of the vessels and baring of circumlinear vessels can be seen in glaucoma as well as in other diseases of the optic nerve. Bayoneting of the vessels can be seen if the rim is absent or very thin. This causes the vessels to pass under the overhanging edge of the cup and then make a sharp bend as they cross the disk surface. This convoluted appearance of the vessels is called 'bayoneting' (Fig. 2.8).

Peripapillary Atrophy

The zone closer to the optic nerve head with retinal pigment epithelium (RPE) and choroidal atrophy and baring of sclera is known as zone-β. The more peripheral zone with only RPE atrophy is called zone-α (Fig. 2.12). A highly significant correlation has been reported between the location of peripapillary atrophy and visual field defects.[23] Changes may represent congenital anomalies, especially in myopic eyes. However, appearance of these changes *de novo* or their presence in small, non-myopic disks should be viewed with suspicion. Peripapillary atrophy may be a focal or circumferential (Figs. 2.6, 2.8 and 2.11).

Retinal Nerve Fiber Layer Abnormalities

Examination of the nerve fiber layer is often useful in detecting early glaucomatous damage with normal disk appearance and normal visual fields. The NRR is formed by axons converging from the retina to the scleral canal. Since the axons are spread out in a thin layer in the retina, even minor losses of the axons can be observed in the retinal nerve fiber layer. In healthy eyes, the nerve fiber layer in the arcuate region appears

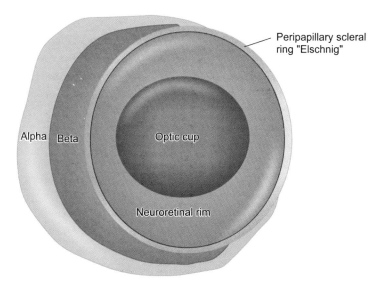

Fig. 2.12: Peripapillary atrophy. The diagram shows atrophic zone closer to the optic nerve head called zone-β and the more peripheral zone called zone-α.

slightly opaque with radially oriented striations. The small retinal blood vessels have a blurred and crosshatched appearance, as they lie buried in the nerve fiber layer. The best way to assess the nerve fiber layer is by doing slit-lamp biomicroscopy through a dilated pupil using red free light, a wide-slit beam and high magnification. In the presence of nerve fiber layer atrophy, the small retinal blood vessels become more clearly visible and appear unusually sharp, clear and well-focused. The fundus in the affected area appears darker and deeper red in contrast to the silvery or opaque hue of the intact nerve fiber layer. Defects may be in the form of a wedge shape arising from the disk margin and widening towards the periphery (Fig. 2.13), or slit-like defects that are narrower than the adjacent blood vessels. While the former may be pathological, the latter are physiological. Diffuse areas of nerve fiber layer atrophy are less common in early glaucoma and more difficult to identify.

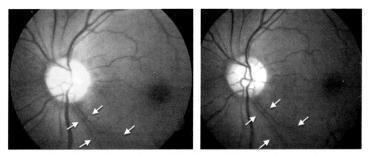

Fig. 2.13: A wedge-shaped retinal nerve fiber layer defect can be seen between arrows. It is more easily made out in red-free photograph.

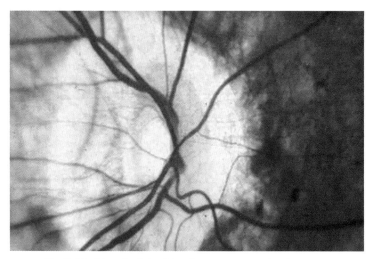

Fig. 2.14: Myopic disk with primary open-angle glaucoma.

Myopic versus Glaucomatous Optic Disk

Myopic disks can present difficulty in evaluation for glaucoma due to the tilted disks, peripapillary atrophy and shallow cupping. One needs to examine carefully the disk to look for changes in the contour of the blood vessels, as well delineate the disk margin from the peripapillary changes (Fig. 2.14).

Differential Diagnosis

In addition to glaucoma, other abnormalities can cause excavation and/or pallor of the optic disk and it is, therefore, important to rule out these possibilities before making the diagnosis of glaucoma:

- *Physiological cupping:* Assessment of the size of the optic disk, careful examination of the NRR and the retinal nerve fiber layer can help distinguish physiological cupping from glaucomatous damage in most cases (Fig. 2.15).

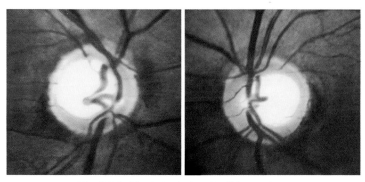

Fig. 2.15: Physiological optic disk cupping.

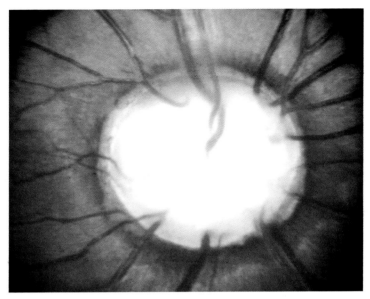

Fig. 2.16: Morning glory optic disk.

- *Optic nerve coloboma:* Optic nerve colobomas typically demonstrate enlargement of the papillary region, partial or complete excavation, blood vessels entering and exiting from the border of the defect and a glistening white surface. The visual field defects can be in the form of generalized constriction, centrocecal scotomas, altitudinal defects, arcuate scotomas, enlargement of the blind spot and ring scotomas that can mimic those found in glaucomatous eyes.

- *Morning glory syndrome:* This is a variant of optic disk coloboma and is characterized by a large excavated disk, central core of white or gray glial tissue surrounded by an elevated annulus of variably pigmented subretinal tissue (Fig. 2.16). The retinal vessels appear to enter and exit from the margins of the disk, are straightened and often sheathed.

- *Congenital optic disk pit:* Congenital optic disk pits appear gray or yellowish white, round or oval, localized depression within the optic nerve (Fig. 2.17). They are located within the temporal aspect of the disk in over half of the cases and centrally in about one-third. Involvement is usually unilateral in about 80% cases and the optic disk is larger on the involved side. Approximately 55–60% of the eyes have a field defect in the form of arcuate scotomas, paracentral scotoma, altitudinal defect, generalized constriction and nasal or temporal steps.[24]

- In the absence of other indicators of congenital anomaly like associated fundus coloboma, the differential diagnosis may be difficult and the absence of progression on follow-up may be the only indicator that the patient has a congenital anomaly and not glaucoma.

- *Anterior ischemic optic neuropathy:* A history of acute visual loss, initial swelling of the optic disk, absence of marked cupping, presence

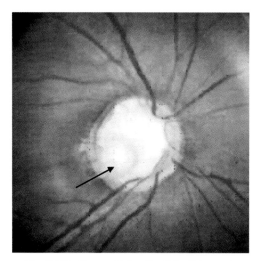

Fig. 2.17: Congenital optic disk pit (arrow).

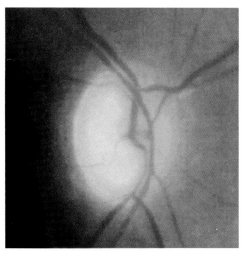

Fig. 2.18: Anterior ischemic optic neuropathy. The optic disk photograph is from a patient with long-standing anterior ischemic optic neuropathy (AION) mimicking typical glaucomatous cupping.

of centrocecal scotoma or altitudinal defects, rise in erythrocyte sedimentation rate (ESR) can help differentiate it from glaucoma. In the late stages the cupping in some cases may be exactly the same as is seen in glaucoma (Fig. 2.18).

- *Neurological causes:* Younger age, unusual history of onset and progression, normal IOP and pallor of the NRR disproportionate to cupping should arouse suspicion of a neurological disorder causing optic disk damage (Fig. 2.19). Presence of visual field defects that respect vertical midline and the pattern of the field defects should be able to suggest the possible site of the intracranial lesion.[25]

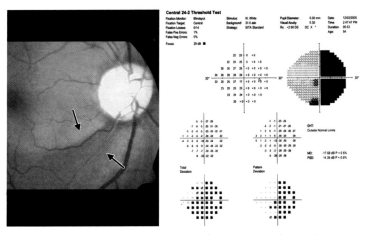

Fig. 2.19: Optic disk photograph showing significant cupping, but with disproportionate pallor, with visual field defect showing a temporal hemifield defect suggestive of chiasmal compression.

CONCLUSION

In summary, the optic disk evaluation in glaucoma is best done stereoscopically at the slit-lamp with a dilated pupil using one of the 60 D, 78 D or 90 D lenses. Changes in the NRR, optic disk hemorrhage(s), peripapillary atrophy and nerve fiber layer defect(s) are more important features than the cup–disk ratio. The cup–disk ratio is to be documented and interpreted along with the disk size and not in isolation. One should avoid the urge to instantaneously diagnose glaucoma based on the cup to disk ratio alone. The diagnosis of glaucoma depends on multiple factors including the presence of a visual field defect that correlates with the anatomic changes on the optic nerve head and the peripapillary retina.

REFERENCES

1. Quigley HA, Broman AT. The number of people with glaucoma worldwide in 2010 and 2020. Br J Ophthalmol. 2006;90(3):262-67.
2. Dandona L, Dandona R, Srinivas M, et al. Open-angle glaucoma in an urban population in southern India: the Andhra Pradesh eye disease study. Ophthalmology. 2000;107(9):1702-9.
3. Zangwill LM, Bowd C, Berry CC, et al. Discriminating between normal and glaucomatous eyes using the Heidelberg retina tomograph, GDx nerve fibre analyser and optical coherence tomograph. Arch Ophthalmol. 2001;119(7):985-93.
4. Bowd C, Zangwill LM, Berry CC, et al. Detecting early glaucoma by assessment of retinal nerve fibre layer thickness and visual functions. Invest Ophthalmol Vis Sci. 2001;42(9):1993-2003.
5. Medeiros FA, Zangwill LM, Bowd C, et al. Comparison of the GDx VCC scanning laser polarimeter, HRT II confocal scanning laser ophthalmoscope,

and stratus OCT optical coherence tomograph for the detection of glaucoma. Arch Ophthalmol. 2004:122(6);827-37.

6. Johnson CA, Adams AJ, Casson EJ, et al. Blue-on-yellow perimetry can predict the development of glaucomatous field loss. Arch Ophthalmol. 1993;111(5):645-50.

7. Bayer AU, Maag KP, Erb C. Detection of optic neuropathy in glaucomatous eyes with normal standard visual fields using a battery of short-wavelength automated perimetry and pattern electroretinography. Ophthalmology. 2002;109(5):1350-61.

8. Sample PA, Bosworth CF, Blumenthal EZ, et al. Visual function-specific perimetry for indirect comparison of different ganglion cell populations in glaucoma. Invest Ophthalmol Vis Sci. 2000;41(7):1783-90.

9. Quigley HA, Dunkelberger GR, Green WR. Chronic human glaucoma causing selectively greater loss of larger optic nerve fibers. Ophthalmology. 1988;95(3):357-63.

10. Sommer A, Pollack I, Maumenne AE. Optic disc parameters and onset of glaucomatous field loss. I. Methods and changes in disc morphology. Arch Ophthalmol. 1979;97(8):1444-8.

11. Greaney MJ, Hoffman DC, Garway-Heath DF, et al. Comparison of optic nerve imaging methods to distinguish normal eyes from those with glaucoma. Invest Ophthalmol Vis Sci. 2002;43(1):140-5.

12. Armaly MF, Saydegh RE. The cup/disc ratio. Arch Ophthalmol. 1969;82(2): 191-6.

13. Jonas JB, Zäch FM, Gusek GC, et al. Pseudoglaucomatous physiologic large cups. Am J Ophthalmol. 1989;107(2):137-44.

14. Jonas JB, Fernandez MC, Naumann GO. Glaucomatous optic nerve atrophy in small discs with low cup-to-disc ratios. Ophthalmology. 1990;97(9):1211-5.

15. Garway-Heath DF, Ruben ST, Viswanathan A, et al. Vertical cup/disc ratio in relation to optic disc size: its value in the assessment of the glaucoma suspect. Br J Ophthalmol. 1998;82(10):1118-24.

16. Jonas JB, Dichtl A. Advances in the assessment of the optic disc changes in early glaucoma. Cur Opin Ophthalmol. 1995;6(2):61-6.

17. Jonas JB, Gusek GC, Naumann GO. Optic disc, cup and neuroretinal rim size, configuration, and correlations in normal eyes. Invest Ophthalmol Vis Sci. 1988;29(7):1151-8.

18. Kitazawa Y, Shirato S, Yamamoto T. Optic disc hemorrhage in low-tension glaucoma. Ophthalmology. 1986;93(6):853-7.

19. Jonas JB, Budde WM. Optic nerve head appearance in juvenile-onset chronic high-pressure glaucoma and normal-pressure glaucoma. Ophthalmology. 2000;107:704-11.

20. Jonas JB, Xu L. Optic disc hemorrhages in glaucoma. Am J Ophthalmol 1994; 118(1):1-8.

21. Drance SM, Fairclough M, Butler DM, et al. The importance of disc haemorrhage in the prognosis of chronic open-angle glaucoma. Arch Ophthalmol. 1977:95(2):226-8.

22. Heijl, A. Frequent disc photography and computerized perimetry in eyes with optic disc haemorrhage. Acta Ophthalmol. 1986:64(3):274-81.

23. Jonas JB, Naumann GOH. Parapapillary chorioretinal atrophy in normal and glaucoma eyes. II. Correlations. Invest Ophthalmol Vis Sci. 1989:30(5): 919-26.
24. Brown GC. Congenital fundus abnormalities. In: Duane TD (Ed). Clinical Ophthalmology. Philadelphia, PA: JB Lippincott; 1991.
25. Choudhari NS, Neog A, Fudnawala V, et al. Cupped disc with normal intra-ocular pressure: the long road to avoid misdiagnosis. Indian J Ophthalmol. 2011;59(6):491-7.

3

Peripapillary Atrophy in Glaucoma

Ki Ho Park

Peripapillary chorioretinal atrophy or peripapillary atrophy has been reported to be more frequently present and extensive in eyes with high-tension glaucoma than in healthy eyes.[1-6] It has been suggested that there are significant correlations between the extent or the location of peripapillary atrophy and visual field defects in high-tension glaucoma.[5,7,8] In normal-tension glaucoma, peripapillary atrophy is known to be a significant risk factor for progression of visual field damage,[9,10] and is correlated with structural and functional damage of optic nerve.[11] In spite of numerous evidences there has been some controversy about the association of peripapillary atrophy with glaucoma. In this chapter, the clinical implications of peripapillary atrophy in glaucoma are reviewed.

Peripapillary atrophy has been divided into a central zone (zone beta)—characterized by retinal pigment epithelial loss and choroidal atrophy with visible large choroidal vessels and sclera—and a peripheral zone (zone alpha) with irregular hyper- and hypo-pigmentation.[4-6] Because zone alpha shows less clinical significance in glaucoma than zone beta and the boundary of zone alpha is sometimes unclear, therefore, many articles use the term peripapillary atrophy as zone beta. The peripapillary scleral ring, a thin white band of scleral tissue surrounding the optic nerve head, should not be considered as peripapillary atrophy (Fig. 3.1).

Histologically, peripapillary atrophy areas correspond to areas of choroidal thinning or absence[12] and those without retinal pigment epithelium next to the disk.[12-14] Zone alpha is the equivalent of pigmentary irregularities in the retinal pigment epithelium. In fluorescein angiography, zone beta of peripapillary atrophy does not fluoresce in the choroidal filling phase.[15]

Peripapillary atrophy can also be divided into congenital and acquired atrophy.[12] Congenital peripapillary atrophy is found mainly in oblique

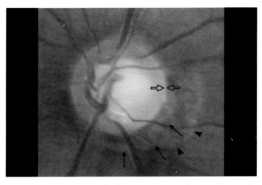

Fig. 3.1: Peripapillary atrophy is divided into a central zone (zone beta, black arrows) characterized by retinal pigment epithelial loss and choroidal atrophy with visible large choroidal vessels and sclera, and a peripheral zone (zone alpha, black arrow heads) with irregular hyper- and hypo-pigmentation. The peripapillary scleral ring (between open arrows), a thin white band of scleral tissue surrounding the optic nerve head, should not be considered as peripapillary atrophy.

implantation of the optic disk.[16] Acquired peripapillary atrophy can develop from both myopia and glaucoma. Myopic peripapillary atrophy develops from temporal disk tilting as the eyeball grows, so the shape of whole contour including temporal peripapillary atrophy margin and nasal disk margin matches the original normal disk shape before the disk tilt occurs (Fig. 3.2). Even though there is some overlapping between the myopic peripapillary atrophy and glaucomatous peripapillary atrophy, the glaucomatous peripapillary atrophy presents, in most cases, infero-temporally or superotemporally outside the normal shape of disk margin (Fig. 3.2).[11]

Zone alpha is present in almost all eyes, while zone beta in about 10–20% of normal eyes.[4-6] Zone alpha and zone beta are significantly larger in eyes with glaucomatous optic nerve damage than in normal eyes.[4-9,11,12,17,18] Additionally, zone beta occurs more often in glaucomatous eyes than in normal eyes.[4-6] In normal-tension glaucoma zone beta is found with a relatively higher frequency (84–97%)[11,19] than in primary open-angle glaucoma.

The simple method of examination is using an ophthalmoscope or with +78 D or +90 D lens at the slit-lamp. Quantitative analysis using digitalized optic disk photographs can be used. Another choice of quantitative analysis is a method using confocal scanning laser ophthalmoscope. The method was first introduced by Park[11] and the software has been developed to measure the area and angular and radial extent of peripapillary atrophy by simply drawing a contour line around the peripapillary atrophy.[19,20]

Numerous previous studies have suggested that in high-tension and normal-tension glaucoma the extent or the location of peripapillary atrophy significantly correlates with the visual field defects.[7-8,11] The location of peripapillary atrophy spatially correlates with the neuroretinal rim loss in the optic nerve head,[5,6,11] peripapillary atrophy is larger in that sector with the more marked loss of neuroretinal rim.

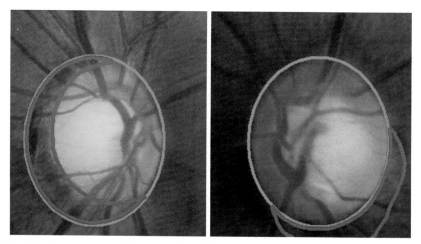

Fig. 3.2: Myopic peripapillary atrophy (left) is developed from temporal disc tilting as the eyeball grows, so the shape of whole contour (green) including temporal peripapillary atrophy margin (red) and nasal disc margin matches the original normal disc shape (green) before the disc tilt had occurred. Even though there is some overlapping between the myopic peripapillary atrophy and glaucomatous peripapillary atrophy (right), the glaucomatous peripapillary atrophy presents in most cases inferotemporally (red) or superotemporally outside the normal shape (green) of disc margin.

Ahn et al.[20] investigated the correlation between disk hemorrhage and peripapillary atrophy in glaucoma patients. They found a significantly larger zone beta in the hemorrhagic eyes than in the contralateral nonhemorrhagic eyes (Fig. 3.3). The frequency of zone beta was higher and the neuroretinal rim was smaller in the hemorrhagic eye. A multivariate regression analysis revealed that peripapillary atrophy area was an independent significant factor associated with disk hemorrhage. They concluded that peripapillary atrophy is closely associated with the disk hemorrhage in glaucoma patients independent of a small neuroretinal rim area.

A study had been performed by Honrubia and Calonge on 549 eyes belonging to three different groups: normal population, ocular hypertension and glaucoma.[21] A highly significant association was observed between the presence of peripapillary atrophy and the presence of defects in the retinal nerve fiber layer (RNFL), as well as between the intensity of peripapillary atrophy and defects in the RNFL. This association was statistically significant in the population of ocular hypertensives ($p = 0.0360$) but not in the population of eyes considered normal. While it was not a direct relationship between peripapillary atrophy and RNFL defect, Sugiyama et al.[22] demonstrated that disk hemorrhage is associated with RNFL defect in location and the size of peripapillary atrophy in normal-tension glaucoma. These studies suggested a close relationship between peripapillary atrophy, disk hemorrhage and RNFL defects.

Park et al.[11] investigated the ability of parameters of peripapillary atrophy to differentiate normal-tension glaucoma from glaucoma-like disks.

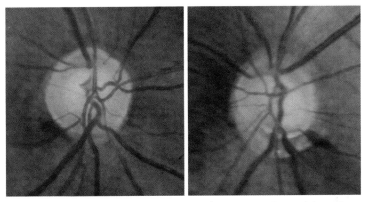

Fig. 3.3: A 36-year-old male normal-tension glaucoma patient with unilateral disc hemorrhage in his left eye (right). The size of peripapillary atrophy is larger in the eye with disc hemorrhage (right) than in contralateral nonhemorrhagic right eye (left). Neuroretinal rim narrowing and retinal nerve fiber layer defect in the sector of largest peripapillary atrophy can be detected as well (right).

Thirty-three eyes of 33 patients with glaucoma-like disks without evidence of visual field defects and RNFL defects, and 33 eyes of 33 patients with normal-tension glaucoma, matched for age and intraocular pressure, were enrolled. The authors found that the area of peripapillary atrophy zone beta, atrophy-to-disk area ratio and angular and radial extent of zone beta measured by confocal scanning laser ophthalmoscope [Heidelberg retina tomograph (HRT)] were significantly larger in normal-tension glaucoma patients. In a multiple logistic regression analysis, the size of zone beta showed a significant difference between the normal-tension glaucoma group and glaucoma-like disk group. The authors concluded that measurement of peripapillary atrophy by HRT can be a useful additional tool to differentiate normal-tension glaucoma from glaucoma-like disks.

There is a considerable evidence that the peripapillary atrophy is a risk factor for glaucoma, relatively less affected by high intraocular pressure. Studies using regression analysis of survival data based on the Cox proportional hazard model found that peripapillary atrophy was one of the significant risk factors influencing progression of visual field damage in normal-tension glaucoma.[9,10,23] Buus and Anderson[24] reported a higher frequency (64%) and greater extent of peripapillary atrophy in normal-tension glaucoma than ocular hypertension (34%). Supporting this finding is the fact that the zone beta in high-tension glaucoma is larger in eyes with relatively lower IOP than in those with higher IOP.[6] Using a high-tension glaucoma model in monkeys, Derick et al.[25] reported that the presence of, or change in, peripapillary atrophy was not significantly associated with the IOP-induced optic nerve damage.

Enlargement of peripapillary atrophy has been studied by several investigators. In a retrospective review of 127 glaucoma patients and 49 control individuals, Rockwood and Anderson[26] observed peripapillary abnormality in the form of retinal pigment epithelium changes in 21% of the glaucoma patients with progressive glaucomatous cupping and in 4% of normal control subjects. Uchida et al.[27] demonstrated that 37% of 75 glaucoma patients had a progressive peripapillary atrophy within 8 years of follow-up; 64% of 33 eyes with progressive disk damage compared to 17% of 42 eyes without progressive disk damage showing an association between increasing peripapillary atrophy and progressive glaucoma. Kwon et al.[28] also observed an enlargement of peripapillary atrophy, however, with a lower rate: 3 (6%) in 51 eyes treated for primary open-angle glaucoma during a follow-up of at least 9 years.

The morphologic characteristics of peripapillary atrophy are different among various types of glaucoma. The peripapillary atrophy zone beta is significantly larger in eyes with highly myopic primary open-angle glaucoma (exceeding –8 D) compared with those with less myopic or normal refractive errors.[29] In primary open-angle glaucoma, increased fundus tessellation is associated with larger peripapillary atrophy and lower intraocular pressure.[30] Zone beta is significantly smallest in juvenile-onset primary open-angle glaucoma.[31] Some studies suggested that peripapillary atrophy is larger in size in normal-tension glaucoma than in primary open-angle glaucoma[17] while others reported that eyes with normal-tension glaucoma and eyes with primary open-angle glaucoma do not differ in peripapillary atrophy.[32] Primary angle-closure glaucoma has lower prevalence of peripapillary atrophy and smaller peripapillary atrophy-to-disk area ratio compared to those in primary open-angle glaucoma.[33]

Peripapillary atrophy is associated with the optic nerve damage because the prelaminar portion of the optic nerve head receives its main blood supply from the peripapillary choroid via branches of short posterior ciliary arteries with characteristic sectoral distribution,[34-38] the absence or dysfunction of that centripetal branch in the sector of peripapillary atrophy will cause ischemic optic nerve head damage in that segment.[36-38] Previous studies have shown that the visual field defects and the optic nerve head damage are associated with the location of peripapillary atrophy.[7,8,11] Peripapillary atrophy is significantly associated with disk hemorrhage,[20,22,39] a well-known localized risk factor for glaucoma progression. Thus, peripapillary atrophy may represent a local vascular insufficiency in that area and in the corresponding segment of the optic nerve head,[1,9] thereby acting as a local vascular risk factor for the development of optic nerve head damage in normal-tension glaucoma. Another mechanism, but not proven, is that the area with peripapillary atrophy does not have blood-retinal barrier due to loss of RPE, so any vasoactive substances released from the area may increase vasospasm within the area and induce focal ischemia of the optic nerve tissues.[40]

Peripapillary atrophy is found more frequently and is larger in glaucomatous eyes compared to normal eyes. The size and extent of glaucomatous field defect correlates with functional and structural damage of the optic nerve. Further, it may help differentiating normal-tension glaucoma from glaucoma-like optic disks. It is a risk factor for glaucoma progression, especially in normal-tension glaucoma. Its close relationship with disk hemorrhage suggests a probable role of localized vascular insufficiency as the cause for glaucomatous damage remains to be proven with further study.

REFERENCES

1. Primrose J. Early signs of the glaucomatous disc. Br J Ophthalmol. 1971;55(12): 820-5.
2. Wilensky JT, Kolker AE. Peripapillary changes in glaucoma. Am J Ophthalmol. 1976;81(3):341-5.
3. Geijssen HC, Greve EL. The spectrum of primary open angle glaucoma. I: Senile sclerotic glaucoma versus high tension glaucoma. Ophthalmic Surg. 1987;18(3):207-13.
4. Jonas JB, Nguyen XN, Gusek GC, et al. Parapapillary chorioretinal atrophy in normal and glaucoma eyes. I. Morphometric data. Invest Ophthalmol Vis Sci. 1989;30(5):908-18.
5. Jonas JB, Naumann GO. Parapapillary chorioretinal atrophy in normal and glaucoma eyes. II. Correlations. Invest Ophthalmol Vis Sci. 1989;30(5):919-26.
6. Jonas JB, Fernandez MC, Naumann GO. Glaucomatous parapapillary atrophy. Occurrence and correlations. Arch Ophthalmol. 1992;110(2):214-22.
7. Anderson DR. Correlation of the peripapillary anatomy with the disc damage and field abnormalities in glaucoma. In: Greve EL, Heijl A (Eds). Fifth International Visual Field Symposium, 1982. The Hague: Dr W Junk, 1983;1-10 (Doc Ophthalmol Proc Ser; 35).
8. Heijl A, Samander C. Peripapillary atrophy and glaucomatous visual field defects. In: Heijl A, Greve EL, (Eds). Sixth International Visual Field Symposium, 1984. Dordrecht: Dr W Junk, 1985;403-7 (Doc Ophthalmol Proc Ser; 42).
9. Geijssen HC. Studies on Normal Pressure Glaucoma. New York: Kugler Publications; 1991.
10. Araie M, Sekine M, Suzuki Y, et al. Factors contributing to the progression of visual field damage in eyes with normal-tension glaucoma. Ophthalmology. 1994;101:1440-44.
11. Park KH, Tomita G, Liou SY, et al. Correlation between peripapillary atrophy and optic nerve damage in normal-tension glaucoma. Ophthalmology. 1996;103(11):1899-1906.
12. Fantes FE, Anderson DR. Clinical histologic correlation of human peripapillary anatomy. Ophthalmology. 1989;96(1):20-5.
13. Kubota T, Jonas JB, Naumann GO. Direct clinico-histological correlation of parapapillary chorioretinal atrophy. Br J Ophthalmol. 1993;77(2):103-6.
14. Jonas JB, Königsreuther KA, Naumann GO. Optic disc histomorphometry in normal eyes and eyes with secondary angle-closure glaucoma. II. Parapapillary region. Graefes Arch Clin Exp Ophthalmol. 1992;230(2):134-9.
15. Hayreh SS, Walker WM. Fluorescent fundus photography in glaucoma. Am J Ophthalmol. 1967;63(5):982-9.
16. Nevarez J, Rockwood EJ, Anderson DR. The configuration of peripapillary tissue in unilateral glaucoma. Arch Ophthalmol. 1988;106(7):901-3.

17. Tezel G, Kass MA, Kolker AE, et al. Comparative optic disc analysis in normal pressure glaucoma, primary open-angle glaucoma, and ocular hypertension. Ophthalmology. 1996;103(12):2105-13.
18. Tuulonen A, Jonas JB, Välimaki S, et al. Interobserver variation in the measurements of peripapillary atrophy in glaucoma. Ophthalmology. 1996;103(3): 535-41.
19. Park KH, Park SJ, Lee YJ, et al. Ability of peripapillary atrophy parameters to differentiate normal-tension glaucoma from glaucomalike disc. J Glaucoma. 2001;10(2):95-101.
20. Ahn JK, Kang JH, Park KH. Correlation between a disc hemorrhage and peripapillary atrophy in glaucoma patients with a unilateral disc hemorrhage. J Glaucoma. 2004;13(1):9-14.
21. Honrubia F, Calonge B. Evaluation of the nerve fiber layer and peripapillary atrophy in ocular hypertension. Int Ophthalmol. 1989;13(1-2):57-62.
22. Sugiyama K, Tomita G, Kitazawa Y, et al. The associations of optic disc hemorrhage with retinal nerve fiber layer defect and peripapillary atrophy in normal-tension glaucoma. Ophthalmology. 1997;104(11):1926-33.
23. Daugeliene L, Yamamoto T, Kitazawa Y. Risk factors for visual field damage progression in normal-tension glaucoma eyes. Graefes Arch Clin Exp Ophthalmol. 1999;237(2):105-8.
24. Buus DR, Anderson DR. Peripapillary crescents and halos in normal-tension glaucoma and ocular hypertension. Ophthalmology. 1989;96(1):16-9.
25. Derick RJ, Pasquale LR, Pease ME, et al. A clinical study of peripapillary crescents of the optic disc in chronic experimental glaucoma in monkey eyes. Arch Ophthalmol. 1994;112(6):846-50.
26. Rockwood EJ, Anderson DR. Acquired peripapillary changes and progression in glaucoma. Graefes Arch Clin Exp Ophthalmol. 1988;226(6):510-5.
27. Uchida H, Ugurlu S, Caprioli J. Increasing peripapillary atrophy is associated with progressive glaucoma. Ophthalmology. 1998;105(8):1541-5.
28. Kwon YH, Kim YI, Pereira ML, et al. Rate of optic disc cup progression in treated primary open-angle glaucoma. J Glaucoma. 2003;12(5):409-16.
29. Jonas JB, Dichtl A. Optic disc morphology in myopic primary open-angle glaucoma. Graefes Arch Clin Exp Ophthalmol. 1997;235(10):627-33.
30. Jonas JB, Gründler A. Optic disc morphology in "age-related atrophic glaucoma." Graefes Arch Clin Exp Ophthalmol. 1996;234(12):744-9.
31. Jonas JB, Gründler A. Optic disc morphology in juvenile primary open-angle glaucoma. Graefes Arch Clin Exp Ophthalmol. 1996;234(12):750-4.
32. Jonas JB, Xu L. Parapapillary chorioretinal atrophy in normal-pressure glaucoma. Am J Ophthalmol. 1993; 115(4):501-5.
33. Uchida H, Yamamoto T, Tomita G, et al. Peripapillary atrophy in primary angle-closure glaucoma: a comparative study with primary open-angle glaucoma. Am J Ophthalmol. 1999;127(2):121-8.
34. Lieberman MF, Maumenee AE, Green WR. Histologic studies of the vasculature of the anterior optic nerve. Am J Ophthalmol. 1976;82(3):405-23.
35. Anderson DR, Braverman S. Reevaluation of optic disk vasculature. Am J Ophthalmol. 1976;82(2):165-74.

36. Hayreh SS. Blood supply of the optic nerve head and its role in optic atrophy, glaucoma, and oedema of the optic disc. Br J Ophthalmol. 1969;53(11):721-48.

37. Hayreh SS. Blood supply of the anterior optic nerve. In: Ritch R, Shields MB, Krupin T (Eds). The Glaucomas. St. Louis: CV Mosby; 1989.

38. Hayreh SS. The 1994 Von Sallman Lecture. The optic nerve head circulation in health and disease. Exp Eye Res. 1995;61(3):259-72.

39. Hayakawa T, Sugiyama K, Tomita G, et al. Correlation of the peripapillary atrophy area with optic disc cupping and disc hemorrhage. J Glaucoma. 1998;7(5): 306-11.

40. Rankin SJ, Drance SM. Peripapillary focal retinal arteriolar narrowing in open angle glaucoma. J Glaucoma. 1996;5(1):22-8.

Perimetry in Glaucoma

Rangaraj NR

VISUAL FIELD

Perimerty is the evaluation of visual function at a given instance of time. Static and kinetic perimetry are different ways to plot the visual fields. The stimuli in static perimetry are at fixed locations and vary in intensity to plot the visual field. The kinetic perimetry has different sizes of stimulus moving from not seeing to seeing to plot the visual fields. This chapter discusses static perimetry, which is now widely used in clinical applications. The characteristic pattern of visual field loss makes many eye conditions like glaucoma, optic nerve diseases and neurological alter the visual function in a characteristic pattern, which makes computer-assisted perimetry a valuable tool for diagnosis and follow-up (Figs. 4.1 and 4.2). Visual field testing compliments other parameters like intraocular pressure and structure changes in the optic nerve head in decision making as in glaucoma to chart progression of the disease.

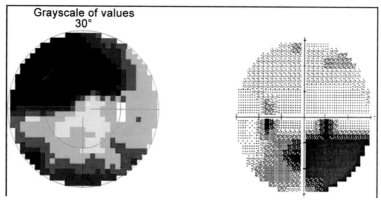

Fig. 4.1: Gray/color scale.

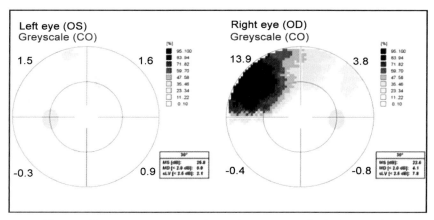

Fig. 4.2: Two on one representation with age matched color/gray scale.

The central 30 visual field examination using white on white automated static perimetry is currently the gold standard in evaluation, management and follow-up of glaucoma.

DEFINITION, TERMINOLOGIES AND PRINCIPLES IN VISUAL FIELD PERIMETRY

Visual field is the area seen when the eye is steadily fixated at a point at that instant. Hence the visual field could vary in a subtle area within the normality for the age matched population. Visual field is always measured with standard conditions of background illumination and color. The size of the stimulus varies in a kinetic perimetry from 1 to 5, with size 3 being fixed for routine static perimetry with age matched database.

Static perimetry tests the subject's ability to perceive the faintest light presented in a given location in the tested area of visual field. Differential light sensitivity is the perception of least difference between the stimulus light and the background illumination. Differential light sensitivity in effect measures the least difference between the stimuli and the background illumination.

Visual field when measured for diagnosis, follow-up and comparison is done under standard conditions of color, and background illumination that is fixed for a particular machine. Stimulus size may vary for normal estimations and for low vision conditions.

The patient's threshold is defined as the stimulus luminance, which is perceived for a given background illumination, with a probability of 50% chance of seeing or not seeing which is described by the frequency of seeing curve (FOSC) as function of stimulus luminance. Threshold is expressed in decibel (dB) scale in clinical practice. In reality, the threshold is not a fixed point; it fluctuates during the test when it is being conducted and over long periods of time at the same test points. The FOSC is very steep normally; this is due to the consistency of response to the projected light stimulus during visual field examination. This ability to perceive the 50% threshold illumination is very sharp in normal individual at all test points in the visual field, about 4 dB bandwidth (Fig. 4.3). The test points which are abnormal due to disease show inconsistency of response and the bandwidth of response becomes more than 4 dB, which makes the FOSC flat (Fig. 4.4). Generalized depression of the field causes the FOSC shift to the right but remains steep.

The standard testing conditions in perimetry data are obtained from one visit to the next. This consistent data obtained during each visit help in

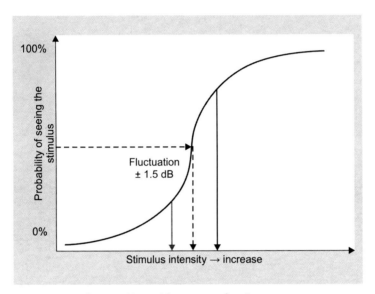

Fig. 4.3: Normal frequency of seeing curve..

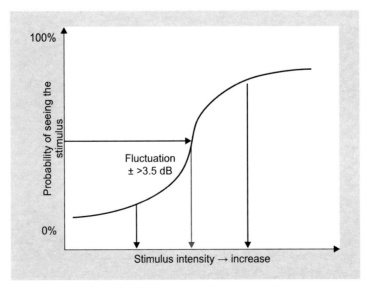

Fig. 4.4: Flat frequency of seeing curve.

follow-up and comparison to be made with age related normals. These standard test conditions are adopted in the widely used Octopus and Humphrey perimeters. The clinically relevant test conditions are the background illumination, size and duration of stimulus.

Background illumination affects the shape of the hill of vision. Lower background illumination in static perimetry increases the dynamic range and highlights areas of depressed sensitivity better because of the flatter slope of the hill of vision (Fig. 4.5). The drawback of lower background illumination is longer period of adaptation for the patient before the test is started. The Goldmann kinetic perimetry uses a 31.4 asb as the background illumination. The direct projection perimeters like the Octopus 300 and 600 use background illumination of 31.5 asb, hence can be used in normal clinic lighting conditions with little influence on adaptation time.

The stimulus exposure time is 100 ms in the Octopus perimeter, which is time enough to reach temporal summation of the stimulus luminance. Any exposure longer than 200 ms will provoke fixation reflex and give erroneous results (Fig. 4.6). Setting the stimulus interval takes into consideration the

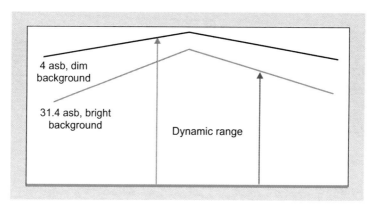

Fig. 4.5: Dynamic range with low and high background illumination.

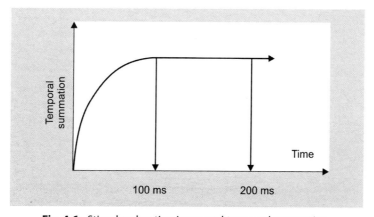

Fig. 4.6: Stimulus duration in ms and temporal summation.

'no' answer and the next stimulus. The adaptive stimulus presentation keeps track of the average time of response and proceeds with the completion of the test either faster or slower. The normal stimulus interval is set between 1.5 and 4 seconds.

MEASUREMENT STRATEGIES

It is important to understand that the 'how' of testing is the strategy and the 'where' is the program or the set of test points being tested. The choice of test strategies is offered in the Octopus 300/900 series perimeter to meet the different clinical situations of diagnosis and follow-up. The two main testing procedures offered across all perimeters are the screening tests (qualitative) and the quantitative tests as offered by the full threshold tests in the 4-2-1 dB steps.

Traditional screening strategies give qualitative results in a yes or no format to save time to get a general idea of the visual field to help in looking for an expected pattern of visual field loss expected in the particular disease process. New strategies like tendency-oriented perimetry (TOP) and dynamic give quantitative results in the same time. The two-zone testing and screening strategies are of only academic value now.

The widely used perimeters, which offer the normal full threshold testing strategy, are the dynamic strategy (Weber), TOP, Swedish Interactive Thresholding Algorithm (SITA) fast and standard as the main testing strategies. Classical normal full threshold strategy introduced by Flammer in the 1970s still forms the basis of automated perimetry.

Normal Testing Strategy

The normal strategy is the basis of all new strategies. Understanding the normal strategy makes visual field interpretation logical. Normal traditional full threshold tests all points in a random manner in steps of decreasing luminance such that a yes or no answer is obtained to the least amount of stimulus at all test points. The perimetry being computerized helps in correlating all the randomized stimulus intensities and answers in a printout. To make things easy for the patient and duration of test shorter, testing starts at one point in each of four visual field quadrants called anchor points. The anchor points test the general slope of the hill of vision to the age-corrected normal values. The visual field determination starts from this approximate hill of vision test points from the expected age-corrected minus 4 dB. A 'no' answer drops the stimulus luminance by 6 dB if the first response to a minus 4 dB start is negative. A brighter light stimulus is projected which is 8 dB less to quickly approach the depressed sensitivity of the test point. Once the anchor points are determined further testing in a 4-2-1 dB step approach at each of the predetermined test points are determined from the data obtained from

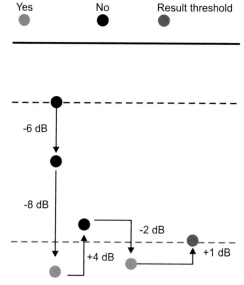

Fig. 4.7: Schematic representation of 4-2-1 bracketing strategy.

the estimated hill of vision rather than starting from normal hill of vision values which would make the testing tedious. This is approximately five questions per test point hence sensitive enough to detect shallow pathology. Normal strategy takes about 15–18 minutes per eye to complete a visual field examination (Fig. 4.7).

Shorter and smarter new strategies minimize the effects of physical and retinal fatigue. Octopus perimeter provides the dynamic strategy and TOP. The Humphrey provides the perimeter strategies SITA fast and SITA standard.

Dynamic Test Strategy

Weber introduced the dynamic strategy of visual field testing. The stimulus luminance step size (bracketing) adapts to the slope of the FOSC. When the depth of the defect is deep the step size increases from increments steps of 2 to 10 dB to achieve final calculated value from the last two tested values. The accuracy obtained with this test is comparable to the regular full threshold test with a 4-2-1 dB strategy. This strategy provides quantitative data, which may be represented as the gray scale, Bebie curve and global indices. Quantitative values are useful for follow-up and to track changes over time. The test duration is about 40–50% in severely depressed fields and 30–40% in marginally depressed fields when compared to normal threshold. Short-term fluctuation values may also be calculated by retesting all locations in the second phase if additional information is needed. Dynamic strategy provides data of the visual field comparable to the regular full threshold determination done in four stages (Figs. 4.8A and B).

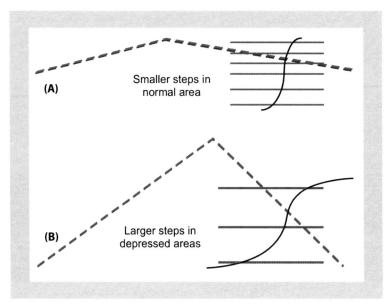

Figs. 4.8A and B: (A) Smaller steps in normal test locations. (B) Larger steps in depressed areas.

Tendency-oriented Perimetry

TOP strategy, introduced by González de la Rosa, reduces the time taken to complete the visual field analysis by 80% to the time taken by normal threshold. TOP takes into consideration the neighboring test locations when the results are interpreted. TOP strategy can be applied to all test methods like blue on yellow and flicker or programs like macular-M2. The neighboring zones in visual field exhibit a topographical interdependence; this establishes a tendency between adjacent points under examination.

TOP evaluates every 'yes' and 'no' in two ways, the location under test is evaluated for the differential sensitivity, which is called the vertical bracketing and the neighboring points are also adjusted by interpolation. A yes answer at the test location will influence the neighboring point positively and a no answer will influence the neighboring point negatively on the dB scale. In regular full threshold perimetry every test location is tested at least four to six times before arrival at the final value of differential sensitivity. A single answer in TOP is adjusted five times from the results of the neighboring test locations in the grid for final results.

These steps may be in either direction to determine the final threshold of dl sensitivity (Fig. 4.9). Grayscales show a rounded effect in TOP compared to regular threshold grayscale values because of the adjustments of the neighboring points. Hence the average sensitivity values obtained may be a little 'shallow' compared with regular threshold testing (Fig. 4.10). This difference is not of any significance when the parameter in follow-up is

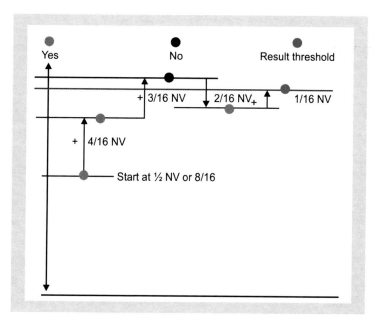

Fig. 4.9: Schematic representation of the bracketing in TOP.

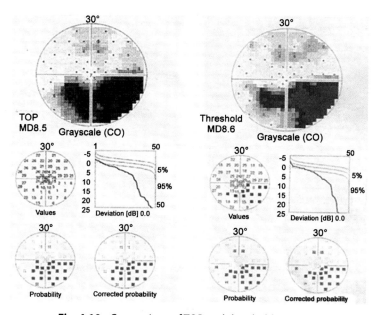

Fig. 4.10: Comparison of TOP and threshold strategy.

only changes over time, since the pathology is already established and the patient compliance is improved for follow-up testing. Note the difference in MD values of only 0.1 between the two strategies (Fig. 4.10). The gray/color scale shows some spread and shallowness of the color scale in the TOP strategy.

Swedish Interactive Thresholding Algorithm

The SITA strategy optimizes with reduction in time up to 50% without loss of quality of the visual field examination and reduced fatigue for the patient. In the software tests each point to the known predetermined value of threshold is expected. Hence a constant modeling of the normal visual field and glaucomatous defects are calculated. This triggers the testing at a location at the predetermined threshold value to stop. These values are also affected by the neighboring points and location along the nerve fiber layer. The false positive and negatives are calculated values and save time. SITA strategy is very glaucoma-specific. SITA standard is based on bracketing strategy and favored on Humphrey visual field analyzer by clinician. To even further reduce the time, the SITA fast based on FASTPAC is available. SITA standard is used for glaucoma baseline and progression analysis.

Qualitative 2 Level Testing

With the introduction of faster full threshold testing, these screening tests are almost obsolete. 2-level testing uses a maximum of two questions per location and provides a simple quantification of the tested location. The test starts with a stimulus –4 dB less than the age corrected value. A 'yes' answer sums up the test result of that location. A 'no' answer provides the same location the brightest stimuli and a 'yes' tags the test location as relative defect. A 'no' to the brightest stimulus is classified as an absolute defect. The usual time taken for 2 level quantitative testing is around 5 minutes which is more than some of the quantitative test procedures.

PROGRAM AND TEST POINTS

Programs are the fixed locations in the visual fields where the stimuli are presented in a random fashion. The Octopus and Humphrey perimeters have almost similar programs.

Octopus G1/G2 Programs

The two programs are identical in the central 30° consisting of 59 test point locations and differ only in the peripheral 15 additional points tested between the 30° and 60° in G2. The G2 is a program optimized for Octopus 900 series perimeter. The G1 program test locations respect the topography of the nerve fiber layer and are weighted to detect the nasal step in glaucoma (Fig. 4.11A). The foveal and paracentral areas have resolution of 2.8° in the G1/G2 programs compared to 4.2° resolution in a classical Program 32 test location. The increased resolution in the foveal area gives a good follow-up when there is a fixation threat, without the need of an additional visual field test for the fovea. Depressed areas have a high false-negative behavior because of a flatter FOSC and extend the test duration.

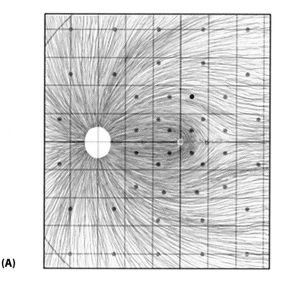

(A)

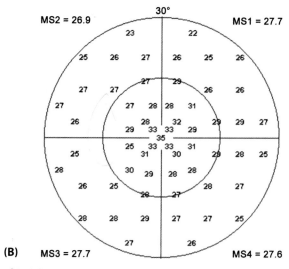

(B)

Figs. 4.11A and B: (A) G1 test points superimposed on the nerve fiber layer. (B) Typical G1 locations of test points.

All strategies can run on the G1 and G2 program (Fig. 4.11B). Most clinical needs are satisfied with the 300/600 series Octopus perimeter. The extra test points between 30° and 60° of testing do not give additional information but only confirm what is seen in the central 30° field.

Programs 32, 30-2 and 24-2

This is the classic 'off-axis' program introduced by Octopus and later by the Humphrey perimeter as the 30-2 program. There are 76 test locations in a grid pattern with a resolution of 6°. This program is not related to the topography of the nerve fiber layer or pathology with both eyes having identical pattern of test locations. The area where the blind spot appears marks the right and left eye. The program 32 is still an option, since old follow-up with Octopus was done with this program. It may also be used in neurological cases where this program defines the vertical and horizontal meridians well. The 24-2 does not test the peripheral points but retains only the temporal points (nasal step) to reduce the time taken for the strategy to complete the test (Fig. 4.12).

Macular Programs

The macular programs were designed for detection and follow-up of central and paracentral visual field defects in patients with neurological diseases, drug toxicity, macular or peri-macular diseases. This is available in both popular perimeters. (Fig. 4.13).

The M2 program has 45 test locations, which are tested in two stages consisting of the central 4° and the area between 4 and 9°. The 45 test locations in the central 4° gives a 0.7° resolution with a Goldmann Size III, which is 0.43° in diameter (Fig. 4.13). The additional 36 test locations situated in the outer 4–9° gives this program the highest resolution in the central 10° of the visual

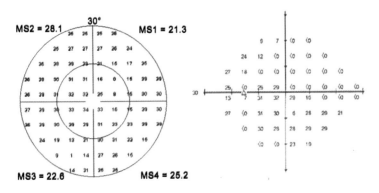

Fig. 4.12: Test point locations in the P32, the 30-2 program 24-2.

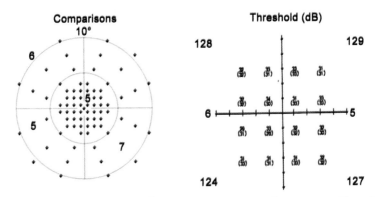

Fig. 4.13: Test point locations in the M2 (Octopus) and macular programs (Humphrey).

field. The M2 program can be run using the TOP, dynamic or normal strategy to define the visual field pathology in question.

The macular program in Humphrey visual field analyzer tests the central 16 points which are thresholded to improve reliability and repeatability. The 10-2 provides the higher threshold central only test points in the Humphrey perimeter.

Macular and central programs are used to detect split fixation in advance visual field defects in glaucoma and central scotomas due to drug toxicity.

SYSTEMATIC INTERPRETATION OF A SINGLE FIELD REPORT

The seven-in-one printout contains the raw results from the visual field examination and easy to read statistical data interpreting the results in a clinic setting. The single field printout presents the relevant statistical calculations, images, graphs, plots and indices on a single page. (Figs. 4.14A and B).

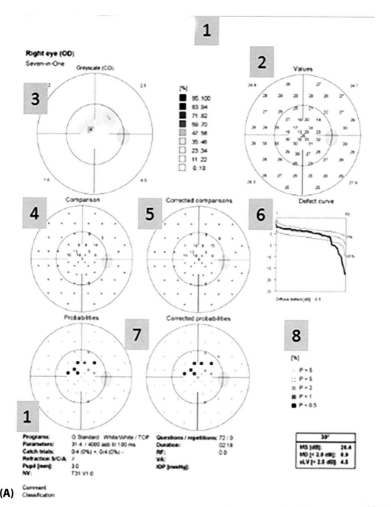

(A)

(Contd.)

(Contd.)

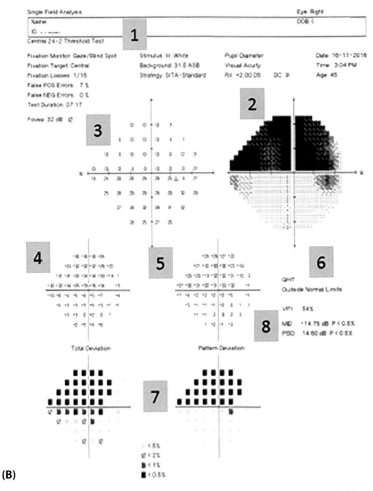

(B)

Figs. 4.14A and B: (A) Octopus single field report. (B) Humphrey single field report.

The seven in one report is interpreted in the following order:

1. *Patient and examination data:* The patient name, age, details of the examination strategy and program. The refractive error, pupil size along with the reliability indices of the test conducted provides the references from which the final interpretation is done. Fixation losses in Octopus are automatic based on image analysis. The Humphrey has a gaze tracking at the bottom of the report with upward lines indicating gaze error of more than 10°. Lines downward indicating a blink.

2. *The Octopus value table and the measured values in the Humphrey:* These are the measured values of the test conducted. All further statistical and graphical details are derived from this set of raw data.

3. *Grayscale (in color or in B/W):* The gray scale is a graphic representation of the pattern of visual field defects for the doctor that can be used to

explain the nature of the problem to the patient. This representation is derived from the raw values. The Octopus perimeter gives an option of representation from the comparison to define the area of pathology.

4. *Comparison table and total deviation:* They represent the local difference between the measured values and the normal age-matched values. This representation highlights the area of pathology at a glance in numbers away from normal. A '+' indicates a normal between -2 and $+2$ deviation in an Octopus printout.

5. *Corrected comparison and pattern deviation table:* They shows the defects discounting any uniform depression caused by a cataract or refractive errors.

6. *Cumulative defect (Bebie) curve:* An arrangement of all tested data points from the highest value to least from left to right, which is overlaid on a statistically age corrected normal for comparison. The diffuse defect is the overall decrease in sensitivity due to uniform loss, e.g., cataract and refractive errors. The topography of the defect is not provided. The glaucoma hemifield test (GHT) gives plain language results of the comparison on five paired mirror image zones in the upper and lower hemi fields.

7. *Probability plots:* Graphical representation of the probability or the statistical significance of a defect in comparison to the age-matched individuals and grayscale representation minus the diffuse defect in the corrected comparisons and the pattern deviation plots. These plots are derived from the total deviation, pattern deviation, comparison and corrected comparison. The probability symbols are easy to read, for example, a test location displaying a black spot indicates less than 0.5% normal population have this as normal.

8. *Visual field indices:* Condenses the visual field results in a few numbers. Octopus has the following indices: mean sensitivity (MS) is the patient's arithmetic mean of the measured raw values. Mean defect (MD) is patient corrected values for the age match. This age correction makes MD independent of age. sLV is square root of loss variance. This index provides a measure of variability across the visual field. Humphrey printouts have similar indices: mean deviation (MD) shows how much on an average the whole field deviates from normal age match. Pattern standard deviation (PSD) highlights irregularities in the visual field caused by localized defects. PSD is sensitive for early and moderate defects only. Visual field index (VFD) is derived from PSD, which is less affected with the presence of cataract and provides a correlation to the ganglion cell loss. VFI is 100% in normal and 0% in perimetric blindness.

INTERPRETING VISUAL FIELD CHANGE

Visual field testing has been used as end point and as an outcome measure in large trials like the collaborative initial glaucoma treatment study (CIGTS) and ocular hypertension treatment study (OHTS). The follow-up of patients in these large studies led to development of scoring pathologic test points to standardize and evaluate change in visual fields to indicate the end point for the particular patient in the study. These large studies included patient having primary open angle glaucoma, which hence was used for progression or change and not diagnosis. Visual field provides measurement of test locations with smart strategy and program to evaluate statistically significant deviation from normal populations. It measures the percentage of population having the visual field test point normal e.g., $<5\%$, $<1\%$ and $<0.5\%$. With $>0.5\%$ indicating that a population of $>0.5\%$ will have that test point as normal.

POAG has a specific pattern of loss in sensitivity at test locations at the nasal, paracentral, superior and inferior areas of the visual field. When these areas are flagged as significant with probabilities of $<1\%$, $>1\%$ or $>0.5\%$ the indices, the cumulative defect curve (Octopus), diffuse defect, GHT and VFI (Humphrey) indicate high probability that these test points reflect pathology. The Anderson criteria of 3 or more contagious 'nonedge points' in typical arcuate area on 30-2 program or P32 depressed at p $<5\%$ with at least one point at p $<1\%$, PSD/CPSD @ p $<5\%$, GHT = outside normal limits that

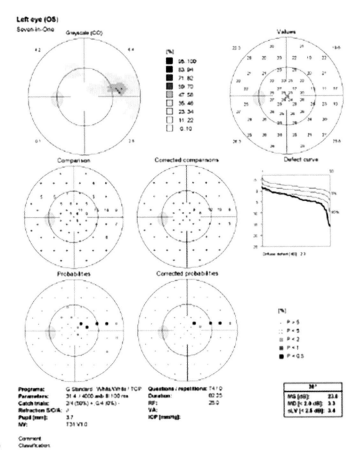

(A)

(Contd.)

(Contd.)

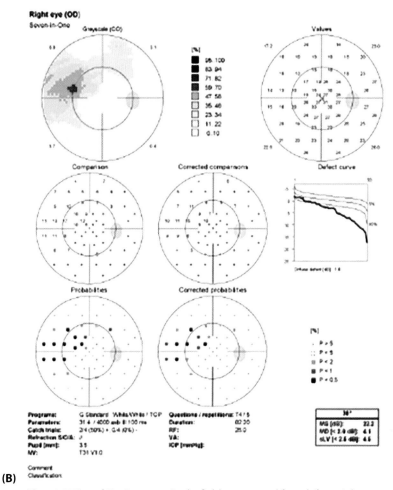

(B)

Figs. 4.15A and B: Octopus single-field report read from left to right.

is demonstrated on 2 field tests are thumb rules that help in summarizing the visual fields clinically for decision making. These criteria are universal to any static automated visual field test results. This reproducible pathology on visual field should also correlate with the structural damage on fundus examination.

Case Example

A 70-year-old male patient presented with gradual and painless defective vision for past one year. His visual acuity was 6/24 NV N12 both eyes. IOP (Applanation) was 24 mm Hg both eyes. The single field, the two on one print-out, fundus picture and OCT gave a structure and function correlation for a diagnosis of cataract and POAG. OCT is not needed to make the diagnosis,

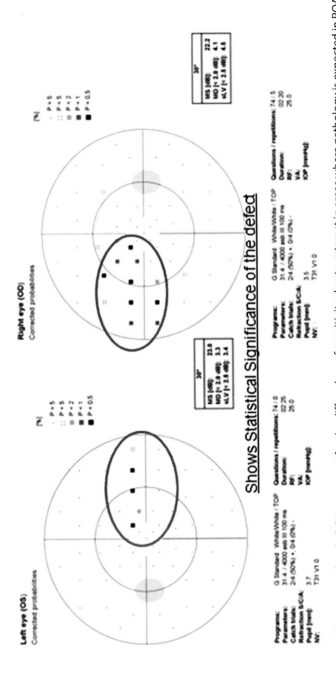

Fig. 4.16: The corrected probabilities account for the diffuse loss of sensitivity due to cataract in areas where pathology is expected in POAG.

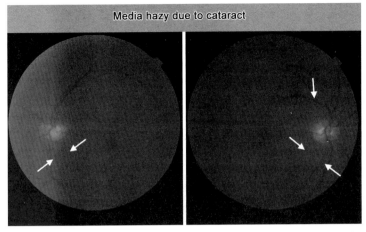

Fig. 4.17: Red free pictures reflecting nerve fiber layer defects correlating the visual field defects despite the cataract haze.

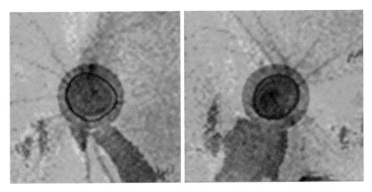

Fig. 4.18: OCT pictures reflecting nerve fiber layer defects correlating the visual field defects despite the cataract haze.

it was included only to display the nerve fiber layer defect despite the media haze. (Figs. 4.15 to 4.18).

ACKNOWLEDGMENT

Figures 4.2 to 4.4, and 4.17A are printed with permission from HAGG-STREIT AG.

BIBLIOGRAPHY

1. Bebie H, Fankhauser F, Spahr J. Static perimetry: strategies. Acta Ophthalmol. (Copenh). 1976;54(3):325-38.
2. Bebie H, Flammer J, Bebie T. The cumulative defect curve: separation of local and diffuse components of visual field damage. Graefes Arch Clin Exp Ophthalmol. 1989;227(1):9-12.

3. Dannheim F. First experiences with the new Octopus G1-program in chronic simple glaucoma. IPS Meeting (1986).
4. Fankhauser F, Koch P, Roulier A. On automation of perimetry. Graefe's Arch Clin Exp Ophthalmol. 1972;184(2):126-50.
5. Flammer J, Drance SM, Fankhauser F, et al. Differential light threshold in automated static perimetry. Factors influencing short-term fluctuations. Arch Ophthalmol. 1984;102(6):876-9.
6. Flammer J, Jenni A, Bebié H, et al. The Octopus glaucoma G1 program. Glaucoma. 1987;9:67-72.
7. Gonzàlez de la Rosa M, Pareja A. Influence of the fatigue effect and the mean deviation measurement in perimetry. Eur J Ophthalmol. 1997;7(1):29-34.
8. Morales J, Weitzmann M, Gonzàlez de la Rosa M. Comparison between tendency oriented perimetry (TOP) and Octopus threshold perimetry. Ophthalmology. 2000;107(1):134-42. Weber J, Klimaschka T. Test time and efficiency of the dynamic strategy in glaucoma perimetry. Ger J Ophthalmol. 1995;4:24-31.

Ultrasound Biomicroscopy in Glaucoma

Kaushik S, Pandav SS

INTRODUCTION

Ophthalmic ultrasound imaging is based on the emission of an acoustic pulse and reception of the pulse after it has been reflected off ocular tissues. It has been used in the form of A- and B-scans for many decades. Ultrasound biomicroscopy (UBM) is a new imaging technique that uses high-frequency ultrasound to produce images of the eye at near microscopic resolution.[1] The use of a higher frequency transducer allows for a more detailed assessment of the anterior ocular structures than was available using the traditional B-scan ultrasound. It also decreases penetration (to only 5 mm), but increases the resolution of the imaged structures. Lateral and axial resolutions are estimated to be 40 and 20 μm, respectively. High-frequency UBM provides high-resolution in vivo imaging of the anterior segment in a noninvasive fashion and can scan through opaque media.[2] In addition to the tissues easily seen using conventional methods (i.e., slit-lamp), such as the cornea, iris, and sclera, structures including the ciliary body and zonule, previously hidden from clinical observation, can be imaged and their morphology assessed. Additionally, pathophysiological changes involving anterior segment architecture can also be evaluated qualitatively and quantitatively.[3]

This chapter will review the various applications of the UBM for glaucoma and illustrate how it can be a useful tool in the management of various conditions.

TECHNOLOGY

The technology for UBM, originally developed by Pavlin, Sherar, and Foster, is based on 50- to 100-MHz transducers incorporated into a B-mode clinical scanner (Fig. 5.1). Higher frequency transducers provide finer resolution of

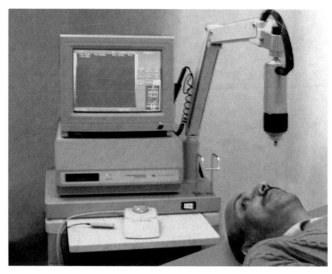

Fig. 5.1: Ultrasound biomicroscopy model P40 (Paradigm Medical Industries).

more superficial structures, whereas lower frequency transducers provide greater depth of penetration with less resolution. The commercially available units operate at 50 MHz and provide lateral and axial physical resolutions of approximately 50 and 25 μm, respectively. Tissue penetration is approximately 4–5 mm. The scanner produces a 5 × 5 mm field with 256 vertical image lines (or A-scans) at a scan rate of 8 frames per second. The real-time image is displayed on a video monitor and can be recorded on videotape for later analysis.

More recent generations of the UBM incorporate the water bath around the probe into a hand piece, which can be applied as the patient is in the sitting position using a coupling gel between the globe and the probe.

IMAGE ACQUISITION

Images are acquired with the patient lying supine. Room illumination, fixation, and accommodative effort affect anterior segment anatomy and should be held constant, particularly when quantitative information is being gathered.

In the Paradigm Instruments UBM, the probe is suspended from a gantry arm to minimize motion artifacts.

In the OTI (Ophthalmic Technologies, Toronto, Canada) device, the probe is small and light enough not to require a suspension arm. Scanning is performed with the patient in the supine position. A plastic eyecup of the appropriate size is inserted between the lids, holding methylcellulose or normal saline coupling medium (Figs. 5.2 and 5.3).

This is uncomfortable and may potentially distort the eye anatomy and angle configuration. This requirement of globe contact renders this instrument minimally invasive and may make it impractical for many clinical situations,

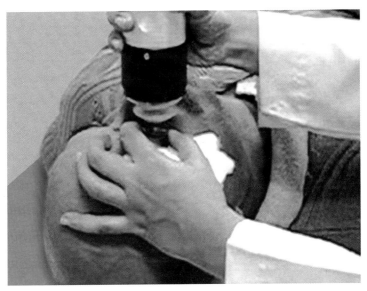

Fig. 5.2: Ultrasound biomicroscopy model P40, with probe in eyecup.

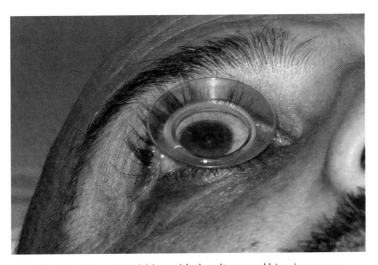

Fig. 5.3: Image acquisition with the ultrasound biomicroscopy.

such as perforating ocular injuries or infective corneal perforations. In addition, a highly skilled operator is needed to obtain high-quality images, and the learning curve of the technique is fairly steep. Also this is one technique where it is preferable and at times may be mandatory for the treating physician to do the procedure himself, since it is imperative to image precisely the area of interest. The high magnification renders general scanning of little use. To maximize the detection of the reflected signal, the transducer should be oriented so that the scanning ultrasound beam strikes the target surface perpendicularly.

CLINICAL APPLICATIONS

Before studying any imaging technique for disease pathology, it is important to know what the normal eye looks like. The normal anterior segment can be imaged very well with the UBM and is illustrated below.

Cornea

Going from anterior to posterior (Fig. 5.4), the first echogenic line structure is the corneal epithelium (a). The next is the Bowman's membrane (b). The stroma is minimally echogenic (c) and is then followed by another echogenic structure—the Descemet's membrane (d).

The Normal Angle of the Anterior Chamber

The normal angle (Fig. 5.5) is seen as the junction between the cornea and sclera where the iris root inserts into the ciliary body. The sclera is normally

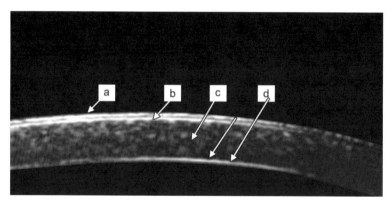

Fig. 5.4: Cornea imaged with the ultrasound biomicroscopy.

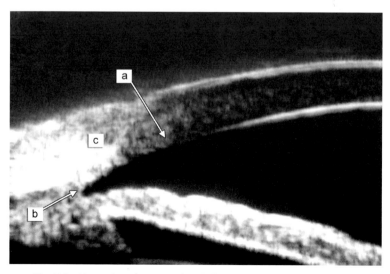

Fig. 5.5: Normal angle imaged with the ultrasound biomicroscopy.

not as echolucent as the cornea owing to the irregular arrangement of the collagen fibers. The junction between the cornea and sclera marks the anterior Schwalbe's line (a). The anterior-most part of the junction between the sclera and the ciliary body band is the scleral spur (b). Identification of the scleral spur is critical to angle assessment using the UBM. The scleral spur is the only constant landmark allowing one to interpret UBM images in terms of the morphologic status of the anterior chamber angle and is the key for analyzing angle pathology. The area between the scleral spur and the anterior Schwalbe's line is the region identified as the trabecular meshwork (TM) (c) on the UBM.

Generally, in the normal eye, the iris has a roughly planar configuration with slight anterior bowing, and the anterior chamber angle is wide and clear. However, morphology of the anterior segment structures alters in response to a variety of physiologic stimuli such as accommodation and lighting.

It is important to maintain a constant testing environment critical for longitudinal comparison.

UBM in Glaucoma

The major applications of the UBM in glaucoma can be summarized under the following headings:
- Angle measurement—quantifying the angle
- Pathophysiology of angle closure
  - Pupillary block glaucoma
  - Plateau iris
- Pigmentary glaucoma
- Pseudoexfoliation
- Goniodysgenesis
- Iridocorneal endothelial (ICE) syndrome
- Ocular trauma
  - Angle recession
  - Iridodialysis
  - Cyclodialysis clefts
  - Occult foreign bodies
- Ciliochoroidal detachment

Angle Assessment

UBM measurement of angle structures maybe influenced by variation in physiological variability. Failure to control accommodation and room illumination can alter the findings when using UBM. Direction of gaze can be standardized by placing markers on the ceiling to optimize orientation of the eye when measuring different quadrants. Other sources of variability are more difficult to control and this technique of angle assessment is inherently subjective in nature.

Quantifying the Angle

It is possible to use the UBM to quantify the width of the angle.[3] It is important to understand some concepts of measurement inherent to the machine properties.

Physical resolution is often confused with measurement precision. However, physical resolution only specifies how close together two objects can be located and yet still be determined to be distinct. It also specifies the smallest object detectable. Measurement precision refers to the width and height of a single pixel on the screen that can be identified by the operator using the screen cursor. Commercially available instruments provide lateral and axial physical resolution of approximately 50 and 25 μm, respectively. The resolution of the Paradigm device is slightly better than that of the OTI device. The theoretical lateral and axial measurement precision on the standard UBM monitor (864×432 pixels) is approximately 6 and 12 μm. Although UBM cannot distinguish two small objects less than 25 μm apart along the axial scanning line, it can still measure the distance between two objects far enough apart (>25 μm, such as corneal thickness, anterior chamber depth) with 12-μm precision.

The UBM measurement software calculates distance and area by counting the number of pixels along the measured line or inside the designated area and multiplies the pixel counts by the theoretical size of the pixel. However, it is still difficult to analyze an image when observers are required to manually place calipers on the areas of interest in order to derive values from each image.

Angle Measurement

Pavlin et al.[3] established various quantitative measurement parameters as standards (Fig. 5.6). The position of the scleral spur is used as a reference point for most of their parameters, because this is the only landmark that can be distinguished consistently in the anterior chamber angle region.

- *The angle-opening distance (AOD):* This is defined as the distance from the corneal endothelium to the anterior iris, perpendicular to a line drawn along the TM, at a given distance from the scleral spur. This is measured at 250 μm (AOD 250), which consistently falls on the TM and 500 μm (AOD 500) from the scleral spur, which measures the angle opening anterior to the TM. The AOD—reflects the amount of relative pupillary block in patients with occludable angles. The AOD 250 is a measure of the angle opening at the level of the posterior TM. AOD 500 is a measure of the angle opening at the level of the anterior Schwalbe's line.
- *The trabecular-ciliary process distance (TCPD):* This is measured from a point on the TM, 500 μm anterior to the scleral spur, extended perpendicularly through the iris to the ciliary process. The TCPD defines the port through which the iris must traverse and has implications as to

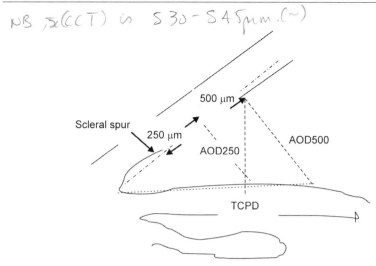

Fig. 5.6: Angle parameters.

the potential maximal angle opening, and defines the space available between the TM and ciliary process. It is a typical feature in an individual eye. It is the sum of three segments: the angle opening 500 μm from the scleral spur; the thickness of the iris at that point, and the width of the ciliary sulcus. An anteriorly placed ciliary process can reduce the peripheral anterior chamber depth and make it susceptible to occlusion.

In a comparative study between UBM and gonioscopy,[4] excellent correlation was found between gonioscopically quantified angles and those quantified by the UBM. There is actually no role of the UBM in quantifying the angle for diagnosing angle closure, but it is of immense help in qualifying the cause of a narrow angle.

Pathophysiology of Angle Closure

- *Pupillary block glaucoma (Figs. 5.7A and B):* Relative pupillary block with aqueous pooling behind the iris can be easily recognized on the UBM. Laser iridotomy is the treatment of choice and adequacy of treatment can be confirmed easily by UBM.[5-8]
- *Plateau iris (Figs. 5.8A to C):* This entity is often difficult to diagnose clinically. The typical gonioscopic features include a comparatively flat iris plane compared to an obvious convexity in pupillary block, and a sharp drop-off of the iris in the periphery. Confirmatory signs include the 'double hump' sign on indentation due to prominent ciliary processes abutting the periphery of the iris against the TM. Often a plateau iris is suspected when there is a persistency of symptoms or raised pressures despite a successful iridotomy. This entity can be beautifully diagnosed by UBM.[9]

In these cases, appropriate treatment is a laser peripheral iridoplasty. The UBM can show adequacy of treatment by demonstrating that the peripheral iris has been pulled away from the TM by the laser contraction burns.

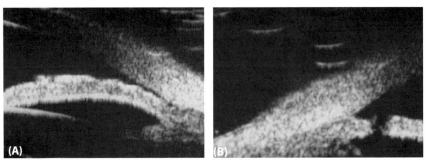

Figs. 5.7A and B: (A) Pupillary block angle closure. (B) Pupillary block angle closure with laser iridotomy.

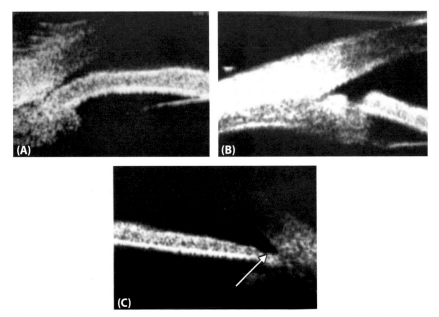

Figs. 5.8A to C: (A) Plateau iris with prominent ciliary process. (B) Plateau iris with patent but ineffective iridotomy. (C) Plateau after laser iridoplasty. Note the peripheral contraction burns.

- *Angle closure with iridociliary cysts (Fig. 5.9):* Isolated iridociliary cysts are an uncommon cause of angle closure. However, they must be suspected especially in young patients with closed angles and no other explainable cause. UBM is probably the only investigation which can demonstrate them objectively.[10]

Pigmentary Glaucoma

Pigmentary glaucoma is now recognized to be caused by a concave iris configuration resulting in a 'reverse pupillary block' where the aqueous dams in from of the iris.[11] This causes the iris to rub against the ciliary processes and

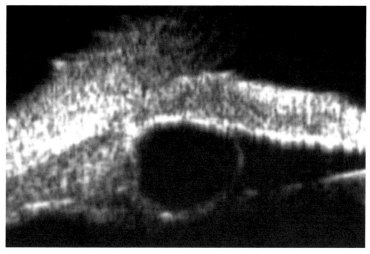

Fig. 5.9: Iridociliary cyst and angle-closure.

zonules (Fig. 5.10A), resulting in pigment dispersion all over the anterior segment including the anterior lens surface, corneal endothelium and TM. With time, this pigment clogs the TM and causes raised pressures and eventually optic nerve head damage. Laser peripheral iridotomy serves to reverse this pathology and the iris flattens, thus relieving the reverse pupillary block (Fig. 5.10B).[12]

Pseudoexfoliation

Pseudoexfoliation is commonly thought to be a cause of secondary open-angle glaucoma. However, in certain situations, angles may be closed. The broken zonules cause the lens to become more spherical and move forward (Fig. 5.11). In this condition, it leads to a secondary angle closure. Usually, by this time, there is significant cataract, and cataract removal would solve the problem. However, in case the lens in clear, a laser iridotomy works very well.

Goniodysgenesis

Goniodysgenesis was also known as mesodermal dysgenesis or anterior segment cleavage syndromes. Current terminology groups these disorders into the spectrum of the Axenfeld–Rieger anomaly. The common features are multiple iris processes, and higher insertion of the iris signifying improper recession of the iris during angle development (Figs. 5.12A and B).

Iridocorneal Endothelial Syndrome

This group of entities comprising Chandler's syndrome, Cogan–Reese syndrome and essential iris atrophy is characterized by a membrane which grows

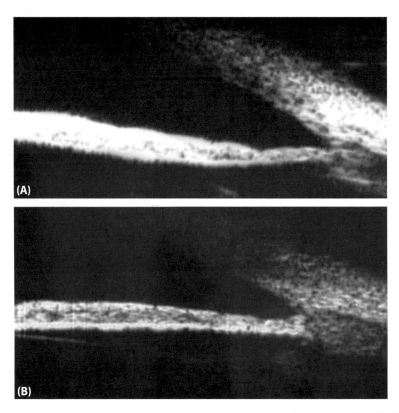

Figs. 5.10A and B: (A) Pigmentary glaucoma with concave iris configuration. (B) Pigmentary glaucoma after laser peripheral iridotomy. Note the flattened iris and resolution of reverse pupillary block.

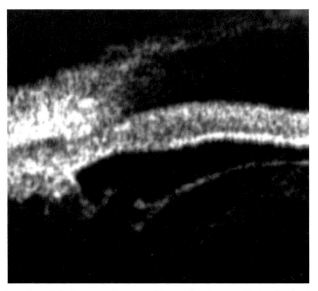

Fig. 5.11: Pseudoexfoliation syndrome with angle closure. Note the broken zonules and spherical lens configuration.

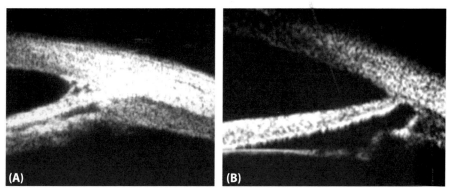

Figs. 5.12A and B: (A) Goniodysgenesis with abnormally prominent iris processes. (B) Goniodysgenesis with abnormally high iris insertion.

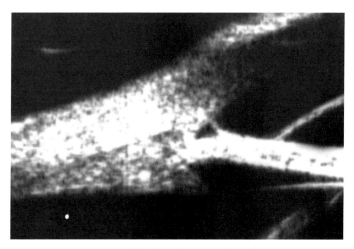

Fig. 5.13: Iridocorneal endothelial (ICE) syndrome with PAS but normal angle of anterior angle.

on to the iris from the corneal endothelium, hence its name. The characteristic features include broad-based peripheral anterior synechiae, but the angle underlying is normal (Fig. 5.13).

Ocular Trauma

- *Angle recession and iridodialysis:* A tear between the longitudinal and circular ciliary muscle can be easily demonstrated on the UBM. Like-wise iridodialysis or separation of the iris from its root can be recognized (Fig. 5.14).
- *Cyclodialysis clefts:* Cyclodialysis clefts may be the cause of unexplained hypotony following trauma. Often difficult to ascertain with gonioscopy, they may be detected by careful examination by the UBM. (Fig. 5.15).[13]

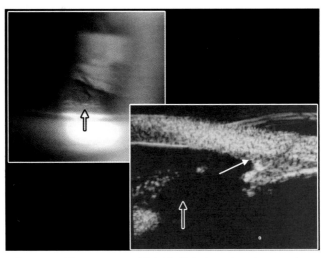

Fig. 5.14: Blunt trauma with iridodialysis and angle recession.

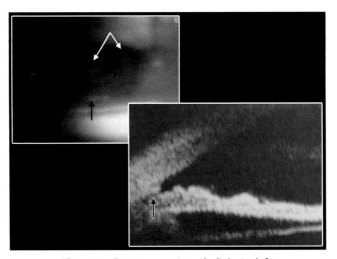

Fig. 5.15: Post-traumatic cyclodialysis cleft.

- *Occult foreign bodies:* Foreign bodies lodged in the iris or ciliary body area can be extremely difficult to localize. The UBM can aid immensely by precisely localizing them to enable their removal with certainty (Fig. 5.16).[14-16]

Ciliochoroidal Detachment

Ciliochoroidal detachment can result in unexplained postoperative hypotony, which may remain undetected by conventional methods of investigations. The UBM, by imaging anterior to the pars plana can pinpoint the cause easily (Fig. 5.17).

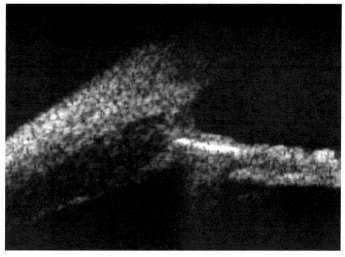

Fig. 5.16: Occult foreign body lodged in the iris stroma, accurately localized by the ultrasound biomicroscopy

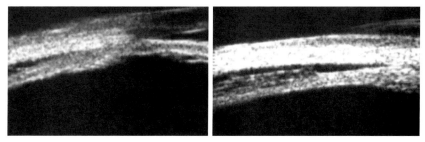

Fig. 5.17: Occult ciliochoroidal detachment following uncomplicated cataract surgery leading to unexplained hypotony postoperatively. Note the fluid in the supraciliary space.

CONCLUSION

UBM technology has become an indispensable tool in qualitative and quantitative assessment of the anterior segment. It has clarified concepts in the pathophysiology of diseases such as pigment dispersion, plateau iris and pseudoexfoliation glaucoma. Future advancements including incorporation of Doppler technology may further enhance the utility of the device in quantitative assessment of the anterior segment.

REFERENCES

1. Pavlin CJ, Sherar MD, Foster FS. Subsurface ultrasound microscopic imaging of the intact eye. Ophthalmology. 1990;97(2):244-50.
2. Pavlin CJ, Harasiewicz K, Sherar MD, et al. Clinical use of ultrasound biomicroscopy. Ophthalmology. 1991;98(3):287-95.

3. Pavlin CJ, Harasiewicz K, Foster FS. Ultrasound biomicroscopy of anterior segment in normal and glaucomatous eyes. Am J Ophthalmol. 1992;113(4):381-9.
4. Kaushik S, Jain R, Pandav SS, et al. Evaluation of the anterior chamber angle in Asian Indian eyes by ultrasound Biomicroscopy and gonioscopy. Indian J Ophthalmol. 2006;54(3):159-63.
5. Kaushik S, Kumar S, Jain R, et al. Ultrasound biomicroscopic quantification of the change in anterior chamber angle following laser peripheral iridotomy in early chronic primary angle closure glaucoma. Eye (Lond). 2007;21(6):735-41.
6. Gazzard G, Friedman DS, Devereux JG, et al. A prospective ultrasound biomicroscopy evaluation of changes in anterior segment morphology after laser iridotomy in Asian eyes. Ophthalmology. 2003;110(3):630-8.
7. Garudadri CS, Chelerkar V, Nutheti R. An ultrasound biomicroscopic study of the anterior segment in Indian eyes with primary angle-closure glaucoma. J Glaucoma. 2002;11(6):502-7.
8. Yoon KC, Won LD, Cho HJ, et al. Ultrasound biomicroscopic changes after laser iridotomy or trabeculectomy in angle closure glaucoma. Korean J Ophthalmol. 2004;18(1):9-14.
9. Kumar RS, Baskaran M, Chew PT, et al. Prevalence of plateau iris in primary angle closure suspects: an ultrasound biomicroscopy study. Ophthalmology. 2008;115(3):430-4.
10. Marigo FA, Finger PT, McCormick SA, et al. Anterior segment implantation cysts. Ultrasound biomicroscopy with histopathologic correlation. Arch Ophthalmol. 1998;116(12):1569-75.
11. Potash SD, Tello C, Liebmann J, et al. Ultrasound biomicroscopy in pigment dispersion syndrome. Ophthalmology. 1994;101(2):332-9.
12. Breingan PJ, Esaki K, Ishikawa H, et al. Iridolenticular contact decreases following laser iridotomy for pigment dispersion syndrome. Arch Ophthalmol. 1999;117(3):325-8.
13. Park M, Kondo T. Ultrasound biomicroscopic findings in a case of cyclodialysis. Ophthalmologica. 1998;212(3):194-7.
14. Kaushik S, Ichhpujani P, Ramasubramanian A, et al. Occult intraocular foreign body: ultrasound biomicroscopy holds the key. Int Ophthalmol. 2008;28(1):71-3.
15. Berinstein DM, Gentile RC, Sidoti PA, et al. Ultrasound biomicroscopy in anterior ocular trauma. Ophthalmic Surg Lasers. 1997;28(3):201-7.
16. Laroche D, Ishikawa H, Greenfield D, et al. Ultrasound biomicroscopic localization and evaluation of intraocular foreign bodies. Acta Ophthalmol Scand. 1998;76(4):491-5.

6

Optical Coherence Tomography in Glaucoma

R Ramakrishnan, Arjit Mitra

INTRODUCTION

Optical coherence tomography (OCT) is a noncontact noninvasive technology providing high-resolution, cross-sectional images of the eye. It is an optical imaging system providing in vivo imaging of the retina analogous to B scan. Its use in retina and glaucoma has been steadily growing. Many studies have been performed, showing its reproducibility and correlation with histological appearance. Its use for glaucoma diagnosis and in vivo capabilities of retinal nerve fiber layer (RNFL) and optic nerve head (ONH) analysis has revolutionized the previous uncertain diagnostic challenges into an accurate and precise diagnosis.

Although visual field assessment has been the gold standard for glaucoma diagnosis, it has been documented that up to 40% of the RNFL may be lost before a defect is apparent on the visual field. The Ocular Hypertension Study (OHTS) showed that 55% of eyes that converted to glaucoma did not have a field defect but only structural changes in the ONH. Identification of structural optic nerve damage is thus very important in the early diagnosis of glaucoma and in monitoring its clinical course. Until recently, assessment of the optic nerve and RNFL has been largely subjective. Variability in the size and appearance of the optic disk of normal eyes complicates the detection of early glaucomatous optic nerve damage. Standard techniques to diagnose and monitor structural changes in glaucoma, have included serial stereoscopic photographs of the optic disk and monochromatic photographs of the RNFL. While these methods provide objective information for comparisons, the interpretation of photographs remains subjective, and variation in photographic assessment among even experienced observers is well documented.[1] Furthermore, qualitative assessment of photographs may not be sensitive to small changes over time, and it is difficult to pick up diffuse damage on these photographs.

New technologies, such as confocal scanning laser ophthalmoscopy (HRT), scanning laser polarimetry (GDxVCC) and OCT[2] have become available that provide quantitative, reproducible and objective measurements of ONH and RNFL thickness.[3] The present chapter will focus on the principles of OCT and its role to diagnose and manage glaucoma patients.

BASIC PRINCIPLES OF OCT

The OCT contains an interferometer that resolves retinal structures by measuring the echo delay time of light that is reflected and backscattered from different microstructural features in retina. OCT is based on the principle of Michelson interferometry. Low-coherence infrared (830 nm) light coupled to a fiber optic travels to a 50/50 beam splitter and is directed through the ocular media to the retina and to a reference mirror, respectively. Light passing through the eye is reflected by structures in different retinal tissue layers. The distance between the beam splitter and reference mirror is continuously varied. When the distance between the light source and retinal tissue is equal to the distance between the light source and reference mirror, the reflected light from the retinal tissue and reference mirror interacts to produce an interference pattern. The interference pattern is detected and then processed into a signal (Fig. 6.1). The signal is analogous to that obtained

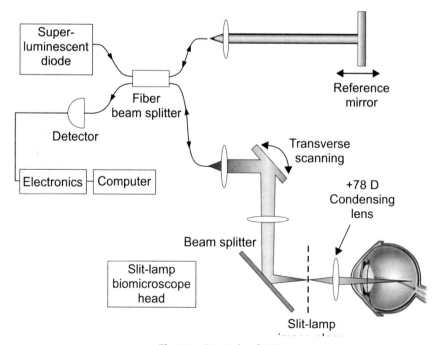

Fig. 6.1: Principle of OCT.

by A-scan ultrasonography using light as a source rather than sound. A two-dimensional (2D) image is built as the light source is moved across the retina. One can think of the image as a series of stacked and aligned A-scans to produce a 2D cross-sectional retinal image that resembles that of a histologic section. This imaging method thus can be considered a form of in vivo histology.

The newer Stratus OCT (OCT 3; Carl Zeiss Inc, Dublin, California, USA) can be used in the absence of dilation in many individuals, and usually requires a 3-mm pupil for adequate visualization. An infrared-sensitive charge-coupled device video camera documents the position of the scanning beam on the retina. The OCT image can be displayed on a gray scale where more highly reflected light is brighter than less highly reflected light. Alternatively, it can be displayed in color whereby different colors correspond to different degrees of reflectivity. On the OCT scanners currently commercially available, highly reflective structures are shown with bright colors (red and yellow), while those with low reflectivity are represented by darker colors (black and blue). Those with intermediate reflectivity appear green.

Current commercial scanners employ a low coherence super luminescent diode source (820 nm). The presently available model Stratus OCT (OCT 3) has a theoretical axial resolution < 10 mm. Ultrahigh resolution research OCT scanners use a titanium sapphire laser that has an ultrabroad spectral bandwidth centered at approximately 800 nm. With these light sources, axial resolution can be increased to 2–3 mm, but these light sources are expensive and have a limited role in routine clinical applications.[4]

Comparison with HRT, GDX AND RTA

Other technologies are available for ONH in aging and nerve fiber layer analysis. The past decade has seen the emergence and refinement of HRT and scanning laser polarimetry (SLP) GDx and the retinal thickness analyzer (RTA).

The major limitation of HRT is that the use of a reference plane is required. For this manual tracing of the ONH margin has to be done by a trained technician or ophthalmologist. As compared to HRT II, OCT does not require a trained technician to mark the points for disk margin. The measurements may be affected by blood vessels. The HRT is useful for scanning the ONH and its use for determining RNFL thickness is limited by axial resolution of the CSLO device.

The SLP device, GDx suffers from high variability in readings due to normal anatomical variations in different eyes as well as presence of pathological changes in different individuals. Some of these sources of error, which adversely affect reliability, include ethnicity and age variations, prior corneal surgeries like LASIK, corneal transplantation, vitreous opacities, motion artifacts and macular structural pathologies.

Comparison with Ultrasound

OCT is the optical equivalent of ultrasound using light reflection as opposed to sound detection of tissues. As compared to ultrasound, it is a noncontact technology, providing for patient comfort and acceptability. As compared to UBM no special sterile materials are needed in OCT.

IMPORTANCE OF OCT IN GLAUCOMA

The management of glaucoma has ideally been based on the combination of intraocular pressure, clinical examination of ONH and visual field testing. Advances in our understanding of glaucoma have contributed to the view that retinal ganglion cell layer death is an early process in glaucoma. This precedes the changes in the visual field by several years. IOP is the only variable currently amenable to treatment. However, owing to the variability, spikes and fluctuation of IOP throughout the day there is a doubt as to the reliability of the isolated IOP values measured days weeks or months apart. The correct value of IOP, as measured by the different types of tonometers, is subject to a lot of debate.

Stereophotographic evaluation as well as serial ophthalmoscopic examinations of the ONH require a skilled observer. However, there is a significant amount of inter-observer variation between different individuals, thus grossly affecting the reliability. Coming to the visual field, the fields presently in vogue, use automated techniques and is a subjective test. The visual fields are prone to short and long-term fluctuations and thus require serial testing over a period of time to obtain reliable fields. The whole process is long drawn out and diagnosis is delayed, resulting in loss of time in instituting management.

From the above we can thus conclude that the diagnosis of glaucoma is delayed and the traditional tests do not provide a reliable diagnosis in time for providing appropriate care. Here comes the role of OCT in glaucoma. It can diagnose glaucoma early and with a certain degree of reliability whereby treatment can be instituted in time.

OCT provides high-resolution measurements and cross-sectional imaging of the retina, optic disk and the RNFL. For glaucoma applications, an operator-determined circular or linear path is scanned around the optic disk to generate a series of 100 axial reflectance profiles. From these, a real-time 2D tomographic image is constructed. The first reflection measurement is the vitreous–internal limiting membrane interface. The highly reflective interface posterior to this is the RPE photoreceptor interface. A threshold of reflectivity between the two is set as the posterior boundary of the RNFL. RNFL and retinal thickness are calculated from these landmarks. Average measurements are given for 12° and 30° sectors. The depth values of the scans are independent of the optical dimensions of the eye, and no reference plane is required. Useful measurements in glaucoma patients are normally made along a circle concentric with the optic disk.

INSTRUMENTATION

The OCT system hardware consists of the patient module, the computer unit, the flat screen video monitor, key board, mouse and color inkjet printer. The hardware mounts on a wheelchair accessible motorized power table.

Procedure

The patient is seated with the chin on the provided chin rest and the forehead against a curved strap. As it is a noninvasive procedure the patient enjoys a great degree of comfort throughout the duration of the test. A pupil diameter of 3.2 mm is recommended by the manufacturer. The room lights are dimmed and in most cases scanning can be done without the need for dilatation. However, in Indian population sometimes the pupillary diameter is inadequate and thus pupillary dilatation is needed. In presence of media opacities pupillary dilatation is a must. Otherwise the signal strength will not be accurate to give a reliable reading. A pupillary size of 3 mm is however adequate for most purposes in presence of a clear optical media. An infrared CCD camera monitors the position of laser beam on the retina. An internal fixation reference beam allows the patient to focus his vision, thereby reducing unwanted movements. A circle of 3.4 mm is used for sampling the RNFL as it has been shown to correlate best with changes in glaucoma.[5] OCT 3 offers highest sampling density of 512 sampling points. The scans are made by linear scans in a spoke pattern configuration. The OCT generates a real-time tomographic section of the tissues from the collected reflectance interferometer data. The anterior reflectance is from the interface between the vitreous and the internal limiting membrane. The posterior limit of the RNFL is the boundary of retinal pigment epithelium (RPE). The ending of RPE at the edges of the optic disk automatically determines the disk margins eliminating observer variations inherent in HRT due to requirement for manually marking disk edges. The cup diameter is measured on a line parallel to the disk line and offset anteriorly by 150 μm and various ONH parameters are automatically calculated. Mean RNFL thickness is calculated using the inbuilt RNFL thickness average analysis protocol.

CLINICAL USES

- To evaluate the RNFL for early (pre-perimetric) glaucoma detection.[6]
- To detect study and follow the macular changes in hypotony induced maculopathy after glaucoma surgery.
- To evaluate cystoid macular edema after combined cataract and glaucoma surgery and use of anti-glaucoma medications.[7]
- To evaluate ONH tomography in glaucoma patients.

SCANS

There are two basic scan patterns: lines and circles. The OCT 3 constructs all 18 scan protocols from line or circle scans. The three most commonly used scans are:

1. *Fast optical disk:* This protocol acquires six 4 mm radial line scans which are designed for the ONH analysis.
2. *Fast RNFL thickness:* This protocol acquires three 3.4 mm diameter circle scans, which are designed for use with the RNFL thickness analyses.
3. *Fast macular thickness map:* It consists of six 6 mm radial lines scans through a common central axis. This protocol is designed for examination of macular thickness as an indicator of glaucoma. It is designed for use with the analyses that measures retinal thickness and to obtain maps of retinal thickness in a circular area centered on the macula.

The analysis protocols assist us with diagnostic analysis of scan images of the posterior segment of the eye. There are 11 quantitative analysis protocols for glaucoma and retina and seven image processing protocols.

DIFFERENT ANALYSIS PROTOCOLS IN GLAUCOMA

Basically, three different analysis protocols are used in glaucoma evaluation. These are the RNFL analysis, the ONH analysis and the macular thickness analysis. The sum of these three analysis protocols provide a comprehensive glaucoma evaluation and help the observer arrive at a diagnosis with a high degree of reliability.

1. *RNFL analysis:* The analysis of RNFL aids in the identification of early glaucomatous damage circular scans of 3.4 mm in diameter around the ONH provide measurement of the RNFL in the peripapillary region. This has been shown to correlate best with changes in glaucoma.[5] The RNFL measurement is graphed in a TSNIT orientation and compared to the age matched normative data.
2. *ONH analysis:* Radial line scans through the optic disk provide cross-sectional information on the degree of cupping and the neuroretinal rim area. The disk margins are identified objectively identified using signal from end of RPE. The key parameters include cup-to-disk ratio and horizontal integrated rim volume.
3. *Macular thickness analysis:* This analysis is based on the fact that a thinning of the macula may reflect glaucomatous loss. The structural analysis of the retinal sublayers reveals macular complications. Cross-sectional view provides visualization and measurement of retinal layers.

RNFL THICKNESS ANALYSIS

Interpretation of RNFL Thickness Average Analysis

OCT offers a variety of RNFL thickness measurements and analysis protocols for use in glaucoma. A fast protocol is used for a rapid analysis but the drawback of a fast protocol is that it may miss out on the finer critical points. The other protocol is a detailed one and is useful for diagnosis and follow-up of ongoing RNFL damage.

- *RNFL thickness protocol (3.4 mm):* It acquires a scan with radius 1.73 mm, centered on the optic disk.
- *Fast RNFL thickness protocol (3.4 mm):* It acquires three fast circular scans. This is a time-efficient scan alignment and placement is required only once.
- *Proportional circle protocol:* This protocol allows measurement of RNFL thickness (RNFLT) around the optic disk along a circular scan, the size of which can be tailored as per individual's need taking into account the size of ONH.
- *Concentric three-ring protocol:* This protocol enables us to measure RNFLT along three equally placed default circular scans of 0.9, 1.81 and 2.71 mm radii. However, the scan radius can be altered according to the need.
- *RNFL thickness protocol (2.27× disk):* This circular RNFLT scan size is 2.27 times the size of the ONH as determined by OCT (ending of RPE is automatically defined as ONH margin by the program). This may be useful as a standardization in research studies for comparison in disparate population, providing normative data and comparing RNFL thickness in various ONH sizes. This may help us to measure RNFLT with accuracy is various disk sizes. [6]
- *RNFL map protocol:* This protocol comprises six circular scans of 1.44, 1.69, 1.90, 2.25, 2.73 and 3.40 mm radii. This gives an overlay view of the RNFLT, around the peripapillary area. RNFL measurement with a circular scan of 1.34 mm radius, centered on the ONH, has been shown to have a maximum reproducibility in glaucomatous patients.[8] Mean RNFL thickness is calculated using the inbuilt RNFL thickness average analysis protocol.

Clinical Interpretation of RNFL Thickness Average Analysis

For understanding purpose the RNFL thickness average analysis printout can be divided into various zones (Fig. 6.2) that include:

Zone 1: Patient ID data

Zone 2: Individual TSNIT curves for each eye presented in comparison with the age-matched normative database.

Zone 3: Overlap of TSNIT curve showing a comparison of 2 eyes.

Zone 4: Circular diagram showing quadrant-wise and clock hour-wise distribution of average RNFL thickness in both eyes.

Zone 5: Data table: It shows various ratios, quadrant averages, and difference among the quadrants and between the 2 eyes. Each value is marked in color to show its level of deviation from the normal values.

Zone 6: Red-free photograph; black and white photographs of 2 eyes taken with the infrared camera are available on the printout. These denote the position of scan circle on the fundus.

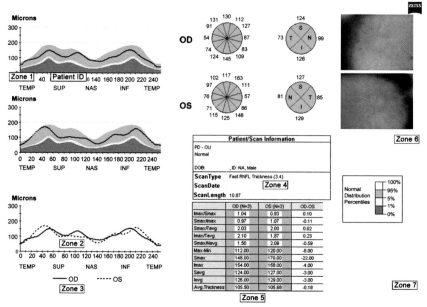

Fig. 6.2: RNFL thickness average analysis scan. Average thickness: The average RNFL thickness along the entire circular scan: Superior average and inferior average (SAVG and IAVG): The average RNFL thickness in the respective 900 of the circular Smax and Imax (superior maximum and inferior maximum): Maximum RNFL thickness recorded in the respective 90° quadrant of the scan. Max–Min: Difference between the maximum and minimum RNFL value along the circular scan.

Zone 7: Percentile distribution color coding: A small box denoting the color coding of percentile distribution of normative database is provided. White and green color represent the distribution within 95%, yellow color representing the areas of RNFL thickness below 5th percentile, and red color representing the areas of RFNFL thickness below 1 percentile. Similar color coding is applicable for the individual TSNIT.

The four ratios provided in the data table are self-explanatory. OCT 3 also enables us to perform a RNFL thickness serial analysis can serially compare up to four scan groups and provide an overview of RNFL thickness change over time. Interpretation of optic disk scan provides ONH analysis.

The newer version of the OCT, OCT 3, allows a detailed quantitative evaluation of the ONH. It is provided with two scan protocols.

OPTIC NERVE HEAD ANALYSIS

Optic disk scan consists of equally placed line scans 4 mm in length, at 30° intervals, centered on the optic disk. The number of lines can be adjusted between 6 and 24 lines.

Fast optic disk scan compresses six optic disk scans into one scan and acquire scan in short time of 1.92 s. The ONH analysis and various ONH parameters are calculated using the inbuilt ONH analysis protocol. This analysis detects the anterior surface of the RNFL and the RPE. The cup perimeter is determined by automatic detection of the reference points. The inbuilt algorithm detects and measures all the features of disk anatomy based on anatomical landmarks, (disk reference points), on each side of the disk where the RPE ends. It locates and measures the disk diameter by tracing a straight line between the disk reference points. The cup diameter is measured on a line parallel to the disk line and offset anteriorly by 150 µm and various ONH parameters are automatically calculated. These parameters include optic disk tomography included average disk area, cup area, rim area (disk area minus the cup area), vertical integrated rim area (VIRA), horizontal integrated rim width (HIRD), cup volume, average cup/disk ratio and horizontal and vertical cup disk ratios.

- *Vertical integrated rim area (Volume):* This estimates the total volume of RNFL tissue in the rim.
- *Horizontal integrated rim width (Area):* It estimates the total rim area and other measurements.

The ONH analysis printout can be divided into various zones (Fig. 6.3) that includes:

Zone 1: Patient ID data

Zone 2: It gives the overview of ONH head analysis along with the composite image figure constructed from all scans and all the important ONH parameters.

Zone 3: Individual radial scan analysis, along with scan image it gives the disk diameter, cup diameter, rim area and rim length in that particular meridian. Overlap of TSNIT curve showing a comparison of 2 eyes.

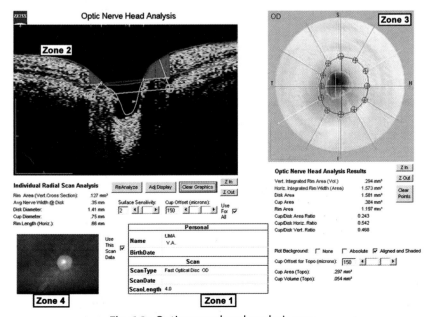

Fig. 6.3: Optic nerve head analysis scan.

Zone 4: Red-free photograph; black and white photograph of the optic disk taken with the infrared camera is also available on the printout.

MACULAR THICKNESS ANALYSIS

Macular Thickness and Macular RNFL Thickness in Glaucoma Eyes

Macula NFL thickness and macular thickness is significantly reduced in glaucoma. Mean macular volume is 7.01 ± 0.42 mm^3 vs 6.57 ± 0.85 mm^3 for normal vs glaucoma eyes, respectively.

The OCT scans are highly informative and show a very high degree of correlation with the slit-lamp – 90 D fundus evaluation and fundus photographs and the Humphrey automated perimetry single field analysis printouts as evident from the following examples (Figs. 6.4 to 6.7).

SD OCT

The first generation OCTs enabled us to get the measurement of the thickness of the RNFL. Numerous studies have since then shown a correspondence between OCT measurements and histological measurements.[9-11] This is the reason why clinicians are studying the RNFL thickness more frequently to aid in early diagnosis of glaucoma and to obtain an accurate assessment of disease progression. The Cirrus^{TM} HD-OCT spectral domain technology is

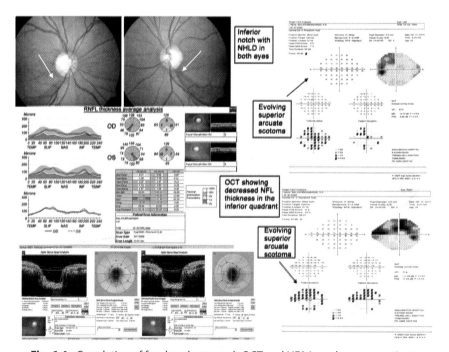

Fig. 6.4: Correlation of fundus photograph OCT and HFA in a glaucoma patient.

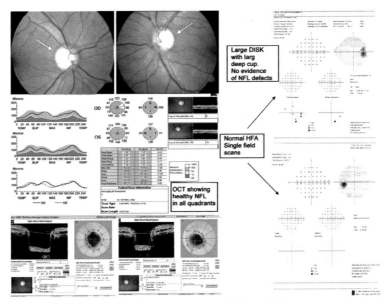

Fig. 6.5: Correlation of fundus photographs, OCT and HFA in a normal patient.

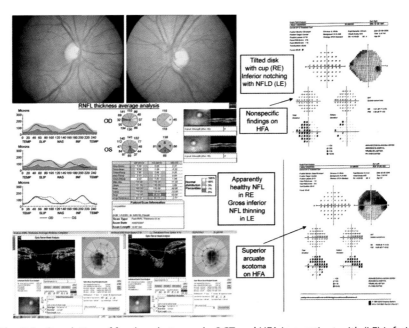

Fig. 6.6: Correlation of fundus photograph, OCT and HFA in a patient with (LE) inferior rim loss.

further advancing the study of glaucoma. It employs a simple, easy-to-use system that allows us to precisely capture and clearly display information about the peripapillary area and the RNFL. The Cirrus™ HD-OCT provides the printout of the two different maps on the same page. The neuroretinal rim thickness map and the RNFL thickness map (Figs. 6.8 to 6.11).

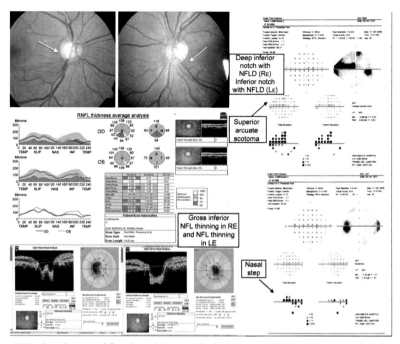

Fig. 6.7: Correlation of fundus photograph, OCT and HFA in a patient with bilateral inferior notching.

OPTIC DISK SCAN

The Cirrus HD-OCT scan of the optic disk captures a 6 × 6 mm cube which is formed from 200 A-scans for each of 200 B-scans. The area within the 6 × 6 mm area is segmented for analysis. From this cube of data the machine automatically identifies the center of the disk and creates a 3.46 mm calculation circle around the disk. The RNFL thickness along the peripapillary circle is analyzed and compared to normative data. Even if the scan was not centered on the optic disk, the RNFL circle analysis will be centered automatically assuring precise registration and excellent repeatability.

FUNDUS IMAGE

The laser scanning ophthalmoscope (LSO) fundus image with OCT fundus image overlay is displayed at the top of the RNFL analysis screen or printout. The location of the calculation circle for the temporal superior or nasal, inferior temporal analysis is shown in red. The operator can reposition the circle for analysis after scan acquisition but this is usually not necessary because the automatic centering is adequate.

RNFL THICKNESS MAP

The RNFL thickness map is based on data calculated over the entire cube. Using a color scale similar to that of a topographical map, cool colors represent

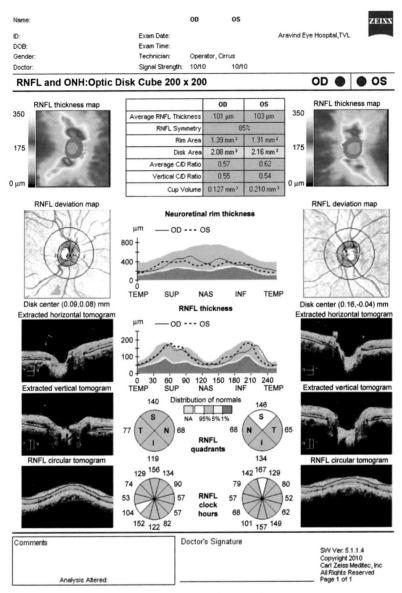

Fig. 6.8: SD OCT scan of a normal patient.

thinner areas and warm colors represent thicker areas. It shows RNFL thickness at each point within the 6 × 6 mm area. The maps exclude the optic disk, which is displayed in dark blue. The color code expresses the thickness from zero (blue) to 350 μm (white).

Deviation Map

The deviation map compared the patients RNFL thickness versus normative data. Data points that are outside normal limits are shown in red and yellow.

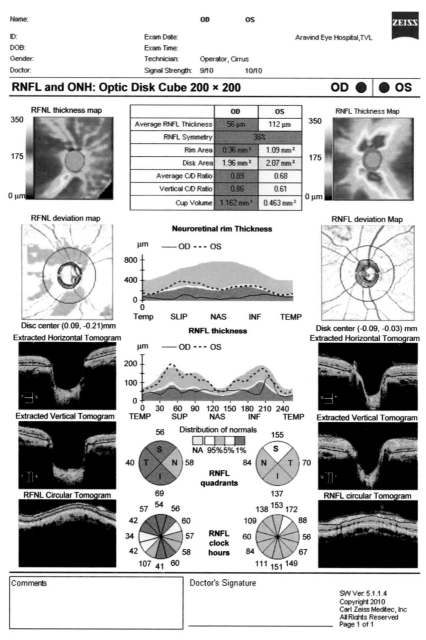

Fig. 6.9: SD OCT scan of a patient showing advanced glaucomatous damage in the right eye.

Average Thickness Values

The RNFL thickness along the TSNIT calculation circle is also illustrated numerically in chart format. The average thickness for all points along the calculation circle is shown for both eyes. Average thickness is also shown for each quadrant and for the clock hours. In each of these charts the patient's

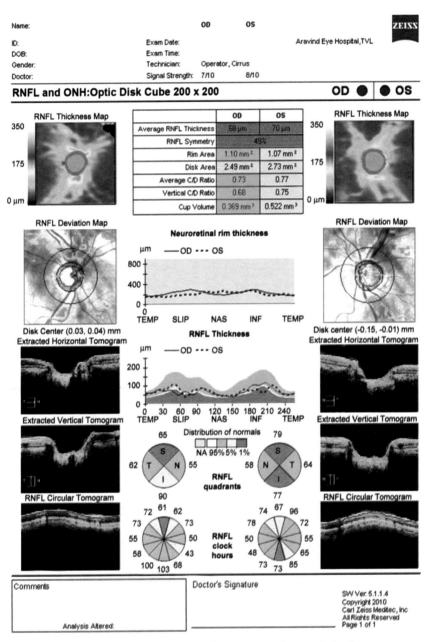

Fig. 6.10: SD OCT scan showing glaucomatous damage in both eyes.

values are compared to normative data. The data table calls out symmetry, which is also compared to normative data.

TSNIT THICKNESS PROFILES

The TSNIT profiles show RNFL thickness at each position along the peripapillary analysis circle and compare these measurements with a normative

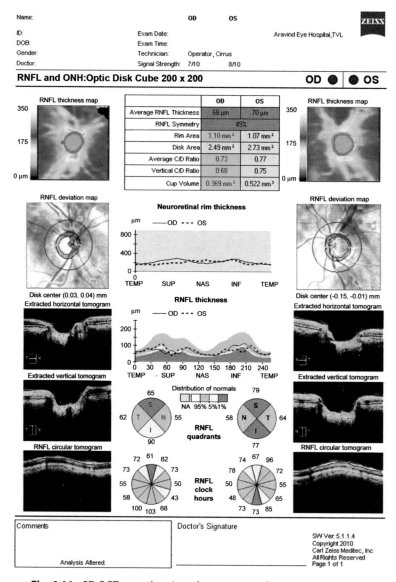

Fig. 6.11: SD OCT scan showing glaucomatous damage in both eyes.

database. They are color coded (white, green, yellow, red) for comparison with the normative RNFL data for subjects of the same age.

NORMATIVE DATABASE

The normative database uses color to indicate the normal distribution percentiles among individuals of the same age as follows:

- *Red*: The lowest 1% of normal measurements fall within the red zone. These readings are considered outside normal limits.
- *Yellow*: The lowest 5% of normal measurements fall within or under the yellow zone.

- *Green*: 90% of all normal measurements fall within the green area.

While interpreting the normative data, we must remember that for each measurement, 1 in 20 normal eyes (5%) will fall below the green zone.

The RNFL normative database helps us identify areas of clinical interest by comparing patient's RNFL thickness measurements with age matched normal subjects. The normative data comparison is available for patients over 18 years of age.

ADVANTAGES OF OCT

- OCT provides objective, quantitative, reproducible measurements of the retina and RNFL thickness.
- In contrast with other imaging techniques, direct measurements of the RNFL are calculated from cross-sectional retinal images.
- Measurements are not affected by refractive status, axial length of the eye, or the presence of early nuclear sclerotic cataracts.
- Structural information is independent of any arbitrarily defined reference plane.
- A single device gives information about the macula, optic disk and RNFL. While OCT provides an objective measurement of nerve fiber layer structure, its clinical use in the early detection and follow-up of glaucoma patients is still under evaluation.

DISADVANTAGES OF OCT

- As with other ocular imaging technology, high cost currently precludes generalized use of the OCT.
- The presence, of posterior subcapsular and cortical cataracts impairs performance, and pupillary dilation is required to obtain acceptable peri-papillary measurements.
- OCT images contain significantly fewer pixels than both SLP and CSLO. Recent evidence suggests that increasing sampling density of OCT scans from 25 points/quadrant to 100 points or more/quadrant provides a less variable representation of RNFL thickness.
- The follow-up for glaucoma requires change analysis techniques that require further development and testing.

NORMATIVE INDIAN DATA

Tewari et al.[7] determined the normative values for macular thickness and volume by OCT 3 in healthy Indian subjects. They evaluated the macula of 170 consecutive, randomly selected normal subjects who were imaged on OCT 3 in this cross-sectional study. OCT parameters of macular thickness were analyzed with baseline variables including age, gender, axial length and refractive error. The average foveal thickness in the population under study was 149.16 ± 21.15 μm. Macular thickness and volume parameters of OCT correlated significantly

(Pearson's correlation coefficient) with age ($r = 0.23$, $P < 0.01$), but not with gender, axial length and refraction. Sony et al.[12] quantified the retinal nerve fiber thickness in normal eyes with OCT. They studied 146 eyes of 146 patients. The average RNFL thickness in this sample population was $104 + 8.51$ μm (95% CI 87.25–121). The RNFL was thickest in inferior quadrant, followed by the superior quadrant, and progressively less in nasal and temporal quadrant. The RNFL was significantly correlated with age but not with gender.

Budenz et al.[13] have recently reported that the RNFL thickness as measured by stratus OCT varies significantly with age, ethnicity, axial length and optic disk area. In summary, they reported that the mean RNFL thickness for the entire population was 100.1 μm (SD 11.6). Thinner RNFL measurements were associated with older age ($P < 0.001$), being Caucasian versus either Hispanic or Asian ($P = 0.006$), greater axial length ($P < 0.001$) or smaller optic disk area ($P = 0.010$). For every decade of increased age, mean RNFL thickness measured thinner by approximately 2.0 μm [95% confidence interval (CI), 1.2–2.8]. For every 1 mm greater axial length the mean RNFL thickness measured thinner by approximately 2.2 μm (95 % CI, 1.1–3.4). For every increase in square mm of optic disk area, mean RNFL thickness increased by approximately 3.3 μm (95% CI, 0.6–5.6). Comparison between ethnic groups revealed that Caucasians had mean RNFL values (98.1 ± 10.09 μm) slightly thinner than those of Hispanics (103.7 ± 11.6 μm) or Asians (105.8 ± 9.2 μm). There was no relationship between RNFL thickness and gender.

In the study done by Ramakrishnan et al.[14] Around 118 Indian patients were evaluated with the help of the Stratus OCT 3000 V 4.0.1. The results revealed that the mean ± standard deviation RNFL thickness for the various quadrants: superior, inferior, nasal, temporal and along the entire circumference along the ONH were 138.2 ± 21.74, 129.1 ± 25.67, 85.71 ± 21, 66.38 ± 17.37, and 104.8 ± 38.81 μm, respectively. There was no significant difference in the measurements between males and females and no significant correlation with respect to age.

THE FUTURE

The pre-perimetric diagnosis of glaucoma is going to be the real challenge for the future. The ultra-high resolution (UHR) OCT is the thing to look forward to for the diagnosis of glaucoma at the earliest. It utilizes $Ti:Al_2O_3$ laser and achieves a much lower resolution of around 2 μm, which is not possible with the currently available OCTs. The studies with UHR OCT have been encouraging.

REFERENCES

1. Varma R, Steinmann WC, Scott IU. Expert agreement in evaluating the optic disc for glaucoma. Ophthalmology. 1992;99:215-21.
2. Daniel M Stein. Imaging in Glaucoma. Ophthalmology Clinics of North America Imaging. Joel S. Schuman, Vol 17, March 2004, Elsevier Saunders; 41-46.

3. Bowd C, Zangwill LM, Berry CC, et al. Detecting early glaucoma by assessment of retinal nerve fiber layer thickness and visual function. Invest Ophthalmol Vis Sci. 2001;42(9):1993-2003.
4. Voo I. Clinical applications of OCT. Ophthalmology Clinics of North America Imaging. Joel S. Schuman, Vol 17, March 2004, Elsevier Saunders; 21-31.
5. Schuman JS, Hee MR, Puliafito CA, et al. Quantification of nerve fiber layer thickness in normal and glaucomatous eyes using optical coherence tomography. Arch Ophthalmol. 1995;113(5):586-96.
6. Jones AL, Sheen NJ, North RV, et al. The Humphrey optical coherence tomography scanner: quantitative analysis and reproducibility study of the normal human retinal nerve fiber layer. Br J Ophthalmol. 2001;85(6): 673-7.
7. Tewari HK, Wagh VB, Sony P, et al. Macular thickness evaluation using the optical coherence tomography in normal Indian eyes. Indian J Ophthalmol. 2004;52(3):199-204.
8. Quigley HA, Addicks EM, Green WR. Optic nerve damage in human glaucoma: III Quantitative correlation of nerve fiber loss and visual field defects in glaucoma, ischemic optic neuropathy, papilledema, and toxic optic neuropathy. Arch Ophthalmol. 1982;100(1):135-46
9. Abbott CJ, McBrien NA, Grünert U, et al. Relationship of the optical coherence tomography signal to underlying retinal histology in the tree shrew (*Tupaia belangeri*). Invest Ophthalmol Vis Sci. 2009;50(1):214-23.
10. Chen TC, Cense B, Miller JW, et al. Histologic correlation of in vivo optical coherence tomography images of the human retina. Am J Ophthalmol. 2006;141(6):1165-8.
11. Gloesmann M, Hermann B, Schubert C, et al. Histological correlation of the pig retina radial statification with ultra high resolution optical coherence tomography. Invest Ophthalmol Vis Sci. 2003;44(4):1696-703.
12. Sony P, Sihota R, Tewari HK, et al. Quantification of the retinal nerve fiber layer thickness in normal Indian eyes with optical coherence tomography. Indian J Ophthalmol. 2004;52(4):303-9.
13. Budenz DL, Anderson DR, Varma R, et al. Determinants of normal retinal nerve fiber layer thickness measured by stratus OCT. Ophthalmology. 2007; 114(6):1046-52.
14. Ramakrishnan R, Mittal S, Ambatkar S, et al. Retinal nerve fibre layer thickness measurements in normal Indian population by optical coherence tomography. Indian J Ophthalmol. 2006;54(1):11-5.

7

Pitfalls in the Diagnosis of Angle-closure Glaucoma

Bhartiya S, Ichhpujani P, Gandhi M, Albis-Donado O

INTRODUCTION

Angle-closure disease is less common than open-angle glaucoma worldwide,[1] but its incidence in certain populations is known to be much higher than previously documented. Also, its impact on quality of life of the patient is more critical due to a greater likelihood of blindness, and higher morbidity rates than in patients with open-angle glaucomas. An accurate and timely diagnosis is therefore essential, in order to prevent progression to irreversible visual field loss.

CLASSIFICATION

As a result of population research in regions where angle-closure glaucoma is a major cause of blindness, the definition of angle-closure glaucoma has undergone revision. For more uniform reporting, and to improve the understanding of the mechanisms of angle closure, PJ Foster and colleagues proposed a new terminology, which has been recognized as the International Society of Geographical and Epidemiological Ophthalmology (ISGEO) Classification.[2] As per this classification, the primary group is subdivided according to conceptual stages in natural history of angle closure of glaucoma into primary angle-closure suspect (PACS), primary angle closure (PAC) without optic neuropathy and primary angle-closure glaucoma (PACG) with neuropathy. Previously used terminology such as chronic, intermittent and subacute ACG has become obsolete.

- *PACS:* Irido-trabecular contact (ITC) with normal optic disc and visual field. IOP is normal and PAS is absent (Fig. 7.1).
- *PAC:* ITC + either raised IOP, PAS (Fig. 7.2) or signs of past attack of angle closure such as glaucomflecken or typical symptoms.

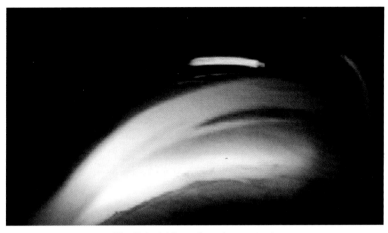

Fig. 7.1: Irido-trabecular contact.

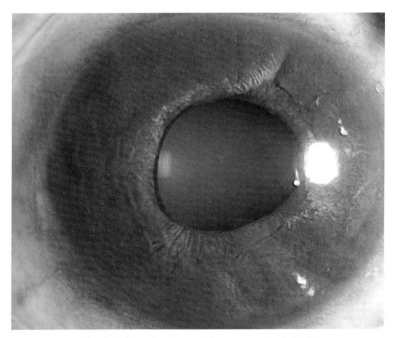

Fig. 7.2: Iris whorling, sphincter atrophy in PAC.

- *PACG:* ITC + structural glaucomatous changes in optic nerve + visual field loss.

Acute Primary Angle Closure

This presents with classic signs and symptoms. Patients have markedly elevated IOP, gonioscopy reveals the angle is closed, circumciliary congestion, the cornea is frequently cloudy, and the patient complains of eye pain and may have nausea and vomiting (Fig. 7.3).

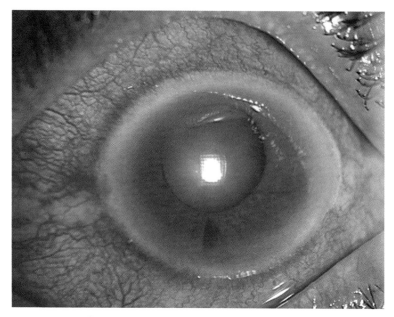

Fig. 7.3: Acute attack of primary angle closure.

This system is the basis for the American Academy of Ophthalmology Primary Angle Closure Preferred Practice Pattern Guideline and is consistent with the World Glaucoma Association consensus on angle-closure glaucoma.

MECHANISMS

Pathologic mechanisms for angle closure exist because of primary anatomic variations in the size, position and relationship of the anterior segment structures (cornea, iris, ciliary body, lens)[3,4] or occur *secondary* to other acquired ocular pathology. These include trabecular obstruction with contraction of neovascular, inflammatory or proliferative fibrocellular membranes, crowding of the angle, plateau iris and lens induced glaucomas.

- *Pupillary block:* The most common mechanism of PAC is pupillary block. Contact between the iris and the lens at the pupillary margin increases resistance to the flow of aqueous into the anterior chamber. When the pressure in the posterior chamber exceeds that in the anterior chamber, the peripheral and midperipheral iris moves forward and contacts the trabecular meshwork resulting in aqueous blockage at two levels: the pupillary margin and the trabecular meshwork.
- *Plateau Iris:* In plateau iris syndrome, the ciliary body is anteriorly positioned or rotated forward, resulting in the anterior displacement of the peripheral iris into the angle. The condition is characterized by either persistent angle closure or angle closure and elevated IOP upon pupillary dilation despite the presence of a patent iridotomy or iridectomy.

- *Recent concepts:* Position of the entire iris relative to the meshwork and volume of iris determines the likelihood of appositional angle closure. Recent quantitative measurements of the iris and angle with anterior segment optical coherence tomography (ASOCT) taking the pupil size into account showed that the angle's narrowing on dilation is partially due to changes in iris volume. As the pupil constricts, the iris gets fatter, swelling with more aqueous humor water and then loses volume on dilation, much like a sponge.[3] Eyes with ACG lose less iris volume on dilation, making angle closure more likely. This physiological risk factor may vary ethnically, providing one explanation for racial differences in ACG.

Another dynamic, physiological risk factor in ACG is choroidal expansion. In small eyes predisposed to angle closure, an expansion in choroidal volume would increase resistance in the iris/lens channel, thereby intensifying pupillary block by moving the lens forward. There are many known situations in which choroidal expansion causes secondary angle closure (e.g., choroidal hemorrhage, topiramate-induced, or Valsalva), but recent research has found choroidal expansion in eyes with primary ACG.

Secondary Causes

There are several secondary causes of angle closure that involve relative and absolute pupillary block. In phacomorphic glaucoma, the mass effect of a thickened or intumescent cataract pushes the iris forward and causes pathological angle narrowing. Forward displacement of the lens in ectopia lentis or microspherophakia can also push the iris forward and shallow the angle. Absolute pupillary block occurs when there is no movement of aqueous through the pupil because of 360° posterior synechiae between the iris and a crystalline lens, an intraocular lens, capsular remnants or the vitreous face. In secondary angle-closure glaucoma without pupillary block, angle closure is due to either contraction of an inflammatory, hemorrhagic or vascular membrane in the angle leading to PAS, or forward displacement of the lens-iris diaphragm, often associated with ciliary body swelling and anterior rotation.

STRONG INDEX OF SUSPICION: RISK FACTORS AND HISTORY

The presenting features of eyes with angle closure vary widely. Eyes with PAC are those with at least 180° of closed or occludable angle on darkroom gonioscopy, no peripheral anterior synechiae (PAS), no signs of angle closure attacks, normal IOP and normal optic nerves. These cases may need close follow-up, but an early laser peripheral iridotomy (LPI) should be considered if the patient has had symptoms such as episodic morning headaches or recurrent subconjunctival haemorrhages (both indicative of episodic elevated

IOP), has a family history positive for angle-closure glaucoma, is part of a high-risk population or has little chance of returning for regular check-ups.

PACG eyes also have closed or occludable angles, along with optic nerve cupping and/or atrophy (sectorial or diffuse), PAS (appositional or permanent), elevated IOP.

Angle closure is more frequently seen in women. An estimated 70% of cases are seen in the female population, and the most likely explanation is a combination of shallower anterior chambers and shorter axial lengths in women.[1]

Age is an important risk factor for developing PAC and PACG. The increase in lens volume with age is the most probable cause. Studies of prevalence of occludable angles in Asian populations show increased risk at 54.3 years, and the prevalence of definite angle closure glaucoma increases at 58 years, so less than 4 years separate PAC from ACG.[5]

Ocular anatomic characteristics that predispose to angle closure are shorter axial length (PACG eyes are about 1 mm shorter than normal eyes) and hyperopia, occludable angles, shallower anterior chambers, thicker lenses, a greater proportion between lens thickness and axial length and a smaller distance between the pupillary border and the lens.[5]

Genetic factors play a major role in PACG. In an Inuit population, the risk of developing angle closure glaucoma in first-degree relatives was reported to be 3.5 times higher.[6] Similarities in axial length and anterior chamber depth (ACD) in first-degree relatives of angle-closure patients indicate that at least some ACG risk anatomical characteristics can be partially heritable. He et al. found that the heritability of ACD and drainage angle width in Chinese twins could be as high as 70–90%.[7]

In a nutshell, the risk factors for PAC are female gender, increasing age, East Asian ethnicity, shallow anterior chamber, shorter axial length, and genetic factors.

CLINICAL EXAMINATION AND PITFALLS

Some subtle signs of previous intermittent sub-acute attacks may help in refining the diagnosis and on deciding on LPI or other forms of angle widening treatments (chronic pilocarpine, laser iridoplasty or even clear-lens phacoemulsification/cataract extraction).

Slit lamp Findings

- *Pupillary ruff:* The partial or total loss of the pupillary ruff is a frequent finding in eyes with previous episodes of angle closure (especially in those with pupillary block), but it can also be found in eyes with pseudoexfoliation (PEX). The pupillary border will have a translucent halo on retro-illumination in cases with PEX, and not in those with pure

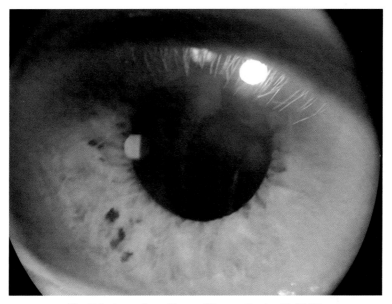

Fig. 7.4: Loss of pupillary ruff in a patient with PACG.

angle-closure (Fig. 7.4). However, a patient may have both entities at the same time. In fact, PEX is considered as a risk factor for PACG because it causes zonular weakness that facilitates forward lens displacement.[8]

- *Pigmentation:* Pigment dispersion may also be present. It can be as subtle as some diffuse pigment granules on the endothelium or on the iris looking as spilled pepper, or it can be heavily laden on all anterior segment structures.
- *Iris atrophy:* Iris atrophy can be seen as patches of iris discoloration, usually near the pupillary border (but it can also be present as a loss of pigment in the peripheral iris folds, or a circumferential atrophy (Fig. 7.5), more frequent in the inferior quadrants.
- *Cellular reaction:* A little bit of flare or even some occasional cells may be seen in patients that had a sub-acute attack the night before examination, and their presence in a symptomatic patient should raise our level of suspicion, but they also need a darkroom to be seen since it is such a subtle finding.
- *Van Herrick slit lamp grading:* It can help to screen patients who would require a further evaluation, however alone it may not be sufficient to identify all patients at risk (Fig. 7.6).

Gonioscopy

Gonioscopy, which is the current reference standard, is a subjective assessment and thus there can be interobserver variabilities as well as technique related pitfalls.

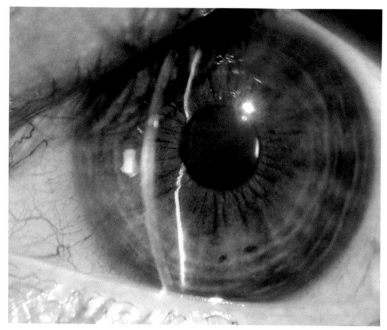

Fig. 7.5: Circumferential atrophy in a patient with chronic angle closure due to ciliary body cysts.

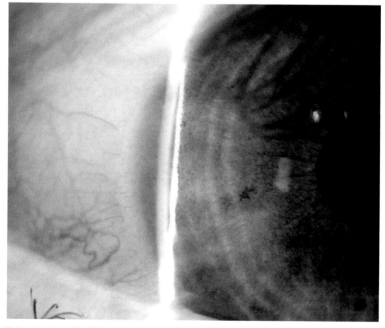

Fig. 7.6: Van Herick of the same patient as in Figure 7.5, the distance between the iris and endothelium varies and becomes smaller in places where cysts are located. In this photograph there is one superior cyst and one inferior cyst at both ends of the line of light on the iris.

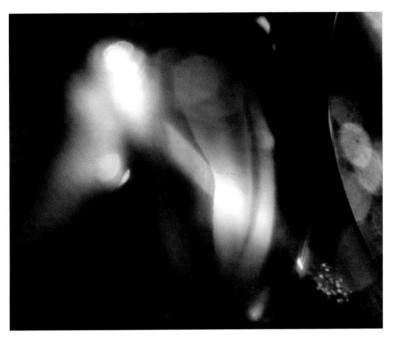

Fig. 7.7: Gonioscopy of the case with ciliary body cysts.

Gonioscopy is done for several reasons—to determine the mechanism of glaucoma, to determine people who are at risk of developing angle closure and to monitor changes in the angle over time for clinical and research purposes. It can also help identify other conditions like neovascularisation, pseudo exfoliation, iris cysts, foreign bodies in the angle and so on (Fig. 7.7).

A simple procedure like a peripheral iridotomy can change the prognosis of the patient with angle closure glaucoma hence it is important that a careful and effective gonioscopy is done to distinguish an open or an occludable angle from angle closure.

Gonioscopy requires practice and understanding of the structures to be seen. Performing this in normal patients will help in identification of the variations from normal. It also requires a cooperative patient. To begin, make sure the patient is comfortably seated and briefed about the procedure.

To avoid making mistakes, it is helpful to follow a standardised technique.

A consensus published by the Association for International Glaucoma Societies proposed a dark-room setting with the illuminating beam of 1 mm to be used. The patient is expected to look straight ahead. This helps in eliminating the effect of illumination of the pupil thereby widening the angle and also avoids artificial opening of the angle by manipulation of the gonio lens. Start the examination in a low magnification to get oriented and then shift to high magnification for detailed examination.[9]

With indentation gonioscopy, it is possible to differentiate between appositional and synechial closure; however, applying too much pressure with lenses, which have a larger base, can compress on the Schwalbe's line and narrow that angle but open the opposite angle. If the gonio lens is not centered on the cornea it can cause fluid displacement and artificially open the angle.

To know the adequate pressure to be applied decrease the pressure to a point that lets the air bubbles get in and then just press enough to make the bubbles escape. Corneal folds and distortion implicate excessive pressure.

An understanding of what a normal anterior chamber angle looks like is essential to differentiating normal angle structures from abnormalities of the angle. A pale featureless angle may appear as closed till a corneal wedge is made to identify the Schwalbe's line. Corneal wedge is helpful even in angles with pigmentation anterior to the Schwalbe's line as in pigmentary glaucomas. Sampaolesi's line tends to be thinner and more granular than pigment at the trabecular meshwork.

For manipulative gonioscopy ask the patient to look towards the mirror when using the Goldman gonio lens to look for synechiae. It also helps identify the creeping angle closures and evidence of past closures. Presence of blotchy pigment, particularly in the superior angle, is a sign of past closure.

Differentiation between iris processes and PAS is important. Iris processes are fine and lacy and do not cross the trabecular meshwork. PAS, on the other hand, are broader and irregular. Iris processes follow the concavity of the recess whereas PAS bridge the underlying structures obscuring the view of the angle structures beneath them. When the patient looks toward the mirror, or during indentation, the PAS drags the iris upward unlike the iris processes that do not inhibit the movement of the iris.

PAS extend beyond the trabecular meshwork up to the Schwalbe's line. Low PAS do not extend to the trabecular meshwork (TM) but may be detectable as localised variation in iris insertion on indentation. These are distinguished from physiological iris insertion variation by their localised nature and greater variability of height. Also comparison between the two eyes can aid in the differentiation.

PAS may also be present in cases of uveitis but those are broad based and are usually more in the inferior angle.

Angle width may vary with age, changes in the lens thickness and disease progression hence gonioscopy should be repeated at least once a year, if not every six months, and whenever the clinical picture and intraocular measurement do not show logical correlation.

Any form of angle measurements (by gonioscopy or imaging) will be invalid if the patient has had pharmacological mydriasis. All cycloplegic and dilating agents will also induce angle widening due to their effect on the longitudinal portion of the cilliary muscle. The more physiological way of assessing dynamic angle changes is to perform measurements during dark and light conditions, and note or measure all changes.

Knowledge and practice can help in doing a good gonioscopy, which can help in a better management of patients.

Intraocular Pressure and Fluctuation

The spontaneous variation in intraocular pressure is known to follow a conserved circadian pattern in both glaucomatous and non-glaucomatous eyes. There is considerable agreement between glaucomatologists that on monitoring 24 hour IOP, significantly higher peak pressures and wider fluctuation have been reported outside the typical office hours often resulting in changes in the management protocol of open-angle glaucoma patients. The diurnal fluctuation of IOP has been reported to be similar in PACG and POAG patients.[10,11]

Baskaran et al. investigated diurnal IOP fluctuations in eyes with various subtypes of angle-closure disease between 8:00 am and 5:00 pm using noncontact air-puff tonometry. They reported IOP fluctuation increases with severity of the angle-closure disease, being significantly higher in PACG (5.4 ± 2.4 mm Hg) and PAC (4.5 ± 2.3 mm Hg) subjects compared with PACS subjects (3.7 ± 1.2 mm Hg) and normal controls (3.8 ± 1.1 mm Hg), with highest IOP found in the early morning.[12]

Sihota et al., on the other hand, reported more IOP peaks in afternoon hours for PACG subjects; when IOP was recorded between 7 am and 10 pm. They reported a diurnal fluctuation of >8 mm Hg seen in 30%, >6 mm Hg in 85% eyes with PCACG, with the difference between POAG and PCACG not being significant statistically.[10]

In a study conducted by two of the authors (SB, PI; unpublished data, presented at APGC, Bali), on angle closure patients post LPI, the mean fluctuation in IOP was found to significantly increase with increase in disease severity, being 4.39 ± 1.47; 5.52 ± 2.29 and 7.38 ± 2.83 mm Hg for PACS, PAC and PACG, respectively. A significant difference between the mean diurnal IOP, and peak diurnal IOP was also noted between the three groups, with a strong correlation between peak IOP and fluctuation (Fig. 7.8).

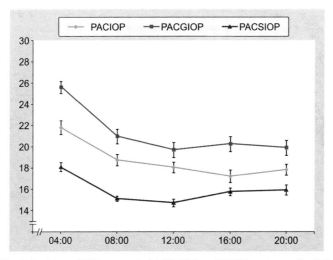

Fig. 7.8: Diurnal IOP curves in PACS, PAC and PACG patients after LPI.

Seventy percent of PACS and PACG and 50% of PAC patients had off office hours peaks (not necessarily >21 mm Hg), emphasizing the need for diurnal variation curves in these patients.

As many as one-fourth of the patients had above normal IOPs despite good office hour IOP control; being 40% (18/44) of those with PAC/PACG. It is also of great clinical relevance that 73 IOP peaks were noted at 4 am.

The SENSIMED Triggerfish® disposable contact lens sensor, CLS, (Sensimed, Lausanne, Switzerland; Class IIa device CE-mark) has led to a paradigm shift in the management of IOP fluctuation, representing the transition from single measurements of IOP during clinic hours to continuous 24 hour IOP monitoring.[13-15]

The device measures the changes in corneal curvature and circumference at the limbus, as a surrogate to changes in IOP, a relationship that has been validated in vitroby Leonardi et al.[16,17]

There is sufficient evidence to show that the device can record IOP fluctuations in real-life situations for up to 24 hour and remains active during undisturbed sleep, acquiring as many as 300 data points during a 30 second period, every 5 minutes, providing a total of 288 measurements over a 24 hour period.

Evaluation of PAC and PACG patients before and after LPI using the SENSIMED Triggerfish CLS by one of the authors (SB) has shown considerable variation in IOP response in terms of fluctuation, with several patients showing a decrease in fluctuation (Fig. 7.9), while others show no difference following LPI (Fig. 7.10) (unpublished data).

Therefore, in the evaluation and management of angle closure glaucoma, IOP variation assessment diurnal variation curve may help pick up IOP peaks and fluctuation, before as well as after LPI. This becomes increasingly relevant in those cases in which patients continue to progress even after apparently well-controlled eye pressures after LPI, on random IOP recordings.

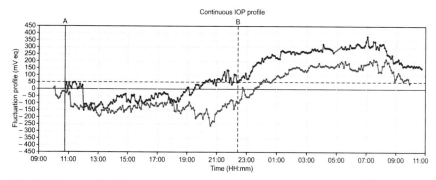

Fig. 7.9: Twenty-four-hour monitoring curve, using SENSIMED Triggerfish® disposable contact lens sensor, CLS blue before, yellow after LPI, in PACG patient. Both curves show marked nocturnal rise in IOP, however, the peak and fluctuation after LPI is less than before LPI (Fig. 7.10).

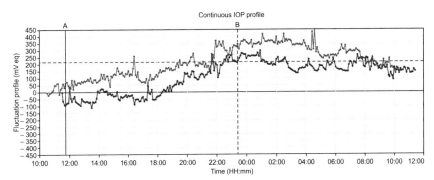

Fig. 7.10: SENSIMED Triggerfish® 24-hour monitoring curve, blue before, yellow after LPI, in PACG patient. Both curves show marked nocturnal rise in IOP, however, the peak and fluctuation after LPI is higher than before LPI.

Anterio Segmnet Optical Coherence Tomography

Anterior segment OCT (AS-OCT) has been in development since 1994, first using the wavelengths used for retinal scans (830–870 nm). Using the time-domain technology, a longer 1320 nm wavelength was used to increase tissue penetration and better visualize opaque structures.

Many spectral-domain posterior OCT machines have had optical and software adaptations to make them capable of performing AS-OCT, so the availability of this technology has increased exponentially, although it isn't necessarily being used in every practice.

One of the main advantages of AS-OCT is the ability to perform dark-adapted angle measurements: since the light source is in the infrared range, the pupil will not constrict, so a better visualization of the dynamic relationship between the iris and the trabecular meshwork during dark-induced mydriasis is possible. This is an important consideration, since even dark-room dynamic gonioscopy is prone to artificially open the angle with the lens and/or with the beam of light, and requires a significant amount of patient collaboration. In contrast, AS-OCT is a purely noncontact procedure, so the vast majority of patients can better tolerate it.

Angle measurements should be done both in dark and light conditions. The amount of time that should pass between light and dark-adapted measurements should be kept short, so the pupil dilator muscles make the first, more pronounced response, before dark-adapted retinal changes are complete.

Although tissue penetration and therefore visualization of structures behind the iris is limited, AS-OCT also permits a qualitative assessment of iris shape and position. When angle closure is related to relative pupillary block, an anterior bowing of the iris can be easily seen (Figs. 7.11A and B).

When the main mechanism is a plateau iris configuration (PIC), the iris has a flat disposition, but the most peripheral portion can be seen surpassing the position of Schlemm's canal or even the trabecular meshwork and Schwalbe's line (Figs. 7.12A and B).

Cornea angle

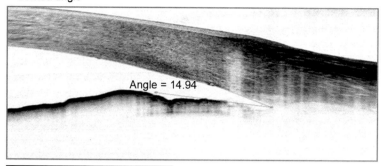

Angle = 14.94

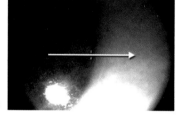

(A)

Cornea angle

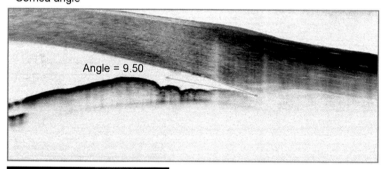

Angle = 9.50

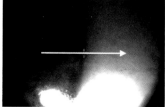

(B)

Figs. 7.11A and B: (A) An eye under light-room conditions, a very small space can be identified between the trabecular meshwork (easily identified by the position of the scleral spur and Schlemm's canal) and the peripheral iris. (B) Same eye in dark-room conditions, the iris has almost complete contact with the trabecular meshwork at this particular position. The infrared picture shows dark-adapted partial pupil dilation. The iris is anteriorly convex due to a relative pupillary block.

AS-OCT is still evolving. A newer swept-source technology permits 3D reconstruction of the anterior segment, using longer wavelengths, and a combination of a time-domain mirrors and Fourier transforms, with much faster acquisition times than the initial AS-OCT.

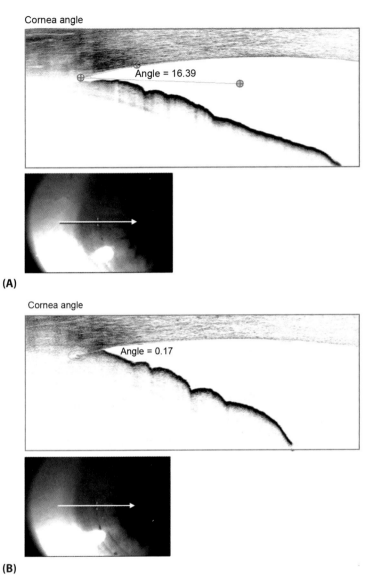

Figs. 7.12A and B: (A) An eye with plateau iris configuration under light-room conditions. The angle recess is patent, but the shape of the peripheral iris is typical. The ciliary processes cannot be seen. (B) Same eye in dark-room conditions, the iris has full contact with the trabecular meshwork. The infrared picture shows dark-adapted pupil dilation. The iris did not increase in convexity, so this might be an angle-closure with predominant plateau component and little pupillary block.

Ultrasound Biomicroscopy

Ultrasound biomicroscopy (UBM) offers an objective investigation for assessing the relationship of the peripheral iris with the ciliary processes.

The UBM criteria used for diagnosis of plateau iris in most of the studies include presence of all the following findings in two or more quadrants:

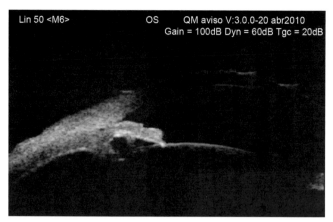

Fig. 7.13: UBM of a case of ciliary body cysts causing angle closure.
Courtesy: Dr Mariana Mayorquin-Ruiz.

anteriorly directed ciliary process supporting the peripheral iris, steep rise of the iris root from its point of insertion, followed by a downward angulation from the corneoscleral wall, a central flat iris plane, absent ciliary sulcus, and irido-angle contact in the same quadrant. But a central flat iris plane may also be seen in cases of pupillary block glaucoma after a peripheral iridotomy. The prevalence of PIC in cases of PACG has been seen in 31–60% of cases.[18]

Anteriorly positioned ciliary processes have also been seen in cases with open angles after LPI. It has been postulated that the presence of an anteriorly placed ciliary process alone does not cause plateau iris. Sakata and colleagues have reported an absent ciliary sulcus and long ciliary processes in 32% of the normal eyes.[19,20]

About 30% of the cases with PACG have plateau iris in the Indian population. Hence it has been suggested that UBM should be performed in all eyes with PACG where the angles fail to open after peripheral iridotomy, as plateau iris is a major cause for angle closure in these cases.

Other situations where UBM is especially useful are angle closures due to ciliary body cysts (Fig. 7.13) or those with phacomorphic glaucoma (Fig. 7.14), since it allows for a better visualization of structures behind the iris than AS-OCT.

The size of the immersion cup is important, since a small eye cup can indent the cornea, resulting in artifactitious angle widening.[21]

Visual Fields

There are many unanswered questions as regards the natural course and mechanisms of the optic nerve and visual field damage in angle-closure glaucoma. Angle-closure glaucoma is typically a high-pressure disease and factors other than the IOP seem less likely to be involved, at least during earlier stages of the disease. Therefore, structure–function relationships in ACG may not be the same as in POAG.[22]

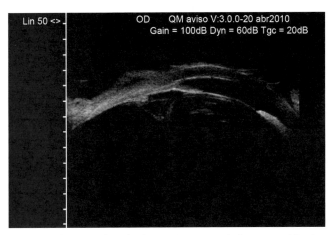

Fig. 7.14: UBM of a case of angle closure in a case of phacomorphic glaucoma.
Courtesy: Dr Mariana Mayorquin-Ruiz.

An automated perimetry study comparing visual field changes of POAG and CACG showed differences between these types of glaucoma. They compared field changes between 11 POAG patients and 14 disease severity-matched CACG patients, and found that CACG showed a more diffuse field loss than did POAG.[22]

Liu and colleagues described the defect patterns on automated visual field throughout the severity groups of angle closure disease. They found a trend of involvement from predominantly the nasal area in the mild group, to the nasal and arcuate areas in the moderate group, and finally to the entire hemifield in the severe and end-stage groups.[23]

Bonomi et al. found that the peripheral nasal upper quadrant was the most frequently affected area at 36–48 hours after remission of single acute angle-closure glaucoma attack.[24]

Diffuse field depression has been reported to be more common after episodes of acute ACG.[25]

CONCLUSION

The diagnosis of acute PAC is mainly clinical. Diagnosis requires a careful history to assess risk factors, slit lamp examination including IOP and gonioscopy. Further investigations required include visual fields, ganglion cell complex OCT, optic nerve and fibres OCT, UBM, AS-OCT, axial length and lens thickness.

REFERENCES

1. Quigley HA, Broman AT. The number of people with glaucoma worldwide in 2010 and 2020. Br J Ophthalmol. 2006;90(3):262–7.
2. Foster PJ, Buhrmann R, Quigley HA, et al. The definition and classification of glaucoma in prevalence surveys. Br J Ophthalmol. 2002;86(2):238-42.

3. Quigley HA. The iris is a sponge: a cause of angle closure. Ophthalmology. 2010;117(1):1-2.

4. Arora KS, Jefferys JL, Maul EA, et al. The choroid is thicker in angle closure than in open angle and control eyes. Invest Ophthalmol Vis Sci. 2012; 53(12):7813-8.

5. George R, Paul PG, Baskaran M, et al. Ocular biometry in occludable angles and angle closure glaucoma: a population based survey. Br J Ophthalmol. 2003;87(4):399-402.

6. Van Ren GH, Arkell SM, Charlton W, et al. Primary angle-closure glaucoma among Alaskan Eskimos. Doc Ophthalmol. 1988;70(2-3):265-76.

7. He M. Angle-closure glaucoma: risk factors. In: Giaconi J, Law S, Caprioli J (Eds.). Pearls of Glaucoma Management. Berlin: Springer-Verlag; 2010. pp. 415-9.

8. Siriwardena D, Arora AK, Fraser SG, et al. Misdiagnosis of acute angle closure glaucoma. Age Ageing. 1996;25(6):421-3.

9. Smith SD, Kuldev S, Shan C, et al. Evaluation of the anterior chamber angle in glaucoma. Ophthalmology. 2013;120(10):1985-97.

10. Sihota R, Saxena R, Gogoi M, et al. A comparison of the circadian rhythm of intraocular pressure in primary chronic angle closure glaucoma, primary open angle glaucoma and normal eyes. Indian J Ophthalmol. 2005;53(4): 243-7.

11. Mansouri K, Weinreb R. Continuous 24-hour intraocular pressure monitoring for glaucoma: time for a paradigm change. Swiss Med Wkly. 2012;142: w13545.

12. Baskaran M, Kumar RS, Govindasamy CV, et al. Diurnal intraocular pressure fluctuation and associated risk factors in eyes with angle closure. Ophthalmology. 2009;116(12):2300-4.

13. Mansouri K, Shaarawy T. Continuous intraocular pressure monitoring with a wireless ocular telemetry sensor: initial clinical experience in patients with open angle glaucoma. Br J Ophthalmol. 2011;95(5):627-9.

14. Mansouri K, Medeiros FA, Ali Tafreshi BS, et al. Continuous 24-hour monitoring of intraocular pressure patterns with a contact lens. Sensor safety, tolerability, and reproducibility in patients with glaucoma. Arch Ophthalmol. 2012;130(12):1534-9.

15. Mansouri K, Weinreb RN. Meeting an unmet need in glaucoma: continuous 24-h monitoring of intraocular pressure. Expert Rev Med Device. 2012;9(3):225-31.

16. Hjortdal JO, Jensen PK. In vitro measurement of corneal strain, thickness, and curvature using digital image processing. Acta Ophthalmol Scand. 1995;73(1):5–11.

17. Leonardi M, Leuenberger P, Bertrand D, et al. First steps toward noninvasive intraocular pressure monitoring with a sensing contact lens. Invest Ophthalmol Vis Sci. 2004;45(9):3113-7.

18. He M, Friedman DS, Ge J, et al. Laser peripheral iridotomy in primary angle-closure suspects: Biometric and gonioscopic outcomes: The Liwan Eye Study. Ophthalmology. 2007;114:494-500.

19. Garudadri CS, Chelerkar V, Nutheti R. An ultrasound biomicroscopic study of the anterior segment in Indian eyes with primary angle-closure glaucoma. J Glaucoma. 2002;11:502-7.

20. Sakata LM, Sakata K, Susanna R Jr, et al. Long ciliary processes with no ciliary sulcus and appositional angle closure assessed by ultrasound biomicroscopy. J Glaucoma. 2006;15(5):371-9.
21. Ishikawa H, Inazumi K, Liebmann JM, et al. Inadvertent corneal indentation can cause artifactitious widening of the iridocorneal angle on ultrasound biomicroscopy. Ophthal Surg Lasers. 2000;31(4):342-5.
22. Kim YY, Nam DH, Jung HR. Comparison of visual field defects between primary open-angle glaucoma and chronic primary angle-closure glaucoma in the early or moderate stage of the disease. Korean J Ophthalmol. 2001;15(1): 27–31.
23. Liu CJ, Chou JC, Hsu WM, et al. Patterns of visual field defects in chronic angle-closure glaucoma with different disease severity. Ophthalmology. 2003; 110(10):1890-4.
24. Bonomi L, Marraffa M, Marchini G, et al. Perimetric defects after a single acute angle-closure glaucoma attack. Graefes Arch Clin Exp Ophthalmol. 1999;237:908–914
25. Douglas GR, Drance SM, Schulzer M. The visual field and nerve head in angle-closure glaucoma (A comparison of the effects of acute and chronic angle closure). Arch Ophthalmol. 1975;93(6):409–41.

8

Uveitic Glaucoma

Malarchelvi P, Aparna AC, Murali A, Nivean M

INTRODUCTION

Uveitic glaucoma is one of the dreadful complications of intraocular inflammation. The association of uveitis with glaucoma in a patient with arthritic iritis was reported first by Joseph Beer in 1813.[1] The prevalence of uveitic glaucoma is reported to be between 5 and 19%.[2,3] The prevalence depends upon the chronological age of the patient, the anatomical location of inflammation, etiology, the chronicity and severity of the disease and prolonged steroid use. In general, old age, anterior uveitis, chronic inflammation, and steroid responders are related with increased prevalence of uveitic glaucoma. Uveitic entities like Fuch's heterochromic uveitis, Posner–Schlossman syndrome, herpetic uveitis and juvenile idiopathic arthritis (JIA) are associated with more risks of developing glaucoma.[4]

There are two important entities: uveitic ocular hypertension and uveitic glaucoma. In uveitic ocular hypertension, patients have uveitis and raised intraocular pressure (IOP) with no demonstrable glaucomatous optic neuropathy or visual field defects. In uveitic glaucoma, patients have uveitis, raised IOP, glaucomatous optic neuropathy, and/or visual field defects.

The IOP can be normal, low or high in patients with uveitis. In acute uveitis, the IOP may be initially low due to hyposecretion of aqueous and increased uveoscleral outflow.[5] Very low IOP on presentation may be seen in ciliary detachment and exudative retinal detachment as in cases of sympathetic ophthalmia and Vogt–Koyanagi–Harada (VKH) syndrome. Eventually due to chronic progressive inflammation there can be ciliary body atrophy, resulting in hypotony and phthisis bulbi.[6]

In most patients with acute uveitis, optic disk remains normal and proper control of inflammation will normalize the IOP and prevent permanent tissue damage and development of glaucoma.

Secondary glaucoma due to uveitis may be due to multiple complex mechanisms. It may be:

- Open angle glaucoma
- Angle closure glaucoma
- Steroid induced glaucoma
- Combined mechanism causing secondary glaucoma

PATHOGENESIS

Secondary Open-angle Glaucoma

- Uveitis causes increased vascular permeability and breakdown of blood aqueous barrier, resulting in elevated levels of proteins in the aqueous humor. This mechanical effect of high viscosity increases the outflow resistance and causes defective drainage through the trabecular meshwork (TM).[7]
- An influx of inflammatory cells that secrete inflammatory mediators like prostaglandins and cytokines occurs shortly after the protein influx in uveitic eyes. The inflammatory cells will increase the IOP by clogging the TM and Schlemm's canal (SC), creating mechanical obstruction and increasing the outflow resistance.
- The risk of IOP rise is more in granulomatous uveitis because of the infiltration of large inflammatory cells like macrophages and lymphocytes compared with non-granulomatous uveitis, in which the cellular infiltrate is more of polymorphonuclear cells.[6] Clogging of the TM by these inflammatory cells, proteins, fibrin and cellular debris elevates the IOP.
- Chronic, severe recurrent forms of uveitis can cause permanent structural damage to the TM by causing injury to the trabecular endothelial cells or scarring of the TM and SC.[8]
- Uveitis causes increased prostaglandin levels in the aqueous humor, which may enhance the ocular signs of inflammation like vasodilatation, increased vascular permeability, and miosis.[9,10] As prostaglandins disrupts the blood aqueous barrier, it increases the influx of aqueous proteins, cytokines, and inflammatory cells, which can again increase the IOP.
- Trabeculitis is the inflammation of the TM. It is commonly associated with viral uveitis. Presence of keratic precipitates on the TM can be seen in gonioscopy. Trabecular lamellae swelling and trabecular endothelial cell dysfunction with decreased phagocytic activity results in narrowing of the pores and obstruction of theTM,[8] resulting in elevated IOP.
- Trabecular obstruction can be contributed by enzymes like Rho-kinase and angiotensin-converting enzyme. Rho-kinase enzyme controls the cellular contraction and formation of focal adhesions. Increased levels of Rho-kinase in TM and SC cells in uveitis also enhances the outflow resistance.[11]

Secondary Angle-closure Glaucoma

The mechanism of secondary angle closure in uveitic glaucoma is due to structural changes associated with inflammation and post-inflammation. It can be due to pupillary block and nonpupillary block mechanisms.

- Pupillary block occurs in uveitis when the pupil becomes secluded by 360° annular synechiae or by an inflammatory membrane across the pupil. In this scenario, there is no flow of aqueous from the posterior to the anterior chamber causing bowing of the iris forward, resulting in the formation of iris bombé. Iris bombé formation in the uveitic eye with ongoing inflammation can cause severe elevation of IOP by synechial angle closure due to the formation of peripheral anterior synechiae (PAS).
- Nonpupillary block angle closure glaucoma occurs in ciliochoroidal effusions, which may cause forward rotation of the ciliary body. This type of uveitic glaucoma is seen in VKH syndrome, sympathetic ophthalmia, and posterior scleritis.[6,12]
- PAS is formed by the organisation of the inflammatory exudates that pulls the iris towards the TM. PAS is more common in iridocyclitis and granulomatous uveitis. These adhesions impair the outflow of aqueous humor through the drainage channels. The iris adhesions are usually broad covering a large area of the angle making its presence significant in the pathogenesis of glaucoma.
- Neovascularization of iris due to chronic inflammation and later fibrovascular contraction causes synechial angle closure glaucoma.

Steroid-induced Glaucoma

Corticosteroid-induced glaucoma occurs in 18–36% of patients.[13,14] Ocular hypertension from steroid administration is dependent on the potency of steroid, structure of the corticosteroid compound, frequency of administration, route of delivery, duration of treatment, and susceptibility of the patient.

IOP elevation in susceptible patients is mediated by more than one mechanism.[15,16] Steroid-induced glaucoma occurs due to glycosaminoglycans accumulation in the TM and reduction in trabecular outflow facility by altering the endothelial cells in the meshwork. An interesting effect of TM exposure to steroids is the induction of myocilin mRNA expression. This protein is intimately involved with increased outflow resistance.

Patients who are more prone to steroid-induced ocular hypertension include primary open angle glaucoma, glaucoma suspects, family history of glaucoma, children, patients with myopia, diabetes, and connective tissue diseases.[16]

Combined Mechanism Causing Secondary Glaucoma in Uveitis

Combined mechanism glaucoma is seen in chronic uveitis, uveitis associated with JIA, sarcoidosis, sympathetic ophthalmia and VKH syndrome. Glaucoma in arthritis associated uveitis occurs with open angle or due to pupillary block mechanism and may be associated with steroid-induced glaucoma. VKH and sympathetic ophthalmia can be associated with nonpupillary block angle closure glaucoma along with steroid-induced glaucoma.

SPECIFIC UVEITIC ENTITIES WITH GLAUCOMA

Arthritis-associated Uveitis

Prevalence of JIA-associated uveitis was reported by Sim et al. as 11.4%.[17] It is typically bilateral, nongranulomatous anterior uveitis. The disease has a chronic course and the eye appears white in spite of severe inflammation. The complications that cause significant visual loss in children with JIA associated iridocyclitis include cataracts, band keratopathy, and glaucoma. Glaucoma in children with JIA associated uveitis is noted in 14–27%.[18]

HLA-B27-associated anterior uveitis represents a distinct clinical entity, more common in young adults between 20 and 40 years. It is strongly associated with sero-negative arthritis like ankylosing spondylitis, psoriatic arthritis, and inflammatory bowel disease.[19]

Glaucoma in arthritis-associated uveitis occurs with open angle or due to pupillary block mechanism.

Fuchs' Heterochromic Iridocyclitis

Fuchs in 1906 first described this clinical condition. The uveitis is chronic low-grade anterior. It is typically unilateral, but in 13% of the patients it is reported as a bilateral condition.[20] Slit lamp examination classically shows fine, stellate-shaped, scattered keratic precipitates with no posterior synechiae and heterochromia iridis (Figs. 8.1A and B). Microhyphema after paracentesis called Amsler's sign is typical of Fuchs' heterochromic iridocyclitis (FHU) and related to the presence of anomalous blood vessels in the angle. IOP rise is noted in 13–60% of the patients.[21] Inflammatory membranes in the angle, mononuclear inflammatory cells, abnormal vessels that can cause

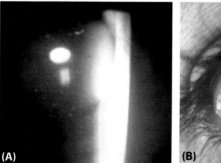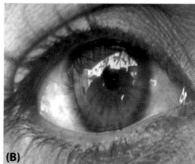

Figs. 8.1A and B: (A) The scattered diffuse stellate keratic precipitates in FHU. (B) Heterochromia of iris in FHU.

hemorrhages, trabeculitis and collapse of the SC result in secondary open angle glaucoma.[22] Initially, the glaucoma responds to medical treatment but surgical intervention is usually required to control the IOP.

Glaucomatocyclitic Crisis (Posner–Schlossman Syndrome)

Posner and Schlossman first described this clinical condition in 1948. It is characterized by recurrent attacks of unilateral acute anterior uveitis associated with increased IOP in the range of 40–60 mm Hg. The pathogenesis remains unknown, but viral infections (Herpes simplex virus and Cytomegalo virus)[23] and gastrointestinal diseases are reported to be associated. Slit lamp examination shows fine, small, fresh keratic precipitates. IOP rise is due to inflammatory changes in the TM, increased levels of prostaglandins in aqueous humor and is associated with open angle glaucoma. The prostaglandin levels in the aqueous humor correlates with level of IOP spike. IOP returns to normal in between the attacks. Chronic recurrent disease is associated with development of glaucomatous disk changes and field defects, which occur in about 25% of cases.[24] The glaucoma responds well to topical steroids and antiglaucoma medications.

Herpetic Keratouveitis

Herpetic uveitis presents as unilateral, acute anterior uveitis. Hyphema and fibrin deposition is noted in severe cases. Sectorial iris atrophy is characteristic of herpetic iritis.[25] The presence of stromal opacities in the cornea are typical of herpetic stromal keratouveitis. Patients may present with classic vesicular lesions in the dermatomal distribution (Figs. 8.2A and B). Secondary glaucoma is the most common complication in patients with herpetic uveitis. Patients with herpes simplex keratouveitis had shown IOP elevation in 28% and glaucomatous damage in 10%. Increase in IOP is attributed to the increased aqueous viscosity, trabeculitis and obstruction of TM due to inflammatory debris.

Intermediate Uveitis

The primary site of the inflammation in intermediate uveitis is the vitreous and the peripheral retina. Mild-to-moderate anterior chamber inflammation is usually present. Posterior synechiae and PAS are commonly seen.[26,27] Snow ball opacities in the vitreous and snow banking (Fig. 8.3) at the pars plana are typical features of intermediate uveitis. It is associated with glaucoma in 7–8% of patients.[28] IOP elevation occurs secondary to synechiae formation, iris bombé or rubeosis iridis.

Sarcoid Uveitis

Sarcoidosis is a multisystem inflammatory disorder. It is more common in females and in blacks.[29] Sarcoidosis causes granulomatous panuveitis. Ocular

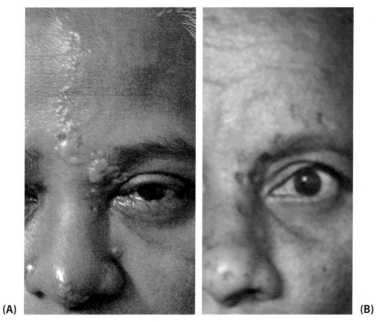

(A)   **(B)**

Figs. 8.2A and B: Active and healed skin lesions in the classic dermatome distribution in a patient with HZO.

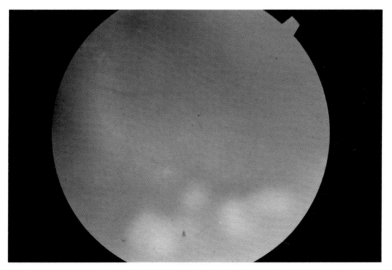

Fig. 8.3: Snowbanking in a patient with intermediate uveitis.

Courtesy: Dr Jyotirmay Biswas.

findings include mutton fat keratic precipitates, Bussaca and Koeppe's nodules, snow ball opacities in the vitreous (Fig. 8.4), retinal periphlebitis, optic nerve head granuloma and orbital and lacrimal gland involvement. Glaucoma is seen in 11% of the patients.[30] Uveitic glaucoma is due to obstruction of TM by the inflammatory cells, cellular debris and nodules and rarely due to iris and angle neovascularization.

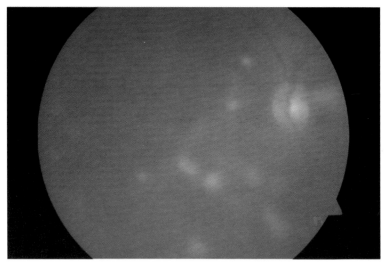

Fig. 8.4: Snowball opacities in a patient with sarcoid uveitis.

Courtesy: Dr Jyotirmay Biswas.

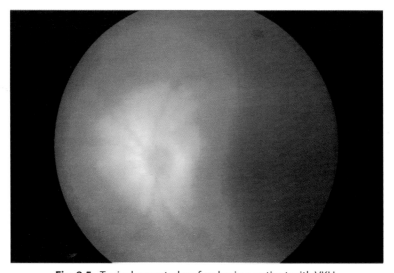

Fig. 8.5: Typical sunset glow fundus in a patient with VKH.

Vogt Koyanagi Harada Syndrome

It is a chronic granulomatous disease, which presents as bilateral panuveitis with dermatologic and central nervous system manifestations. In a study by Pandey et al., the prevalence of glaucoma in patients with VKH syndrome at presentation was 15.8%. The glaucoma was associated with open-angle glaucoma in 64.8%, angle closure in 29.6% and combined in 5.6%.[31] Open-angle glaucoma results due to TM obstruction and nonpupillary block angle closure glaucoma due to ciliochoroidal effusion.[32] Figure 8.5 shows the typical sunset glow fundus in a patient with VKH.

Sympathetic Ophthalmia

Sympathetic ophthalmia is a condition where ocular inflammation occurs secondary to penetrating trauma or surgery to the fellow eye. Granulomatous panuveitis is the classic presentation of sympathetic ophthalmia. Whitish-yellow lesions suggestive of Dalen-Fuchs nodules are seen in the choroid. Elevated IOP is due to inflammatory cell blockage of the TM and histopathological studies revealed cellular infiltration of the iris and ciliary body suggestive of immune reaction.[33]

Grant's Syndrome

Glaucoma associated with precipitates on TM was first described by Chandler and Grant. It is an acute onset bilateral open-angle glaucoma, affecting patients above 50 years of age. Uveitis is evident only by keratic precipitates on the TM or as PAS. Gonioscopy reveals gray-to-yellowish inflammatory precipitates on the TM. Response to topical steroids is good but the condition is not responsive to antiglaucoma medications.[34]

Schwartz-Matsuo Syndrome

Schwartz-Matsuo syndrome consists of retinal detachment, uveitis and glaucoma. The rise in IOP is reported to occur due to blockage of TM by inflammatory cells and also photoreceptor outer segments.[35,36]

Scleritis

Scleritis, especially anterior scleritis, may be associated with glaucoma. The patients (12–46%) with posterior scleritis show increased IOP.[37] Unilateral acute angle closure glaucoma could be the presenting feature of scleritis.[38,39] Glaucoma develops due to permanent damage to the TM, elevated episcleral venous pressure and choroidal effusion with subsequent angle closure glaucoma. Figure 8.6 shows uveitic eye associated with necrotising scleritis in a patient with Wegener's granulomatosis.

CLINICAL WORK-UP IN UVEITIC GLAUCOMA

A complete detailed history, meticulous ophthalmic examination and appropriate ancillary tests should be done in patients with uveitic glaucoma. Identification of the etiological diagnosis of uveitis is important to understand the pathogenesis of glaucoma and to design the treatment protocol.

Slit-lamp Examination

Slit-lamp examination is important to establish the anatomical location of inflammation, assess the degree of inflammation and the type of

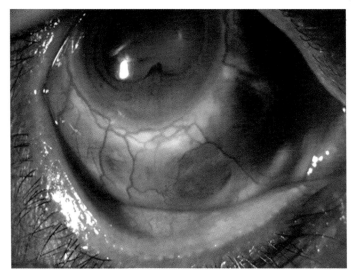

Fig. 8.6: Uveitic glaucoma associated with necrotizing scleritis in a patient with Wegener's granulomatosis.

Courtesy: Dr Jyotirmay Biswas.

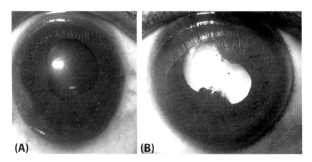

(A)   **(B)**

Figs. 8.7A and B: Broad-based posterior synechiae in an uveitic eye.

inflammatory reaction (granulomatous or non-granulomatous). The structural changes in the ocular architecture caused by the inflammatory exudation such as posterior synechiae (Figs. 8.7A and B), and PAS should also be noted.

A detailed slit lamp examination can detect important clinical signs that may guide us to make the etiological diagnosis (Table 8.1). Central keratic precipitates (Fig. 8.8), Descemet's membrane folds, stromal opacities and sector iris atrophy are seen in viral uveitis. Inflammatory signs like mutton-fat keratic precipitates and iris nodules (Fig. 8.9) may indicate the etiology of granulomatous uveitis like sarcoidosis, VKH and sympathetic ophthalmia. If the slit lamp examination shows fine, diffuse, scattered, stellate-shaped keratic precipitates with mild unilateral anterior uveitis, no posterior synechiae, heterochromia of iris, the etiology may be Fuchs' heterochromic uveitis. Formation of iris bombé and PAS indicates chronic uve-

Table 8.1: Slit-lamp findings that aid in the etiological diagnosis in patients with uveitic glaucoma.

Clinical signs	Diagnosis
Central keratic precipitates Descemet's membrane folds Stromal Sector iris atrophy Hyphema	Viral uveitis
Granulomatous uveitis	Sarcoidosis Vogt-Koyanagi-Harada syndrome Sympathetic ophthalmia
Fine, stellate-shaped keratic precipitates scattered throughout the cornea Iris heterochromia No posterior synechiae	Fuchs' heterochromic iridocyclitis
Iris bombé Peripheral anterior synechiae	Chronic uveitis
Leaking Morgagnian cataract	Lens-induced uveitis and glaucoma

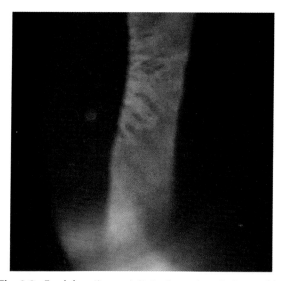

Fig. 8.8: Fresh keratic precipitates in acute anterior uveitis.

itis. Leaking Morgagnian cataract (Figs. 8.10A and B) indicates lens induced uveitis and glaucoma.

Gonioscopy

Gonioscopy is the most critical part of ophthalmic examination in patients with uveitic glaucoma. It has to be done with a gonio lens that indents the

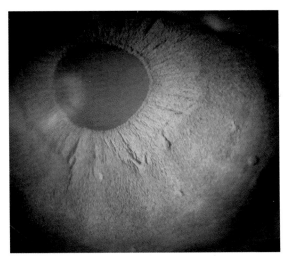

Fig. 8.9: Iris nodules in a patient with granulamatous uveitis.

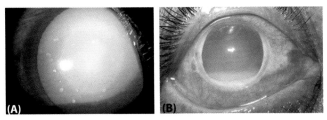

Figs. 8.10A and B: (A) Slit-lamp photograph of Morgagnian cataract. (B) Clinical photo of phacolytic glaucoma.

central cornea and pushes the aqueous into the angle. Gonioscopic examination reveals whether it is open angle or closed angle glaucoma, which is important to plan the treatment protocol. Presence of PAS, keratic precipitates, angle recession, new vessels, lens matter or silicone oil can aid in the etiological diagnosis (Table 8.2). Figure 8.11 shows a gonioscopic picture of an open angle. Figure 8.12A shows PAS and Figure 8.12B shows synechial angle closure in an uveitic eye.

Fundus Examination

The fundus examination should be carefully done. It gives diagnostic clues. Presence of retinochoroiditis may be due to toxoplasmosis. Clinical signs of vitritis, retinal vasculitis and periphlebitis suggest the diagnosis of sarcoidosis. Presence of exudative retinal detachment suggests the diagnosis of VKH or sympathetic ophthalmia (Table 8.3). Structural changes suggestive of glaucomatous optic neuropathy should be evaluated. Presence of optic disk edema or macular edema as a consequence of chronic uveitis should also be evaluated.

Table 8.2: Gonioscopic findings that aid in the etiological diagnosis in uveitic glaucoma patients.

Clinical signs	Diagnosis
Peripheral anterior synechiae	Chronic uveitis
Keratic precipitates, nodules	Sarcoidosis
Angle recession	Traumatic uveitis *look for supertemporal*
Foreign body	*retinal dialysis*
Lens matter in the angle	Lens protein uveitis
Silicone oil	Post retinal detachment surgery

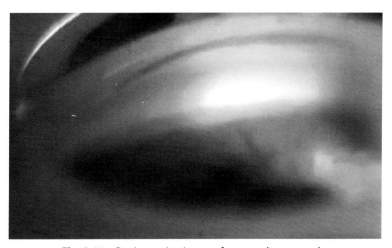

Fig. 8.11: Gonioscopic picture of a normal open angle.

Applanation Tonometry

Applanation tonometry has to be done during every visit.

Visual Field Assessment

Visual field assessment provides useful information regarding the glaucomatous status of the eye. This investigation should be done during the quiescent periods of uveitis.

Optical Coherence Tomography

Optical coherence tomography (OCT) provides information about the retinal nerve fiber layer (RNFL) changes in glaucoma. OCT must be performed during quiescent periods of uveitis. RNFL measurements may facilitate early detection of disk damage even before visual field changes occur and aid in identifying the group of patients who need more aggressive treatment for IOP

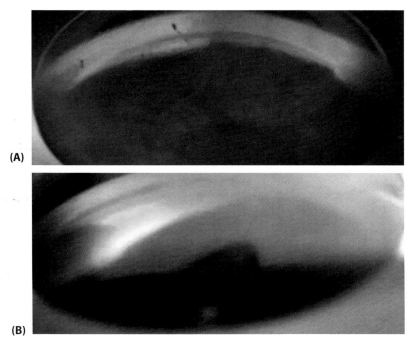

Figs. 8.12A and B: (A) Gonioscopic picture of broad-based peripheral anterior synechiae in a patient with uveitic glaucoma. (B) Gonioscopic picture of synechial angle closure in a patient with uveitic glaucoma.

Table 8.3: Fundus findings that aid in the etiological diagnosis in uveitic glaucoma patients. Optic disc has to be looked for glaucomatous disc changes.

Signs	Diagnosis
Retinochoroiditis	Toxoplasmosis
Exudative retinal detachment	VKH, sympathetic ophthalmia
Vitritis, retinal vasculitis, perivascular sheathing	Sarcoidosis

control. OCT has also become the standard investigation to confirm the diagnosis of macular edema.

Figure 8.13 displays the color fundus photograph of an uveitic glaucomatous eye showing a superior wedge-shaped RNFL defect with thinning of superior and inferior neuroretinal rim. Visual field shows inferior arcuate scotoma with areas of depressed sensitivity along the superior area. OCT of optic nerve head shows reduction in superior and inferior RNFL thickness with depressed.

B-scan Ultrasonography

B-scan is useful to assess the posterior segment in opaque media and to rule out retinal detachment in patients with very low IOP.

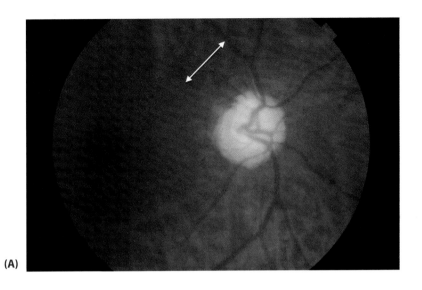

(A)

Fixation monitor:	Blind spot	Stimulus:	III. White	Date: Apr 13, 2016
Fixation target:	central	Background:	31.5 asb	Time: 12:16 PM
Fixation losses:	0/18	Sreategy:	SITA-standard	Age: 64
False POS errors:	0%	Pupil diameter:	3.0 mm
False NEG errors:	0%	Visual acuity:	6/9
Test duration:	08:06	Rx: +2.75 DS
Fovea:	Off

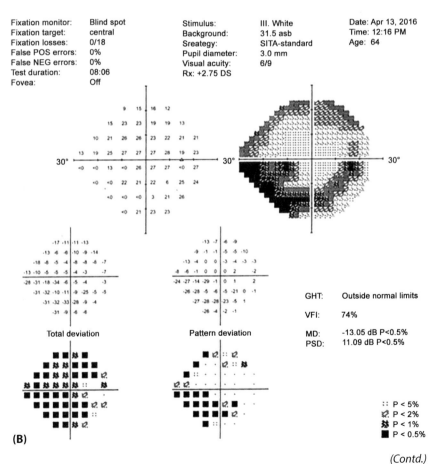

Total deviation

Pattern deviation

GHT: Outside normal limits

VFI: 74%

MD: -13.05 dB P<0.5%
PSD: 11.09 dB P<0.5%

:: P < 5%
Ⅻ P < 2%
⅍ P < 1%
■ P < 0.5%

(B)

(Contd.)

(Contd.)

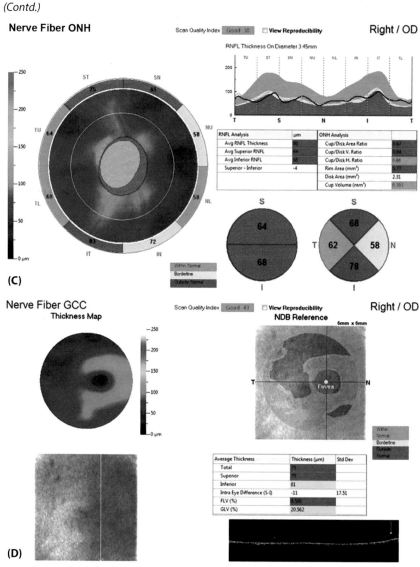

Figs. 8.13A to D: Fundus photo of a uveitic glaucoma eye showing a superior wedge-shaped RNFL defect with thinning of superior and inferior neuroretinal rim. Visual field shows inferior arcuate scotoma with areas of depressed sensitivity along the superior area. OCT ONH analysis shows reduction in superior and inferior RNFL thickness with depressed TSNIT graph and corresponding reduction of GCC thickness.

Ultrasound Biomicroscopy

Ultrasound biomicroscopy (UBM) provides valuable information regarding the ciliary body and iridocorneal angle (Table 8.4). Presence of forward rotation of ciliary body, choroidal thickening and cilio-choroidal effusion and are diagnostic features of non-pupillary block angle closure glaucoma.

Table 8.4: UBM findings that aid in the etiological diagnosis in uveitic glaucoma patients.

Clinical signs	Diagnosis
Ciliochoroidal effusion Forward rotation of ciliary body	VKH, sympathetic ophthalmia, scleritis
Ciliary body tumor	Masquerade syndrome

Table 8.5: Challenges in the diagnosis and treatment of eyes with uveitic glaucoma.

Clinical findings	Challenges
Presence of corneal opacity	Difficulty in performing gonioscopy Difficulty in fundus examination and assessment of optic nerve head
Ciliary body tumor, Small pupil Opaque media like complicated cataract vitritis	Difficulty in fundus examination and assessment of optic nerve head
Chronic recurrent uveitis	Closure of LPI Failure of filtering surgery

Anterior Segment Optical Coherence Tomography

Anterior segment optical coherence tomography (AS-OCT) is helpful for evaluating the position and length of glaucoma drainage device tubes and its relationship with the corneal endothelium. It also provides information about the filtering blebs.

There are several challenges in the diagnosis and management of uveitic glaucoma (Table 8.5).

MANAGEMENT OF UVEITIC GLAUCOMA

Objective of Treatment

The foremost objective is to control the inflammatory disease and prevent permanent structural damage to the eye by the use of appropriate anti-inflammatory medications. The secondary objective is the control of IOP, either by medical or surgical therapy. The tertiary objective is to identify and treat the underlying etiology of uveitis.

Medical Treatment

Anti-inflammatory Drugs

Corticosteroids are the most preferred anti-inflammatory drug in the treatment of uveitis. In uveitic glaucoma it is necessary to initiate therapy with stronger topical steroids such as 1% prednisolone acetate, periocular, intravitreal or systemic steroids may be required in refractory patients and in eyes with active posterior segment inflammation.

Immunomodulatory therapy has become an important component in the management of uveitic glaucoma, particularly for eyes refractory to corticosteroid therapy, steroid responders and for patients intolerant to steroids.

Nonsteroidal anti-inflammatory drugs are not usually helpful and can partially block the hypotensive effect of antiglaucoma medications like brimonidine and latanoprost.[40,41.]

Cycloplegics

Cycloplegics like 1% atropine or 5% homatropine are indicated in the treatment of acute iridocyclitis except in FHU to relieve the pain and discomfort associated with ciliary muscle and iris sphincter spasm. It prevents and breaks the posterior synechiae formation, thereby prevents the structural damage to the ocular tissues that can contribute to increased IOP. In case of PAS with permanent angle closure, cycloplegics are contraindicated.

Antiglaucoma Medications

Adequate control of inflammation usually normalizes the IOP. The phase of IOP spike in the course of uveitis aids in the mode of glaucoma management. Patients with increased IOP only during the acute inflammation can be effectively controlled by antiglaucoma medications, whereas patients with postinflammatory structural damage and chronic glaucoma may require surgical intervention. In steroid responders, weaker steroids or immunomodulatory therapy can be considered.

Nonselective beta-blockers are the first line of anti-glaucoma medication to control IOP in uveitic glaucoma, in patients without systemic contraindications.

The second line of therapy for increased IOP may be systemic carbonic anhydrase inhibitors (CAI) such as acetazolamide followed by topical alpha agonists. Oral CAI has been reported to prevent and reduce cystoid macular edema, which is the common cause of visual loss in uveitic eyes.[42]

The IOP-lowering effect of topical CAI varies greatly in an inflamed eye.[43] Corneal decompensation can occur in patients with underlying endothelial compromise and it is better to avoid topical CAI in these patients. Topical CAI are unlikely to reduce cystoids macular edema as oral CAI because sufficient concentration probably does not reach the retina.

Granulomatous iridocyclitis has been reported as a late adverse effect of treatment with brimonidine, the commonly used alpha agonists.[43]

Pilocarpine, epinephrine and epinephrine prodrugs are medications that are pro-inflammatory and must be avoided in the treatment of active uveitis.[44]

Miotics should be avoided in uveitic glaucoma due to its potential to enhance the formation of posterior synechiae. It increases the spasm of ciliary muscle and worsens the inflammation by disrupting the blood aqueous barrier.

Prostaglandin analogs may have a pro-inflammatory effect. A few cases are reported with exacerbation of anterior uveitis, recurrence of herpetic keratitis and formation of cystoids macular edema.[45] Hence use of prostaglandin analogs in uveitic glaucoma has to be taken with extreme caution in eyes with resolved or controlled uveitis.

Systemic hyperosmotic medications like oral glycerol or intravenous mannitol can be given in patients with marked elevation of IOP as in acute angle closure glaucoma.

Laser Procedures

Laser Peripheral Iridotomy

Laser peripheral iridotomy is the treatment of choice for eyes with acute angle closure due to pupillary block. The inflammatory response following laser procedure tends to be more in uveitic eyes and hence pre- and post-laser corticosteroid treatment is essential. Nd:YAG laser delivers less energy and induces less postprocedure inflammation. The laser iridotomies are prone to higher risk of closure particularly in eyes with active inflammation. Hence at least two big iridotomies are recommended[47] (Fig. 8.14). To reduce the risk of endothelial damage, laser iridotomy should be avoided in eyes with severe active uveitis, corneal edema or in the areas of PAS.

When laser iridotomies cannot be done or not successful, surgical iridectomy can be performed. This procedure can cause increased inflammation, hence topical and oral steroids are recommended in the perioperative

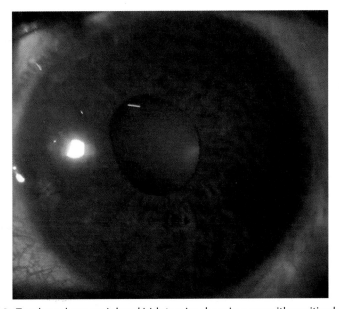

Fig. 8.14: Two large laser peripheral iridotomies done in a eye with uveitic glaucoma.

period. Surgical iridectomy is reported to be successful in uveitic eyes with PAS that involves <75% of the angle.[8]

Argon Laser Trabeculoplasty

Argon laser trabeculoplasty is not recommended as a treatment strategy in uveitic glaucoma because the thermal energy and the laser-induced inflammation may further damage the already injured TM.

Selective Laser Trabeculoplasty

Selective laser trabeculoplasty (SLT) can be considered as an alternate treatment in a quiet eye with uveitic glaucoma. SLT induces least inflammation and does not change the structural integrity of the TM, which is very important in the treatment of uveitic glaucoma, where permanent alterations in the structure can contribute to glaucoma.[46]

Surgical Management

Surgical therapy is indicated in uveitic glaucoma, when there is uncontrolled IOP in spite of maximal tolerated medical therapy.

The prerequisite for an elective surgical intervention is that the eye should be quiet with no active inflammation for a period of three months. In patients with recurrent uveitis, perioperative systemic (0.5–1 mg/kg/day) and topical steroid coverage is recommended to prevent intraocular inflammation and conjunctival inflammatory cells,[40] which can accelerate the wound healing causing failure of surgery.

The choice of surgical procedure depends on the patient's age, pathophysiology of the disease, inflammatory activity of the eye, previous ocular surgeries, conjunctival scarring, surgeon experience and postoperative IOP goal.

Trabeculectomy

Trabeculectomy (Fig. 8.15) is the treatment of choice in uveitic glaucoma when the IOP is not controlled in spite of maximum tolerated medical therapy, in eyes with minimal conjunctival scarring, and in well-controlled uveitis. Conventional trabeculectomy without antiproliferative agents have a lesser chance of success due to accelerated wound healing.[47] Hence the use of mitomycin C, 5-Fluorouracil and biological agents like Ologen are recommended. Uveitic eyes are at risk for postoperative hypotony; therefore it is recommended to suture the sclera flap tightly.

The most common complications after trabeculectomy in patients with uveitic glaucoma are recurrent inflammation and hypotony. Meticulous control of inflammation preoperatively and vigilant monitoring for reactivation is mandatory.

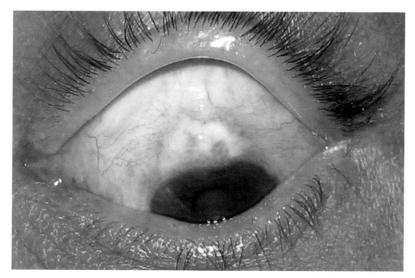

Fig. 8.15: Filtering bleb in a patient with uveitic glaucoma.

Glaucoma Drainage Devices

Glaucoma drainage devices (GDD) (Fig. 8.16) are indicated in uveitic eyes with conjunctival scarring, in active disease, failed trabeculectomy. They are designed to redirect the aqueous to the posterior reservoir. Even in eyes with active uveitis, success rate of upto 57% have been reported.[48] Higher success rates have been reported with the use of conventional anti-inflammatory therapy, primarily with steroids.[49]

Drainage implants with unidirectional valves like Ahmed glaucoma valve (AGV) may be safer than nonvalved Baerveldt implant, because of the

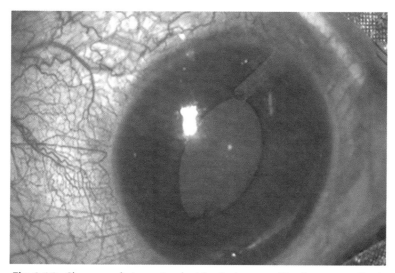

Fig. 8.16: Glaucoma drainage implant in situ in an uveitic glaucoma patient.

lower risk of immediate postoperative hypotony. Success rates of AGV in uveitic glaucoma were reported to be 77% and 50% after follow-up of 1 and 4 years respectively.[50] Transient hypotony, encapsulated bleb, hyphema, occlusion of the tube by inflammatory materials and corneal decompensation are some of the complications associated with GDD in uveitic glaucoma eyes.

Ex-PRESS Mini-glaucoma Shunt

The Ex-PRESS filtration device is a metallic implant. It provides an artificial channel to drain the aqueous into the subconjunctival space. This technology is less invasive procedure. Sclerectomy or peripheral iridectomy is not done in Ex-PRESS shunt procedure, hence there is less chance of inflammation and blockage of the inner ostium by fibrin, blood, or iris.

In a small preliminary case series of 5 patients, Lee et al. reported the efficacy and safety of the Ex-PRESS glaucoma filtration device with mitomycin C in uveitic glaucoma. The qualified success rates was 100% after 6 months follow-up. Postoperative hypotony occurred in 20% of cases due to ciliary shutdown.[51] Larger study trials are warranted to establish the long-term safety and efficacy of the Ex-PRESS in uveitic glaucoma treatment.

Subconjunctival Antivascular Endothelial Growth Factor

Subconjunctival bevacizumab can be used to moderate the wound healing after glaucoma surgery. There are no published data on the efficacy and safety of bevacizumab, intraoperative use as an adjunct to trabeculectomy in uveitic glaucoma.[5] They act by retarding scarring by preventing neovascularisation that enhances the inflammation and promotes failure of the surgical procedure.

Canaloplasty

The canaloplasty surgery consists of 360° of visco-dilation followed by a tension suture. The principle of this surgery is to expand and maintain the patency of the Schelmm's canal and increase the previously reduced intertrabecular spaces, thereby improving the outflow facility of eyes with uveitic glaucoma. A recent retrospective study of 19 eyes of 15 patients was conducted to evaluate the efficacy of this surgical procedure in University of Montreal in herpetic, noninfectious idiopathic uveitic glaucoma.[52] The study revealed that it was completely successful in 74% of cases, partial success in 11% and failure in 16%.

Management of Non-pupillary Block Angle-closure Glaucoma

In uveitic glaucoma eyes in which the angle closure mechanism is caused by ciliary body forward rotation without the evidence of pupillary block, laser iridotomy or surgical iridectomy are not useful. This condition is best treated with immunomodulatory therapy and aqueous suppressants. A surgical filtering procedure is recommended in cases of failure to medical treatment.

Cataract and Uveitic Glaucoma Surgery

Cataract is commonly indicated in uveitic patients. Cataract surgery can compromise the success of glaucoma surgery,[53] but combined cataract and glaucoma surgery increases the postoperative inflammation and may be less successful than isolated procedures.[54]

If combined surgery is indicated, adequate control of inflammation is mandatory pre- and postoperatively. The use of antimetabolites reduces the proliferative response.[55] A meticulous surgical procedure can increase the chance of surgical success.

Cyclophotocoagulation

Ciliary body destructive procedures like cyclophotocoagulation in uveitic eyes must be used with extreme caution. The primary disadvantage of this procedure is the induction of severe intraocular inflammation in an already inflamed eye and destruction of the ciliary body eventually leading to hypotony and phthisis bulbi. Therefore, cycloabation is used only in refractory glaucoma as a last resort in eyes with failed surgical procedures with poor visual potential.[56]

Management of raised IOP is highly challenging in uveitic eyes with active inflammation with glaucomatous optic neuropathy. The current strategy of management includes meticulous, comprehensive and aggressive treatment of uveitis. However, adequate control of inflammation and patient compliance can result in good prognosis.

REFERENCES

1. Beer GJ. Die Lehre v.d. Augenkrankheiten. Vienna. 1813;1:633.
2. Merayo-Lloves J, Power WJ, Rodriguez A, et al. Secondary glaucoma in patients with uveitis. Ophthalmologica. 1999;213(5):300-4.
3. Takahashi T, Ohtani S, Miyata K, et al. A clinical evaluation of uveitis-associated secondary glaucoma. Jpn J Ophthalmol. 2002;46(5):556-62.
4. Foster CS, Havrlikova K, Baltatzis S, et al. Secondary glaucoma in patients with juvenile rheumatoid arthritis-associated iridocyclitis. Acta Ophthalmol Scand. 2000;78(5):576-9.
5. Siddique SS, Suelves AM, Baheti U, et al. Glaucoma and uveitis. Surv Ophthalmol. 2013;58(1):1-10.
6. Tran VT, Mermoud A, Herbort CP. Appraisal and management of ocular hypotony and glaucoma associated with uveitis. Int Ophthalmol Clin. 2000; 40(2):175-203.
7. Chiang TS, Thomas RP. Ocular hypertension following infusion of prostaglandin E_1. Arch Ophthalmol. 1972;88(4):418-20.

8. Moorthy RS, Mermoud A, Baerveldt G, et al. Glaucoma associated with uveitis. Surv Ophthalmol. 1997;41(5):361-94.
9. Beitch BR, Easkins KE. The effects of prostaglandins on the intraocular pressure of the rabbit. Br J Pharmacol. 1969;37(1):158-67.
10. Bhattacherjee P. The role of arachidonate metabolites in ocular inflammation. Prog Clin Biol Res. 1989;312:211-27.
11. Rao PV, Deng PF, Kumar J, et al. Modulation of aqueous humor outflow facility by the Rho kinase-specific inhibitor Y-27632. Invest Ophthalmol Vis Sci. 2001;42(5):1029-37.
12. Kishi A, Nao-i N, Sawada A. Ultrasound biomicroscopic findings of acute angle-closure glaucoma in Vogt-Koyanagi-Harada syndrome. Am J Ophthalmol. 1996;122(5):735-7.
13. Kersey JP, Broadway DC. Corticosteroid-induced glaucoma: a review of the literature. Eye (Lond). 2006;20(4):407-16.
14. Razeghinejad MR, Katz LJ. Steroid-induced iatrogenic glaucoma. Ophthalmic Res. 2012;47(2):66-80.
15. Wordingera RJ, Abbot FC. Effects of glucocorticoids on the TM: towards a better understanding of glaucoma. Prog Retin Eye Res. 1999;18(5):629-67.
16. Jones R, Rhee DJ. Corticosteroid induced ocular hypertension and glaucoma: a brief review and update of the literature. Curr Opin Ophthalmol. 2006;17(2): 163-7.
17. Sim KT, Venning HE, Barrett S, et al. Extended oligoarthritis and other risk factors for developing JIA-associated uveitis under ILAR classification and its implication for current screening guideline. Ocul Immunol Inflamm. 2006; 14(6):353-7.
18. Saurenmann RK, Levin AV, Feldman BM, et al. Prevalence, risk factors and outcome of uveitis in juvenile idIOPathic arthritis—a long-term follow up study. Arthritis Rheum. 2007;56(2):647-57.
19. Rosenbaum JT. Uveitis in spondyloarthritis including psoriatic arthritis, ankylosing spondylitis, and inflammatory bowel disease. Clin Rheumatol. 2015; 34(6):999-1002.
20. Kimura SJ, Hogan MJ, Thygeson P. Fuch's syndrome of heterochromic cyclitis. AMA Arch Ophthalmol. 1955;54(2):179-86.
21. Mohamed Q, Zamir E. Update of Fuchs' uveitis syndrome. Curr Opin Ophthalmol. 2005;16(6):356-63.
22. Jones NP. Fuch's hetrochromic uveitis: an update. Surv Opthalmol. 1993; 37(4):253-72.
23. Bloch Michel E, Dussaix E, Sibillat M. Posner Schlossman syndrome. A cytomegalovirus infection. Bull Soc Ophthalmol Fr. 1998;88(1):75-6.
24. Pillai CT, Dua HS, Azuara-Blanco A, et al. Evaluation of corneal endothelium and keratic precipitates by specular microscopy in anterior uveitis. Br J Ophthalmol. 2000;84(12):1367-71.
25. Liesegang TJ. Classification of herpes simplex virus keratitis and anterior uveitis. Cornea. 1999;18(2):127-43.
26. Miserocchi E, Waheed NK, Dios E, et al. Visual outcome in herpes simplex virus and varicella zoster virus uveitis: a clinical evaluation and comparison. Ophthalmology. 2002;109(8):1532-7.

27. Majumder PD, Biswas J. Pediatric uveitis: an update. Oman J Ophthalmol. 2013;6(3):140-50.
28. Nikkhah H, Ramezani A, Ahmadieh H, et al. Childhood pars planitis: clinical features and outcomes. J Ophthalmic Vis Res. 2011;6(4):249-54.
29. Bonfiolli AA, Orefice F. Sarcoidosis. Semin Ophthalmol. 2005;20(3):177-82.
30. Jabs DA, Johns CJ. Ocular involvement in chronic sarcoidosis. Am J Ophthalmol. 1986;102(3):297-301.
31. Pandey A, Balekudaru S. Incidence and management of glaucoma in Vogt-Koyanagi-Harada disease. J Glaucoma. 2016;25(8):674-80.
32. Forster DJ, Rao NA, Hill RA, et al. Incidence and management of glaucoma in Vogt-Koyanagi-Harada syndrome. Ophthalmology. 1993;100(5):613-8.
33. Lubin JR, Albert DM, Weinstein M. Sixty-five years of sympathetic ophthalmia: a clinicopathologic review of 105 cases (1913–1978). Ophthalmology. 1980;87(2):109-21.
34. Roth M, Simon RJ. Glaucoma associated with precipitates on TM. Ophthalmology. 1979;86(9):1613-9.
35. Lambrou FH, Vela MA, Woods W. Obstruction of the TM by retinal rod outer segments. Arch Ophthalmol. 1989;107(5):742-5.
36. Matsuo T. Photoreceptor outer segments in aqueous humor: key to understanding a new syndrome. Surv Ophthalmol. 1994;39(3):211-33.
37. Chen CJ, Harisdangkul V, Parker L. Transient glaucoma associated with anterior diffuse scleritis in relapsing polychondritis. Glaucoma. 1982;4:109.
38. Jain SS, Rao P, Kothari K, et al. Posterior scleritis presenting as unilateral secondary angle-closure glaucoma. Indian J Ophthalmol. 2004;52(3):241-4.
39. Bodh SA, Kumar V, Raina UK, et al. Inflammatory glaucoma. Oman J Ophthalmol. 2011;4(1):3-9.
40. Sung VCT, Barton K. Management of inflammatory glaucoma. Curr Opin Ophthalmol. 2004;15(2):136-40.
41. Sponsel WE, Paris G, Trigo Y, et al. Latanoprost and brimonidine therapeutic and physiologic assessment before and after oral nonsteroidal anti-inflammatory therapy. Am J Ophthalmol. 2002;133(1):11-8.
42. Whitcup SM, Csaky KG, Podgor MJ, et al. A randomized, masked, cross-over trial of acetazolamide for cystoids macular edema in patients with uveitis. Ophthalmology. 1996;103(7):1054-62.
43. Kuchtey RW, Lowder CY, Smith SD. Glaucoma in patients with ocular inflammatory disease. Ophthalmol Clin North Am. 2005;18(3):421-30.
44. Kok H, Barton K. Uveitic glaucoma. Ophthalmol Clin N Am. 2002;15(3):375-87.
45. Wand M, Gilbert CM, Liesegang TJ. Latanoprost and herpes simplex keratitis. Am J Ophthalmol. 1999;127(5):602-4.
46. Ayala M, Landau Högbeck I, Chen E. Inflammation assessment after selective laser trabeculoplasty (SLT) treatment. Acta Ophthalmol. 2011; 89(4): e306-e309.
47. Nobel J, Derko-Dzulynsky L, Rabinoitch T, et al. Outcome of trabeculectomy with intraoperative mitomycin C for uveitic glaucoma. Can J Ophthalmol. 2007;42(1):89-94.

48. Gil-Carrasco F, Salinas-Van Orman E, Recillas-Gispert C, et al. Ahmed valve implant for uncontrolled uveitic glaucoma. Ocul Immunol Inflamm. 1998;6(1): 27-37.
49. Krishna R, Godfrey DG, Budenz DL, et al. Intermediate-term outcomes of 350 mm^2 Baerveldt's glaucoma implants. Ophthalmology. 2001;108(3):621-6.
50. Papadaki TG, Zacharopoulos IP, Pasquale LR, et al. Long-term results of Ahmed glaucoma valve implantation for uveitic glaucoma. Am J Ophthalmol. 2007;144(1):62-9.
51. Lee JWY, Chan JCH, Qing L, et al. Early postoperative results and complications of using the Ex-PRESS shunt in uncontrolled uveitic glaucoma: a case series of preliminary results. J Curr Glaucoma Pract. 2014;8(1):20-4.
52. Kalin-Hajdu E, Hammamji K, Gagne S, et al. Outcome of viscodilation and tensioning of Schelmm's canal for uveitic glaucoma. Can J Ophthalmol. 2014; 49(5):414-9.
53. Rebolleda G, Muñoz-Negrete FJ. Phacoemulsification in eyes with functioning filtering blebs: a prospective study. Ophthalmology. 2002;109(12):2248-55.
54. Kulkarni A, Barton K. Uveitic glaucoma. In: Shaarwy TM, Sherwood MB, Hitching RA, Crowston JG (Eds.). Glaucoma. Medical Diagnosis & Therapy. London; Elsevier Saunders; 2015. pp. 410-24.
55. Park UC, Ahn JK, Park KH, et al. Phacotrabeculectomy with mitomycin C in patients with uveitis. Am J Ophthalmol. 2006;142(6):1005-12.
56. Vernon SA, Koppens JM, Menon GJ, et al. Diode laser cycloablation in adult glaucoma: long-term results of a standard protocol and review of current literature. Clin Exp Ophthalmol. 2006;34(5):411-20.

Phacomorphic Glaucoma

Bhartiya S, Dada T

INTRODUCTION

Phacomorphic glaucoma is defined as a secondary angle-closure glaucoma due to lens intumescence and is characterized by a sudden rise in intraocular pressure (IOP), which can compromise the function of the optic nerve and may lead to irreversible visual loss if not treated in time.

Due to an unequal distribution of eye care facilities and economic constraints, especially in developing countries, many patients with age-related cataracts are not able to get cataract surgery in time and present with phacomorphic glaucoma. In the European races, a gradual shrinkage of lens with deepening of the anterior chamber (AC) occurs with development of cataract and, therefore, occurrence of phacomorphic glaucoma is relatively unusual. On the other hand, cataract in Indians seems to become intumescent rather commonly. The reason for this racial difference in the morphological changes in the cataractous lens is unknown. Phacomorphic glaucoma constitutes 3.91% of all cataract operations done in India where the incidence of cataract surgery far exceeds the total number of surgeries.[1-5]

CLINICAL FEATURES

Symptoms and Signs

Phacomorphic glaucoma is characterized by the complaints of pain and redness in an eye, which has had a progressive painless diminution of vision. Examination findings include injection of conjunctival and episcleral vessels, corneal edema, shallow AC, and intumescent cataractous lens. An asymmetric central shallowing of the AC in the presence of a unilateral mature

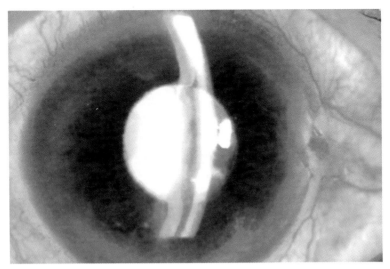

Fig. 9.1: Intumescent lens with shallow AC and circumciliary congestion.

intumescent cataract and elevated IOP are hallmarks of the disease and should immediately alert the examiner to its possibility (Fig. 9.1).

Angra et al.[3] found the mean age at presentation to be 64 years with none occurring below 50 years, thereby concluding that phacomorphic glaucoma is a disease of old age with preponderance between 50 and 60 years. The duration of attack was reported to be related to the type of cataract: lesser with intumescent cataract, whereas no relation could be found with the height of raised IOP. It was found to be three times more common in females. This could be attributed to the lesser attention received by old women in rural India and also anatomically, females having shallower AC depth, thus making them more prone for angle closure .The incidence and rise of IOP were found to be related to the maturity of cataract.[4]

CLINICAL EVALUATION

A thorough examination including the evaluation of corneal clarity and thickness, pupillary reaction, AC inflammation and gonioscopy is mandatory. Specular biomicroscopy, including endothelial counts and morphology for assessment of corneal status and B scan ultrasonography to rule out retinal pathology, must be performed whenever possible, in addition to routine investigations for cataract surgery for determining the intraocular lens (IOL) power.

An endothelial cell loss of 14.8% has been reported by Angra et al. after an attack of phacomorphic glaucoma. In this study, as the preglaucoma endothelial count was not available, they compared the cell count of the fellow eye assuming that the endothelial cell counts in the two eyes are comparable.[3]

Optic disk also shows changes that are significantly related to the duration of attack of glaucoma. Jain et al. reported that nearly all the eyes developed pallor, cupping or atrophy of the disk when the attack lasted for more than 3 weeks. Upto 10 days of attack, a large majority of optic disks (76.2%) retained good color.[5]

MECHANISM

The rise in IOP is caused by a pupillary block mechanism caused by a combination of changes in the size of the lens and the forward displacement of the lens iris diaphragm. Angle closure in phacomorphic glaucoma may be secondary to a pupillary block mechanism, or due to forward displacement of the lens-iris diaphragm. Generally, phacomorphic glaucoma is observed in older patients with senile cataracts, but it can occur in younger patients after a traumatic cataract or a rapidly developing intumescent cataract. If not managed in time, permanent synechial closure of the angle can occur with persistently elevated IOP in spite of removal of the causative cataract.

TREATMENT

Medical therapy should be instituted immediately to lower IOP, control inflammation and salvage any potential vision. Whenever possible, laser peripheral iridotomy should be performed to treat pupillary block in the affected eye, and prophylactically in the fellow eye. Once IOP is controlled medically and the eye is quiet, cataract surgery can be performed. If the patient presents after 72 hours of the onset of symptoms, with synechial angle closure, a combined surgery may have to be performed.[3-5]

It has been reported that these eyes tend to withstand raised IOP for a longer period than expected. At least 54% of the eyes with less than 2 days duration of attack reportedly recovered 6/12 or better vision, whereas only 32% of the eyes recovered this visual acuity if the duration of attack lasted 3–5 days as reported by Jain et al.[5] Thus, as the duration of attack increased there was a progressive decline in the recovery of visual acuity and beyond 3 weeks, visual acuity of only light perception or hand movements may be expected.

Medical Management

Medical management constitutes an important step in the care of phacomorphic glaucoma. Control of the raised IOP is the first line of management of phacomorphic glaucoma, followed by control of the intraocular inflammation and corneal edema.

Maximal preoperative reduction of IOP using systemic hyperosmolar agents (mannitol and glycerol), oral and topical acetazolamide, and topical antiglaucoma medication including beta-blockers and alpha agonists is recommended. Topical steroids may be prescribed to lower inflammation and hypertonic saline for corneal edema.

Angra et al. found that IOP in 37.5% eyes could not be controlled medically. These eyes were found to have extensive peripheral anterior synechiae (PAS), and a longer duration of attack. Visual status also could be improved after medical management; out of the 16 cases, which presented with faulty projection of light, nine cases reversed to have an accurate light projection after bringing down the IOP. They attributed this to the fact that the sudden increase in IOP can lead to a decrease in perfusion pressure and optic nerve ischemia with conduction defects, leading to an inaccurate projection of light, which may be reversed if treated at an early stage with IOP lowering.[3]

Role of Peripheral Iridectomy and Iridoplasty

Most of these cases of intumescent cataract with shallow chambers receive medical attention at a late stage when anterior peripheral synechiae have developed and the closure of angle is either partly or totally structural rather than functional. Therefore, any medical therapy remains only empirical and the only definitive therapy remains the provision of a bypass channel for aqueous outflow.

Tomey et al. reported that in 10 patients treated for phacomorphic glaucoma, by first undergoing neodymium:YAG (Nd:YAG) laser iridotomy, the acute angle-closure glaucoma attack could be reversed or prevented by the iridotomy, before subsequent cataract extraction.[6]

Yip et al. reported that IOP was successfully controlled in 17 eyes (80.75%), with a statistically significant decrease at 2 and 24 h postoperatively of the 21 patients in whom argon laser iridoplasty was performed as the initial step in the management of phacomorphic glaucoma. They concluded that argon laser peripheral iridoplasty (ALPI) is a safe and efficacious measure for the initial management of phacomorphic glaucoma, simultaneously obviating the need to operate in highly inflamed eyes in an emergency setting and achieving satisfactory mid-term visual outcome.[7]

Tham et al. also reported that immediate ALPI, replacing systemic antiglaucomatous medications, appeared to be safe and effective as first-line treatment of acute phacomorphic angle-closure.[8]

Of patients evaluated by Jain et al., 13.95% showed evidence of phacomorphic glaucoma in the opposite eye, 50% of whom had been operated previously and 50% had gone into absolute stage. They, however, did not recommend prophylactic iridectomy on the fellow eyes of these patients because the occurrence of phacomorphic attack seemed to occur almost 10 years later than the acute congestive glaucoma, indicating that it is the swollen cataract per se that is responsible for this attack rather than a narrow angle alone. They were of the opinion that the surgical procedure itself may accelerate the formation of a hydrated cataract. Besides, the presence of an iridectomy was not found to prevent an acute attack in three cases. Thus, it appears that in these cases there is an acute angle closure due to the forward push of the iris root rather than a physiologic pupil block and iris bombe as seen in acute closed angle glaucoma.

Peripheral iridotomy in such a situation may, therefore, be insufficient to prevent an acute attack of phacomorphic glaucoma. Instead these eyes should be kept under observation for development of cataract and cataract extraction should be done before development of the instumescent stage.[5]

Surgical Considerations

The usual surgical treatment recommended for phacomorphic glaucoma is to control the IOP first by medical therapy followed by the definitive treatment by extracting the lens. In case the IOP is not controlled by this, a second stage filtration surgery may be performed. If there is a synechial closure of more than 270° evident preoperatively, a combined cataract and filtration surgery may be the procedure of choice in the first instance.

Preoperative rise of IOP, accuracy of light projection and final visual recovery are significantly related to the duration of glaucoma. A good functional recovery may be obtained if the attack is of a short duration.

In a study by Jain et al., in cases with attack duration more than 20 days only a hand movement or perception of light could be recovered.[5]

Extracapsular Cataract Extraction/Small Incision Cataract Surgery

Extracapsular cataract extraction and manual small incision cataract surgery (SICS) with a sulcus-fixated IOL can be performed but is associated with increased intraoperative and postoperative complications in this condition.[5,9,10] Precautions that must be taken to optimize visual results are as follows:

Care must be taken to control inflammation and IOP preoperatively. Guarded ocular decompression is mandatory. A small pupil often requires the use of sphincterotomy, stretch pupilloplasty, iris hooks or pupillary dilators. Dye-assisted envelop capsulotomy is preferred over can opener technique. Copious use of high viscosity viscoelastic to deepen the AC, and a viscodispersive like Viscoat to protect the corneal endothelium can significantly improve visual outcome. The corneoscleral section must be adequate for the large nucleus. Meticulous cortical cleanup is mandatory to minimize postoperative fibrinoid reaction, together with minimal handling of the iris. Use of heparin surface-modified IOL (HSM PCIOL) placed in the bag is recommended for better visual results.

Prajna et al. reported that patients with age more than 60 years and in whom the glaucoma was present for more than 5 days were at a significantly higher risk of poor visual outcome postoperatively.[10]

PHACOEMULSIFICATION

Following IOP control, clear corneal temporal phacoemulsification is preferred as it leaves the superior site free for a subsequent trabeculectomy, if required.[9] The AC should be deepened by reducing the vitreous pressure by either a vitreous tap,[11] traditional three-port pars plana vitrectomy or 23G/25G sutureless vitrectomy.[12,13]

Operating in a crowded eye, which has a compromised endothelium and high IOP, can lead to a significant risk of complications. Hence, the author has devised the technique of sutureless pars plana limited vitrectomy to lower IOP and deepen the AC prior to phacoemulsification (Figs. 9.2A to D and 9.3A to D).[13]

The corneal endothelium should be protected using Viscoat and chilled balanced salt solution (BSS).

A small pupil is often encountered, which requires the use of sphincterotomy, stretch pupilloplasty, iris hooks or pupillary dilators like Beehlers and Malyugin.

Absence of a fundus glow makes dye-assisted capsulorhexis mandatory.

Rao[14] developed a technique that allows a safe, controlled capsulorhexis in the presence of the shallow AC, increased anterior capsule convexity and high intralenticular pressure seen in eyes with phacomorphic glaucoma. The

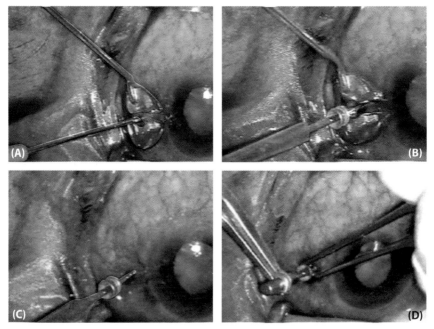

Figs. 9.2A to D: Performance of the 23-gauge vitrectomy. (A) MVR entry is made at the pars plana 3.5 mm from the limbus with an Eckhardt plate in position. (B) The trocar is introduced. (C) The probe is inserted for performing a limited vitrectomy. (D) The entry site is plugged.

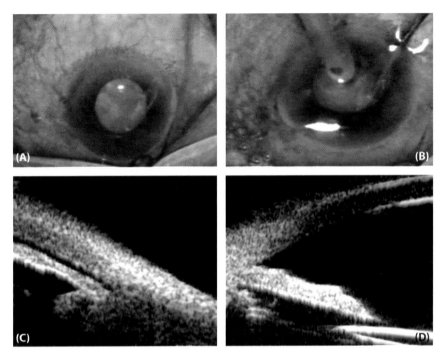

Figs. 9.3A to D: Deepening of the AC following 23 G vitrectomy with phacoemulsification (UBM).

intumescent cataract is decompressed by filling the AC with viscoelastic; a three-gauge needle is then used to aspirate liquid cortex, which facilitates a controlled capsulorhexis. This allows safe phacoemulsification of the cataract and in-the-bag IOL implantation.

A capsular tension ring should be kept handy for management of any zonular dehiscence.

Phacoemulsification should be done in the bag or in the iris plane, using low power and flow rates, with an increased bottle height. Phaco-chop nucleotomy with burst mode, torsional and cold phacoemulsification, which decrease postoperative inflammation and minimize endothelial damage, are preferred.[15]

Careful irrigation aspiration, preferably bimanual, is better in these cases. A hydrophobic, square edge foldable IOL (acrylic) is preferred.[9]

COMBINED SURGERY

Although cataract extraction and PCIOL implantation yield good visual results in phacomorphic glaucoma, a combined glaucoma and cataract surgery results in superior IOP control. Inadequate IOP control with maximal medical therapy (>3 medications) and symptom duration >3–7 days are considered to be an indication for combined surgery.

Trabeculectomy with intraoperative mitomycin C has been found to be more efficacious in lowering IOP in conjunction with phacoemulsification in comparison to its combination with entities, components, couplings and ecosystems (ECCE). Both same site and two-site phacotrabeculectomy have demonstrated similar visual results and IOP reduction.[10,15-18]

The type of conjunctival flap does not influence the final outcome. A fornix-based flap has the advantage of shorter surgical time and faster visual rehabilitation, though it has an increased incidence of bleb leakage.[17] If combined surgery is performed, antifibrotic agents such as mitomycin C must be used.

Ahmed Glaucoma Valve with ECCE

Das et al. reported that ECCE with HSM PCIOL and Ahmed Glaucoma valve (AGV) implantation was performed through two separate incisions in patients diagnosed with phacomorphic glaucoma. A steady control of IOP was maintained in all patients with minimum antiglaucoma medications. Superior preoperative IOP control and shorter phacomorphic attack duration resulted in better postoperative vision.[18]

PROBLEMS IN MANAGING PHACOMORPHIC GLAUCOMA

- Decreased endothelial count
- Corneal edema with decreased visibility
- Anterior chamber inflammation
- Decreased AC depth, less space for instrument maneuver
- Positive lenticular pressure, increased risk of extension of capsulorhexis
- Weak zonules
- Iris prolapse
- Small pupil
- Risk of hemorrhage (expulsive)
- Hard cataract
- Positive vitreous pressure
- Increased chance of posterior capsule tear
- Persistent IOP elevation requiring medical/surgical therapy
- Increased risk of postoperative fibrinoid reaction
- Poor visual outcome due to irreversible optic nerve head (ONH) damage

POSTOPERATIVE REGIMEN

Meticulous postoperative care can improve the visual results even in phacomorphic glaucoma. Potent topical steroids (prednisolone acetate drops 1%) at a frequency of every half to one hourly, with topical antibiotic cover (broad spectrum fourth generation fluoroquinolone) to combat inflammation and prevent infection are imperative. Systemic corticosteroids may be added in patients with severe inflammation.

IOP recordings and control with topical and systemic antiglaucoma therapy is extremely important, especially in cases where a cataract extraction alone has been done. Care of the bleb is mandatory in combined extractions.

Proper refractive correction for both near and distance are essential for visual rehabilitation. Visual fields and ONH evaluation must be carried out as soon as feasible.

The patient must be advised surgery for the other eye, in fact, the patient should preferably not be sent home without surgery on the other eye as these patients often do not have access to health care. In case vitrectomy has been done, peripheral screening to rule out any retinal tear is mandatory.

CONCLUSION

With the advent of superior methods of IOP control, and sophisticated instrumentation for cataract surgery, the visual prognosis in this subset of neglected patients has also become significantly better.

As is true for all other cases of glaucoma, the importance of long-term follow-up to assess IOP control and field loss cannot be over emphasized. Public health education programs to increase awareness and community support, upgradation of eye care delivery services in rural areas for early referral and treatment of cataract cases can help the in primary prevention of this condition.

REFERENCES

1. Pradhan D, Hennig A, Kumar J, et al. A prospective study of 413 cases of lens-induced glaucoma in Nepal. Indian J Ophthalmol. 2001;49(2):103-7.
2. McKibbin M, Gupta A, Atkins AD. Cataract extraction and intraocular lens implantation in eyes with phacomorphic or phacolytic glaucoma. J Cataract Refract Surg. 1996;22(5):633-6.
3. Angra SK, Pradhan R, Garg SP. Cataract induced glaucoma—an insight into management. Indian J Ophthalmol. 1991;39(3):97-101.
4. Verma BMD, Srivastava SK, Rekha. Proc. Acad. Ind. Ophthalmol Soc. 1980;39:316.
5. Jain IS, Gupta A, Dogra MR, et al. Phacomorphic glaucoma—management and visual prognosis. Indian J Ophthalmol. 1983;31(5):648-53.
6. Tomey KF, al-Rajhi AA. Neodymium:YAG laser iridotomy in the initial management of phacomorphic glaucoma. Ophthalmology. 1992;99(5):660-5.
7. Yip PP, Leung WY, Hon CY, et al. Argon laser peripheral iridoplasty in the management of phacomorphic glaucoma. Ophthal Surg Laser Imaging. 2005;36(4):286-91.
8. Tham CC, Lai JS, Poon AS, et al. Immediate argon laser peripheral iridoplasty (ALPI) as initial treatment for acute phacomorphic angle-closure (phacomorphic glaucoma) before cataract extraction: a preliminary study. Eye. 2005;19(7):778-83.
9. Tezel G, Kolker AE, Kass MA, et al. Comparative results of combined procedures for glaucoma and cataract: Extracapsular cataract extraction versus

phacoemulsification and rigid versus foldable intraocular lenses. Ophthalmic Surg Lasers. 1997;28(7):539-50.

10. Prajna NV, Ramakrishnan R, Krishnadas R, Manoharan N. Comparative results of combined procedures for glaucoma and cataract. Indian J Ophthalmol. 1996;44(3):149-55.

11. Chang DF. Pars plana vitreous tap or phacoemulsification in the crowded eye. J Cataract Refract Surg. 2001;27(12):1911-4.

12. Dada T, Kumar S, Gadia R, et al. Sutureless single-port transconjunctival pars plana limited vitrectomy combined with phacoemulsification for management of phacomorphic glaucoma. J Cataract Refract Surg. 2007; 33(6):951-4.

13. Chalam KV, Gupta SK, Agarwal S, et al. Sutureless limited vitrectomy for positive vitreous pressure in cataract surgery. Ophthalmic Surg Lasers Imaging. 2005;36(6):518-22.

14. Rao SK, Padmanabhan P. Capsulorhexis in eyes with phacomorphic glaucoma. J Cataract Refract Surg. 1998;24(7):882-4.

15. Burrato L. Phacoemulsification in glaucomatous eyes. In: Burrato L, Osher RH, Masket S (Eds). Cataract Surgery in Complicated Cases. Thorofare, NJ: Slack Inc.; 2000. p. 182.

16. Kozobolis VP, Siganos CS, Christadoulakis EV, et al. Two site phacotrabeculectomy with intraoperative mitomycin C; Fornix versus limbus based conjunctival openings in fellow eyes. J Cataract Refract Surg. 2002;28(10): 1758-62.

17. Wyse T, Meyer M, Ruderman JM, et al. Combined trabeculectomy and phacoemulsification: a one site versus two sites approach. Am J Ophthalmol. 1998;125(3):334-9.

18. Das JC, Chaudhuri Z, Bhomaj S, et al. Combined extracapsular cataract extraction with Ahmed glaucoma valve implantation in phacomorphic glaucoma. Indian J Ophthalmol. 2002;50(1):25-8.

10

New Insights into Pigment Dispersion Syndrome and Pigmentary Glaucoma

Maris PJG Jr, Bansal RK

HISTORY AND TERMINOLOGY

Over the lifetime of an individual, a certain amount of uveal pigment is chronically dispersed into the anterior segment of the eye. This is perhaps best exemplified by the relatively nonpigmented trabecular meshwork of the infant eye in contrast to the more uniformly pigmented trabecular meshwork of an individual in his eighth or ninth decade of life. Vertical pigment on the corneal epithelium has been described in the literature since the late 1800s.[1] However, it was only in 1940 that Sugar first described pigment dispersion in association with glaucoma in a 29-year-old patient.[2] In 1949, Sugar and Barbour described the features of the condition that is now referred to as 'pigmentary glaucoma (PG)'.[3] Pigmentary glaucoma is a secondary open-angle glaucoma characterized by homogenous brownish pigmentation of the chamber angle, pigment deposition on the corneal endothelium (the 'Krukenberg spindle') and slit-like, radial, midperipheral transillumination defects of the iris. When the anterior chamber findings exist in absence of elevated intraocular pressure (IOP), glaucomatous optic neuropathy or visual field defects, the condition is referred to as pigment dispersion syndrome (PDS).

ETIOLOGY AND PATHOGENESIS

The pathophysiology of PG considers two major mechanisms: (1) The mechanics of pigment dispersion and (2) obstruction of aqueous outflow. Campbell proposed a now widely accepted theory that the rubbing of the posterior iris against packets of lens zonules causes a release of pigment granules from the iris pigment epithelium.[4] The contact between the iris and

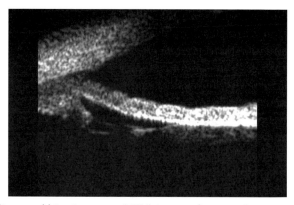

Fig. 10.1: Ultrasound biomicroscopy (UBM) image of an anterior segment showing a deep peripheral iris concavity with iridozonular and iridolenticular contact. (Photo courtesy of Celso Tello, MD).

the zonules is likely accentuated by a posteriorly displaced midperipheral iris. Ultrasound biomicroscopy (UBM) (Fig.10.1) analysis has helped confirm a posterior iris profile in patients with PG and PDS.[5] The distance between the base of the trabecular meshwork and the iris insertion has been shown to be greater in PDS than control eyes.[6] Also, a concave iris profile with a deeper anterior chamber depth has been noted in PDS and PG eyes.[7,8] Yet, a posteriorly directed pressure gradient must exist to cause a posteriorly bowed iris configuration. This suggests that aqueous is moved into the anterior chamber, possibly by the movement of the iris in response to blinking or accommodation. Once in the anterior chamber, the aqueous is prevented from returning to the posterior chamber by a one-way valve effect between the iris and the lens, giving rise to a 'reverse pupillary block' phenomenon.[9] The theory of reverse pupillary block configuration has been supported by Scheimpflug photography of the anterior segment and is eliminated by peripheral iridotomy, miotic therapy and the prevention of blinking.[8,10-12] Recent studies have also implicated corneal biomechanics in the pathogenesis of reverse pupillary block and iridolenticular contact. Patients with PDS have been noted to have flatter curvatures of the anterior and posterior cornea.[13,14] It is theorized that the presence of a flatter cornea in pigment dispersion patients may indirectly contribute to the reverse pupillary block phenomenon during a blink.

Pigment liberation into the anterior chamber offsets the second mechanism responsible for elevated intraocular pressure in PG: the reduction of conventional aqueous outflow. Studies on autopsy eyes have shown that pigment granules accumulate in the trabecular meshwork and can cause significant obstruction to conventional aqueous outflow.[15] In addition to the mechanical slowing of outflow imparted by the presence of pigment granules, the endothelial cells lining the trabecular meshwork likely undergo damage and collapse caused by macrophages phagocytizing the pigment granules. It is this unrelenting process of pigment accumulation in the trabecular meshwork, followed by melanophagocytosis and then subsequent collapse of the trabecular beams and intertrabecular spaces that leads to markedly decreased outflow facility and intractable intraocular pressure elevation.[16,17]

A possible genetic etiology has been suggested in PDS/PG. Mandelkorn and associates reported five families with PDS with several modes of inheritance. They suggested that PDS is inherited in an autosomal dominant or recessive manner with other factors, such as gender, iris color and refractive error, contributing to the clinical manifestation of the condition.[18] In a separate analysis of four affected pedigrees, the gene responsible for PDS was mapped to the telomeric end of the long arm of chromosome 7 (i.e., 7q35–q36).[19]

DEMOGRAPHICS AND SYMPTOMS

The typical PG patient is young, myopic and male, and the presentation is usually bilateral. One study of 108 patients with either PDS or PG showed a preponderance of men (67.6%) compared to women (32.4%).[20] In this study, the men were younger at the time of diagnosis (mean age = 36.7 years) compared to the women (mean age = 43.2 years), and the men were more likely to progress from pigment dispersion to PG. Likewise, the average age of diagnosis for all patients in the study was 38.8 years and is in keeping with other studies that indicate the initial diagnosis of PDS is made between the third and fifth decades.[21-23] Another large study of 799 eyes with PDS showed that when both eyes were affected by glaucoma, the glaucoma was more severe in the eye with the more heavily pigmented chamber angle. Myopia was also noted in the majority (65%) of the patients in that study.[24] PG is encountered primarily in Caucasians, and a very low prevalence has been noted in Black, Hispanic and Asian populations.[20,21,25]

In terms of symptoms, prostaglandins (PGs) and PG are usually asymptomatic entities until PG reaches the advanced-to-end stages. However, even in the early stages of the disease, some patients may report halos after exercise, such as jogging or playing basketball. This is thought to be secondary to increased pigment liberation brought on by an exercise-induced increase in choroidal circulation and choroidal volume and increase in systemic pulse rate, which, in turn, increases cyclical aqueous humor movements and backward bowing of the iris.[11,26] The increased pigment overloads the functional capabilities of the trabecular meshwork and causes a marked elevation in IOP with subsequent symptomatic corneal edema.[27,28] Headache and blurring of vision may also occur in patients with PDS.[22]

CLINICAL EXAM FINDINGS

Despite the relative paucity of symptoms, several features of pigment dispersion can be easily noted on ophthalmic exam. Working anteriorly to

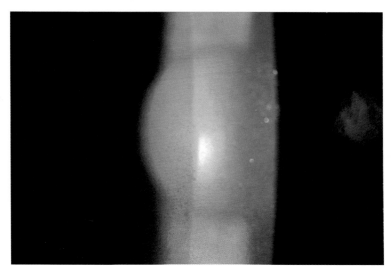

Fig. 10.2: Deposition of pigment on the corneal endothelium, called a Krukenberg's spindle, in a patient with pigmentary glaucoma.

posteriorly, the first findings noted on slit lamp exam is the vertically oriented collection of pigment granules, termed a 'Krukenberg spindle,' on the corneal endothelium (Fig. 10.2). This finding is best noted by focusing a broad beam of light from the slit lamp onto the corneal endothelium. The pattern of the pigment likely represents the vertical meeting of the aqueous convection currents from the left and the right halves of the anterior chamber of the eye.[22] Despite the appearance of pigment on the corneal endothelium, comparisons between the corneas of PDS eyes and matched control eyes have shown no difference in the endothelial cell density or central corneal thickness as measured by specular microscopy and pachymetry, respectively.[29]

A second major diagnostic feature of PDS is midperipheral iris transillumination defects in a radial spoke-like pattern. These defects do not involve the iris sphincter or the iris root and are best observed in retroillumination by projecting the light of the slit lamp through the pupil in a plane perpendicular to the iris.

The third major diagnostic finding of the syndrome is the homogenous dark brown band of pigment for the full circumference of the trabecular meshwork noted on gonioscopy (Fig. 10.3). The pigment may also deposit along Schwalbe's line inferiorly. In addition, careful gonioscopic exam can show the more posterior insertion of the iris and the more concave appearance of the iris face that are typical of PDS.

Once the patient is dilated, pigment can sometimes be seen on the anterior and posterior lens capsule as well as on the lens zonules. Pigment deposited on the posterior lens surface at the junction of the zonules and capsule was first described by Zentmayer in 1938, but is now frequently referred to as a Scheie's stripe.[24,30]

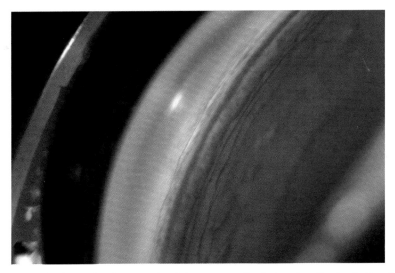

Fig. 10.3: Gonioscopic photograph of the same patient, showing the typically wide-open angle with homogenous, heavy pigmentation of the trabecular meshwork and pigment dusting along Schwalbe's line.

In terms of the posterior segment of the eye, retinal detachments occur more frequently in patients with PDS and PG irrespective of myopic refractive error, and these patients should undergo periodic dilated fundus examinations.[23] In a consecutive case series of 60 patients with PDS, with or without glaucoma, lattice degeneration was present in 20% of patients and full-thickness retinal breaks were noted in 11.7% of patients.[31]

DIFFERENTIAL DIAGNOSIS

There are several other disorders characterized by pigment release into the anterior chamber with associated elevated intraocular pressure. Most of these conditions are unilateral and can be distinguished from PDS and PG by taking a careful history and performing a thorough ophthalmic exam.

- *Pseudoexfoliation syndrome (PXS)*: In this condition, rubbing between the peripupillary iris and mid-peripheral lens leads to pigment deposition. However, this condition is usually distinguished from PDS and PG by the finding of exfoliate material on the lens and pupillary rough and the older age of the patient.
- *Anterior uveitis*: Inflammation of the uveal tract may lead to release of pigment and inflammatory debris in the anterior chamber, but careful gonioscopic exam of these eyes shows that the trabecular meshwork pigmentation is more irregular and is accompanied by occasional peripheral anterior synechiae (PAS). In addition, eyes with uveitis manifest aqueous flare and white cells, keratic precipitates and ciliary flush.
- *Trauma and intraocular surgery*: Trauma can induce anterior segment features suggestive of PG, including increased pigmentation of the

trabecular meshwork, iris atrophy and/or transillumination defects and elevated IOP. Posterior-chamber intraocular lens (IOL) implantation, particularly in cases of complicated cataract extraction, can cause marked pigment dispersion, resulting in heavy pigmentation of the trabecular meshwork and elevated IOP. This occurs secondary to the lens haptics and edges of the optic chafing the posterior surface of the iris, and the transillumination defects typically correspond to these positions. The shedding often stops once all of the pigment has been rubbed off in the localized area.[32] Placement of the IOL in the ciliary sulcus, rather than the capsular bag, or malposition of the IOL in the ciliary sulcus is more likely to produce this phenomenon. Also, it has been noted that plate-haptic IOL's implanted in the ciliary sulcus have more contact with the posterior iris surface than sulcus-placed IOLs with angulated haptics.[33-35]

- *Uveal tumors*: Tumors of the uveal tract can cause secondary glaucoma by means of pigment dispersion and/or direct tumor invasion of the angle. Melanolytic glaucoma occurs when macrophages engulf uveal pigment and block the trabecular meshwork. Recently, Johnson reported a case of a 64-year-old female with a ciliary body melanoma who was erroneously diagnosed with unilateral PG and eventually underwent enucleation.[36]

MANAGEMENT

The natural course of the PDS and PG remains poorly understood and can be unpredictable. There is an early period of active pigment release, and then the disease has been noted to decrease in severity over time or even 'burn-out.' The amelioration of the syndrome over time is believed to occur secondary to the natural enlargement of the crystalline lens, which pushes the peripheral iris forward and partially relives iridozonular touch.[37] There are several reports of arrest of progression or even spontaneous improvement among patients with PG, so therapeutic modalities need to be constantly reassessed when managing this condition.[4,23,25]

- *Initial treatment*: One of the primary goals of treatment, at least during the pigment release stage, should be to minimize iridozonular contact. Miotic agents help to achieve this. Pigment release during exercise has been prevented by pretreatment with pilocarpine drops. Pilocarpine can also cause reversal of iris transillumination defects.[38] The downside of cholinergic drugs, like pilocarpine, lies with their side effects, such as accommodative spasm, induced myopia, poor night vision and the risk for retinal tears and detachment. Weaker strengths of pilocarpine and slow-release formulations, like ocuserts and gels, are often better tolerated. Alpha-1-receptor antagonists, like thymoxamine and dapiprazole, work by relaxing the dilator muscle, leading to pupillary constriction but without affecting accommodation. Theoretically, these agents would be ideal for treating PDS and PG, but they are not typically used. Thymoxamine is not available in the United States because it was never approved by the Federal Drug Administration (FDA) due to its systemic side effect profile. Dapiprazole is available and FDA-approved, but it is not used routinely because of its insufficient action as well as associated side effects, such as conjunctival hyperemia.

- *Recommended medical treatment*: The degree of IOP-lowering and the agents used to achieve it should follow the same guidelines as treatment for primary open-angle glaucoma (POAG). Aqueous suppressants, like beta-blockers and carbonic anhydrase inhibitors, are excellent first-line medical therapies in PG. Prostaglandin analogs can also be useful in medical management. In a 12-month randomized, double-masked study, latanoprost was found to be more effective than timolol in controlling IOP.[39] The investigators suggested that the PG-mediated increase in uveoscleral outflow created an alternate passage for pigment egress, which, in turn, minimized pigment accumulation and overload in the trabecular meshwork. However, their study could not confirm this finding histologically.

- *Laser peripheral iridotomy (LPI)*: David Campbell postulated (presentation at the American Glaucoma Society meeting, San Diego, CA, 1991) that the posterior bowing of the peripheral iris and reverse pupillary block configuration can be overcome with LPI. The flattening of iris after LPI has been observed by many surgeons,[40-42] but the long-term benefits of LPI on IOP control remain disputed.[43,44] In a retrospective analysis of data contributed by members of the American Glaucoma Society, LPI did not result in better IOP control in the long-term (over 2 years) among patients with PG.[45] Therefore, this procedure is most appropriate in patients less than 45 years of age who have well-documented evidence of a concave iris configuration, active pigment release and a well-functioning trabecular meshwork.[46] In cases of a damaged or marginally functioning trabecular meshwork, pigment release following LPI can overload the outflow system and cause acute IOP elevations.

- *Laser trabeculoplasty (LT)*: Laser trabeculoplasty, both argon (ALT) and selective (SLT), is useful in reducing IOP in patients with PG. In a retrospective, long-term study of ALT, the success rate was 80% at one year, 62% at 2 years, and 45% at 6 years. Younger patients had a greater chance of success than did older patients at all time intervals.[47] Due to its ability to selectively target melanin-containing cells of the trabecular meshwork and avoid thermal and coagulative damage to adjacent tissues, SLT is quickly becoming the preferred method of laser trabeculoplasty. However, in a randomized prospective study, SLT was equivalent to ALT in terms of IOP lowering at 1 year.[48] Pressure spikes are not uncommon after laser trabeculoplasty in patients with PG due to the heavy trabecular meshwork pigmentation. Therefore, treatments using lower energy settings and fewer spot applications as well as treating fewer quadrants at one sitting can minimize post-treatment IOP elevations.[49]

- *Surgery*: Just as with most glaucomas, incisional surgery is indicated when medical treatment and laser therapy fails to achieve target IOP. Prior to the widespread use of the PGs analogues, it was estimated that 50% of patients with PG would require surgical intervention.[20] Patients with PG are comparatively young and therefore adjunctive use of anti-fibrotic agents in higher concentrations should be strongly considered. Conversely, one should keep in mind that these patients, in addition to being young and male, are typically myopic and therefore predisposed to postoperative hypotony maculopathy. Likewise, care should be taken to avoid a flat anterior chamber intraoperatively and avoid early postoperative hypotony so as to mitigate against the development of choroidal effusions. Also, as discussed previously, myopic status confers a greater risk of tractional vitreo-retinal complications that may develop postoperatively. Nonpenetrating procedures, such as deep sclerectomy, trabectome or canaloplasty can also be used as primary surgical interventions. Trabectome surgery, in particular, has the benefit of sparing the conjunctiva in the event that a future full-thickness filtration procedure is required for IOP control. However, no data is currently available to compare these nonpenetrating modalities in the surgical management of PG.

SUMMARY

Pigment dispersion syndrome is due to iridolenticular and iridozonlar contact in effected individuals that leads to the liberation of pigment granules, resulting in the hallmark findings of pigment deposits on the corneal endothelium and in the chamber angle as well as iris transillumination defects. When conventional outflow facility becomes overwhelmed and dysfunctional, PG ensues. Pigmentary glaucoma is typically seen in myopic, young adult males. Medical treatment is similar to other forms of open-angle glaucoma. Regarding laser treatment, future research will better elucidate the most efficacious and safe modalities, including laser trabeculoplasty and peripheral iridotomy. Incisional surgical innovations remain ongoing and will hopefully be better tailored to this unique demographic of glaucoma patients.

REFERENCES

1. Krukenberg F. Beiderseitige angeborene melanose der hornhaut. Klin Monatsbl Augenheilkd. 1899;37:254-8.
2. Sugar HS. Concerning the chamber angle. I. Gonioscopy. Am J Ophthalmol. 1940;23:853-66.
3. Sugar HS, Barbour FA. Pigmentary glaucoma: a rare clinical entity. Am J Ophthalmol. 1949;32(1):90-2.
4. Campbell DG. Pigmentary dispersion and glaucoma: a new theory. Arch Ophthalmol. 1979;97(9):1667-72.

5. Kanadani FN, Dorairaj S, Langlieg AM, et al. Ultrasound biomicroscopy in asymmetric pigment dispersion syndrome and pigmentary glaucoma. Arch Ophthalmol. 2006;124(11):1573-76.
6. Sokol J, Stegman Z, Liebman JM, et al. Location of iris insertion in pigment dispersion syndrome. Ophthalmology. 1996;103(2):289-93.
7. Pavlin CJ, Macken P, Trope G, et al. Ultrasound biomicoscopic features of pigmentary glaucoma. Can J Ophthalmol. 1994;29(4):187-92.
8. Potash SD, Tello C, Liebmann JM, et al. Ultrasound biomicroscopy in pigment dispersion syndrome. Ophthalmology. 1994;101(2):332-9.
9. Campbell DG, Schertzer PM. Pathophysiology of pigment dispersion syndrome and pigmentary glaucoma. Curr Opin Ophthalmol. 1995;6(2): 96-101.
10. Doyle JW, Hansen JE, Smith MF, et al. Use of Scheimpflug photography to study iris configuration in patients with pigment dispersion syndrome and pigmentary glaucoma. J Glaucoma. 1995;4(6):398-405.
11. Jensen PK, Nissen O, Kessing SV. Exercise and reversal of papillary block in pigmentary glaucoma. Am J Ophthalmol. 1995;120(1):110-12.
12. Liebmann JM, Tello C, Chew S-J, et al. Prevention of blinking alters iris configuration in pigment dispersion syndrome an in normal eyes. Ophthalmology. 1995;102(3):446-5.
13. Lord FD, Pathanapitoon K, Mikelberg FS. Keratometry and axial length in pigment dispersion: a descriptive case–control study. J Glaucoma. 2001; 10(5):383-85.
14. Yip LW, Sothornwit N, Berkowitz J, et al. A comparison of interocular differences in patients with pigment dispersion syndrome. J Glaucoma. 2009; 18(1):1-5.
15. Grant WM. Experimental aqueous perfusion in enucleated human eyes. Arch Ophthalmol. 1963;69:783-801.
16. Richardson TM, Hutchinson BT, Grant WM. The outflow tract in pigmentary glaucoma: a light and electron microscopic study. Arch Ophthalmol. 1977;95(6):1015-25.
17. Gottanka J, Johnson DH, Grehn F. Histologic findings in pigment dispersion syndrome and pigmentary glaucoma. J Glaucoma. 2006;15(2):142-51.
18. Mandelkorn RM, Hoffman ME, Olander KW, et al. Inheritance and the pigmentary dispersion syndrome. Ophthalmic Paediatr Genet. 1985;6(1-2): 325-31.
19. Anderson JS, Pralea AM, DelBono EA, et al. A gene responsible for the pigment dispersion syndrome maps to chromosome 7q35-q36. Arch Ophthalmol. 1997;115(3):384-8.
20. Farrar SM, Shields MB, Miller KN, et al. Risk factors for the development and severity of glaucoma in patients with pigment dispersion. Am J Ophthalmol. 1989;108(3):223-9.
21. Migliazzo CV, Shaffer RN, Sykin R, et al. Long-term analysis of pigmentary dispersion syndrome and pigmentary glaucoma. Ophthalmology. 1986; 93(12):1528-36.
22. Sugar HS. Pigmentary glaucoma: A 25-year review. Am J Ophthalmol. 1966; 62(3):499-507.

23. Ritch R. Nonproressive low-tension glaucoma with pigmentary dispersion. Am J Ophthalmol. 1982;94(2):190-6.
24. Scheie HG, Cameron JD. Pigment dispersion syndrome: a clinical study. Br J Ophthalmol. 1981;65(4):264-9.
25. Farrar SM, Shields MB. Current concepts in pigmentary glaucoma. Surv Ophthalmol. 1993;37(4):233-52.
26. Speakman JS. Pigment dispersion. Br J Ophthalmol. 1981;65(4):249-51.
27. Haynes WL, Johnson AT, Alward WLM. Inhibition of exercise-induced pigment dispersion in patient with pigment dispersion syndrome. Am J Ophthalmol. 1990:109(5):599-601.
28. Haynes WL, Johnson AT, Alward WLM. Effects of jogging exercise on patients with pigment dispersion syndrome and pigmentary glaucoma. Ophthalmology. 1992;99(7):1096-103.
29. Murrell WJ, Shihab Z, Lamberts DW, et al. The corneal endothelium and central corneal thickness in pigmentary dispersion syndrome. Arch Ophthalmol. 1986;104(6):845-86.
30. Zentmayer W. Association of an annular band of pigment on the posterior capsule of the lens with a Krukenberg spindle. Arch Ophthalmol. 1938; 20:52-7.
31. Weseley P, Liebmann J, Walsh JB, et al. Lattice degeneration of the retina and the pigment dispersion syndrome. Am J Ophthalmol. 1992;114(5):539-43.
32. Samples JR, Van Buskirk EM. Pigmentary glaucoma associated with posterior chamber intraocular lenses. Am J Ophthalmol. 1985;100(3):385-8.
33. Chang SHL, Lim G. Secondary pigmentary glaucoma associated with piggyback intraocular lens implantation. J Cataract Refract Surg. 2004;30(10): 2219-22.
34. Kohnen T, Kook D. Solving intraocular lens-related pigment dispersion syndrome with repositioning of primary sulcus implanted single-piece IOL in the capsular bag. J Cataract Refract Surg. 2009;35(8):1459-63.
35. Apple DJ, Reidy JJ, Googe JM, et al. A comparison of ciliary sulcus and capsular bag fixation of posterior chamber intraocular lenses. Am Intra-Ocular Implant Soc J. 1985:11(1):44-63.
36. Johnson DL, Altaweel MM, Neekhara A, et al. Uveal melanoma masquerading as pigment dispersion syndrome. Arch Ophthalmol. 2008;126(6):868-9.
37. Ritch R, Campbell DG, Camras C. Initial treatment of pigmentary glaucoma. J Glaucoma. 1993;2(1):44-9.
38. Campbell DG. Improvement of pigmentary glaucoma and healing of transillumination defects with mitotic therapy. Invest Ophthalmol Vis Sci (ARVO suppl). 1983;23:173.
39. Mastropasqua L, Carpineto P, Ciancaglini M, et al. A 12-month randomized double-masked study comparing latanoprost with timolol in pigmentary glaucoma. Ophthalmology. 1999;106(3):550-5.
40. Karickhoff JR. Pigmentary dispersion syndrome and pigmentary glaucoma: a new mechanism concept, a new treatment, and a new technique. Ophthal Surg. 1992;23(4):269-77.

41. Carassa RG, Bettin P, Fiore M, et al. Nd:YAG laser iridotomy in pigment dispersion syndrome: an ultrasound biomicoroscopic study. Br J Ophthalmol. 1998;82(2):150-3.
42. Breingan PJ, Esaki K, Ishikawa H, et al. Iridolenticular contact decreases following laser iridotomy for pigment dispersion syndrome. Arch Ophthalmol. 1999;117(3):325-8.
43. Gandolfi SA, Vecchi M. Effect of a YAG laser iridotomy on the intraocular pressure in pigment dispersion syndrome. Ophthalmol. 1996;103(10):1693-5.
44. Wang JC, Liebermann JM, Ritch R. Long-term outcome of argon laser iridotomy in pigment dispersion syndrome. Invest Ophthalmol Vis Sci (Suppl). 2001;42:s560.
45. Reistad CE, Shields MB, Campbell DG, et al. The influence of peripheral iridotomy on the intraocular pressure course in patients with pigmentary glaucoma. J Glaucoma. 2005;14(4):255-9.
46. Gandolfi SA, Ungaro N, Mora P, et al. Pigmentary glaucoma. In Shaarawy TM, Sherwood MB, Hitchings RA, Crowston JG (Eds). Glaucoma: Medical Diagnosis and Therapy. New York: Sauders Elsevier; 2009. Chapter 29. pp. 349-360.
47. Ritch R, Liebmann J, Robin A, et al. Argon laser trabeculoplasty in pigmentary glaucoma. Ophthalmology. 1993;100(6):909-13.
48. Damji KF, Bovell AM, Hodge WG, et al. Selective laser trabeculoplasty versus argon laser trabeculoplasty results from a 1-year randomized clinical trial. Br J Ophthalmol. 2006;90(12):1490-94.
49. Harasymowycz PJ, Papamatheakis DG, Latina M. Selective laser trabeculoplasty (SLT) complicated by intraocular pressure elevation in eyes with heavily pigmented trabecular meshworks. Am J Ophthalmol. 2005;139(6): 1110-3.

11

Exfoliative Glaucoma

Krishnadas R, Malleswari M, Puthuran GV

Exfoliation syndrome is the most common, identifiable cause of open-angle glaucoma.[1] It is an age-related disorder of the extracellular matrix, characterized by excessive production and accumulation of deposits of fibrillar extracellular material in the ocular tissues. Exfoliation deposits are most commonly appreciated in the pupillary border and the anterior lens capsule. Ocular manifestations of exfoliation include angle-closure and open-angle glaucoma, cataract, lens subluxation, and central retinal vein occlusion. Exfoliation syndrome is associated with ocular and systemic hypoxia and apart from glaucoma, predisposes to capsular breaks, zonular dehiscence and vitreous loss during cataract surgery. Other names for XFG are glaucoma capsulare/capsular glaucoma. The glaucoma capsulare was first reported by Lindberg in 1917 in Finland.

There are important differences between the clinical features, course and prognosis of exfoliative glaucoma (XFG) and primary open-angle glaucoma (POAG). The course and prognosis of exfoliative glaucoma is more severe than POAG, with greater 24-h intraocular pressure (IOP) fluctuations, more severe visual field loss and optic nerve damage at the initial diagnosis. It has rapid progression and frequently needs surgical intervention in comparison with POAG. The medical and laser treatment approaches of XFG also significantly differ from that of POAG.

EPIDEMIOLOGY OF EXFOLIATION AND GLAUCOMA

The reported prevalence of exfoliation with and without glaucoma varies widely, reflecting not only true differences in prevalence due to racial, ethnic, geographic and other population differences, but also due to clinical criteria used to diagnose exfoliation, ability of the examiner to detect early/

subtle changes or signs, the method and thoroughness of examination, and prior knowledge or skills of the examiner. Many cases of exfoliation go unreported because of failure to observe the anterior surface of the lens under magnification on a slit-lamp after dilatation. Exfoliation occurs worldwide, though reported prevalence varies extensively. Aasved[2] found prevalence of 6.3%, 4.0% and 4.7% in persons aged over 60 in nursing homes in Norway, England and Germany, respectively. Forsius,[3] looking at persons aged over 60 years in varied groups, found prevalence ranging from 0% in Greenland Eskimos to 21% in Icelanders. The reported prevalence in the United States is generally similar to that in the Western European populations. In the Framingham study, age-specific rates of exfoliation increased from 0.6% for those in the 52–64 years age group to 5% for 75–85 years age group. African Americans are known to have a much lower prevalence of exfoliation than Caucasians.

The prevalence of exfoliation was studied in the rural population of South India.[4] Exfoliation was seen in 308 persons out of 5,150 individuals screened, over the age of 40 with a reported prevalence of approximately 6%. The prevalence showed an increase with age and it was more in men than women. In a yet another rural study in South India,[5] the prevalence of exfoliation was reported to be 3.8%. There was an age-related increase in prevalence but no sex predominance.

The reasons behind true variations in the prevalence of exfoliation form one population to another and within homogenous populations remain unexplained. Geographic distribution patterns are sometimes explained by regional gene pools or environmental INFLUENCES. Populations in lower latitudes (Greece, Iran and Saudi Arabia) develop exfoliation at a younger age. Exposure to sunlight (UV radiation) and dietary factors may play a significant role as well. It has also been observed that in any given population the reported prevalence of exfoliation is much less than that actually found.

In all population studies the prevalence of exfoliation increases with age. Patients with exfoliation who have glaucoma tend to be older than those who do not. Incidence of exfoliation doubles every decade after age 50, although early onset exfoliation has been reported in a few population sub-groups. Although many studies have not found any sex predilection for exfoliation, it has been reported that glaucoma may develop earlier, more frequently and more severely among males than females. Evidences that support a genetic[6] basis for exfoliation and XFG include familial aggregation, transmission in two-generation families, higher concordance rates of disease in monozygotic twins, increased risk of exfoliation in relatives of affected patients and HLA studies. Late-onset and incomplete penetrance make genetic association studies in exfoliation difficult although the disease appears to be inherited as autosomal dominant trait. Recently, sequence variants in the LOXL1 gene,[7] which catalyzes formation of elastin fibers, have been implicated in the pathogenesis of XFG.

Prevalence of Exfoliation in Glaucoma

The prevalence of exfoliation in persons with glaucoma is higher than in age-matched nonglaucomatous population. Reported prevalence varies from 0% to 93% with highest rates in Scandinavia. There is also a high incidence of exfoliation in open-angle glaucoma population in most European countries. In the United States, three series have reported prevalence of exfoliation close to 12% in glaucoma populations. In a study on prevalence of glaucoma in a rural population in South India,[4] exfoliation was present in 26.7% patients with open-angle glaucoma.

Prevalence of Glaucoma in Exfoliation Syndrome

Glaucoma occurs more commonly in eyes with exfoliation than in those without it. In a series of 100 consecutive patients with exfoliation,[8] visual field loss and glaucomatous optic disk damage were detected in 7% and ocular hypertension was observed in 15%. Aasved,[9] for instance, observed elevated IOP with or without glaucoma in 22% of patients with exfoliation as opposed to 1.2% of those without exfoliation. In persons with exfoliation, the risk of developing glaucoma is also cumulative over time. The 5- and 10-year cumulative probabilities of developing glaucoma in exfoliation eyes was 5.3% and 15.4%, respectively,[10] a significantly higher rate than would be expected in a similar population without exfoliation. In this cohort, persons with exfoliation would approximately have 40% chance of either having initially or developing ocular hypertension or glaucoma within 10 years, which translates to a tenfold risk as compared to those without exfoliation, although several persons with exfoliation have been observed not to develop glaucoma over time.

In the study by Arvind[5] et al. in South India, ocular hypertension was detected in 9.3% individuals with exfoliation. Of those with exfoliation 14.8% of the individuals also had narrow, occludable angles and 13% of individuals with exfoliation had disk changes definitive of glaucoma. The study found increased IOP, occludable angles and glaucomatous optic disk changes more frequently in individuals with exfoliation than in persons without evidence of exfoliation. The Aravind Comprehensive Eye Survey,[4] which also studied prevalence of glaucoma in a rural population in South India not ethnically variant from that studied by Arvind[5] et al., definite glaucoma was diagnosed in 7.5% of persons with exfoliation. Individuals with XFG had predominantly open angles. Ocular hypertension was prevalent in 4.22% of exfoliation and the odds ratio of having open-angle glaucoma was higher among those with exfoliation.

Patients with exfoliation syndrome must be followed regularly. A proper examination of the disk should be made at each examination and a color photograph should be taken for future reference. Suspicious disks and pressures should be followed every 4–6 months and normal disks and pressures observed annually or a 2-year interval.

CLINICAL FEATURES

The Crystalline Lens

The most consistent diagnostic feature of exfoliation syndrome is the typical deposits of white material on the anterior lens capsule of the crystalline lens. The classic pattern of exfoliation on the lens capsule consists of three distinct zones, which become distinctly visible on pupillary dilatation: a relatively homogenous central zone, which roughly corresponds to the size of the pupil, a granular peripheral zone and a clear area separating these two. The amount of the exfoliation material on the lens, stage of the disease and the relative position and the size of the pupil determine the variable appearance of these zones on the anterior capsule of the lens. The central zone of exfoliation is a homogenous sheet on the anterior pole of the lens and is slightly smaller (1.5–3.0 mm) than the physiologic pupil (Fig. 11.1). The edges of the central zone are rolled anteriorly, and is absent in about 20–60% of eyes with exfoliation. Computerized image enhancement and Scheimpflug photography increase the visibility of the exfoliation on the lens capsule. The presence of granular with radial striations in the peripheral zone is the most consistent feature (Figs. 11.2 to 11.4). The granularity is due to undisturbed deposition of exfoliation and in eyes treated with miotics with small pupil, granularity may be seen more centrally. Radial nongranular striae in the mid lens surface in fact represent, earlier pregranular stage of exfoliation. To highlight subtle, early deposits of exfoliation, slit-lamp beam is placed 45° to the axis of observation and is focused about 3–4 mm temporal to the center of the lens. Cataracts in exfoliation glaucoma have higher incidence of nuclear opacities compared to cortical or supranuclear opacities. Phacodonesis and

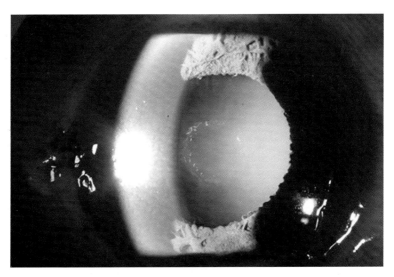

Fig. 11.1: Exfoliation on the anterior lens capsule; relatively homogeneous central zone and a peripheral granular zone with a clear intermediate zone separating the two.

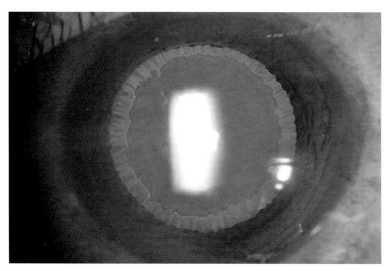

Fig. 11.2: Peripheral granular zone of exfoliation on the lens seen on retroillumination.

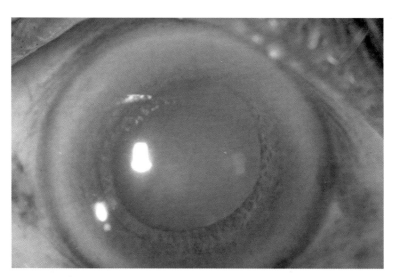

Fig. 11.3: Radial spoke like deposits of exfoliation, an early sign of exfoliation syndrome. Pigments from iris-on the spokes of exfoliation due to constant rubbing of iris on the anterior lens surface.

spontaneous lens dislocation are common with advanced exfoliation and are attributed to zonular weakness and dehiscence. The central zone consists of fibrillin and is composed of loosely arranged and scattered microfibrils, and exfoliation fibers appear to originate by aggregation of microfibrils. The peripheral preequatorial zone is characterized by nodular excrescences on the zonules and their attachment to the anterior lens capsule and this region corresponds to the proliferative zone of the lens epithelium.

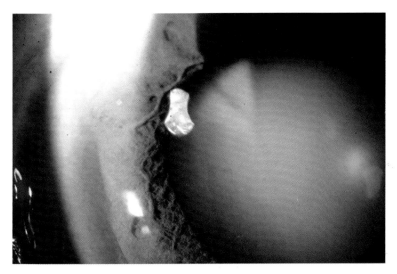

Fig. 11.4: A highly magnified view of the peripheral granular zone on the temporal aspect of the crystalline lens.

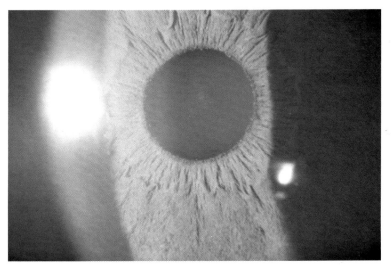

Fig. 11.5: Exfoliation on the iris and pupillary margin is a hallmark of exfoliation syndrome and frequently associated with glaucoma.

Iris

Exfoliation is most prominent on the pupil border next to the crystalline lens. Iris changes could be an early and well-recognized clinical feature. Exfoliation on the pupillary border is not invariable in all eyes with exfoliation and may either be extensive on the pupillary margin or just present sparsely as tiny dots (Fig. 11.5), requiring a high index of suspicion for detection. It has been suggested that coexistent open-angle glaucoma is more likely and severe if the iris has exfoliation. The iris in eyes with exfoliation appears to be more rigid than normal eyes. Pigment loss from iris sphincter with its deposition on the anterior chamber structures is a characteristic hallmark of eyes with exfoliation, loss of pupillary ruff (Fig. 11.6), iris transilluminaton defects (Fig. 11.7), increased trabecular pigmentation and pigmentation of the Schwalbe's line or Sampaolesi's line[11] (Fig. 11.8). Histologically, iris vessel lumen is frequently found to be narrowed and occasionally is obliterated with complete degeneration of the vessel wall. Fluorescein angiographic studies have shown partial occlusion of radial iris capillaries associated with

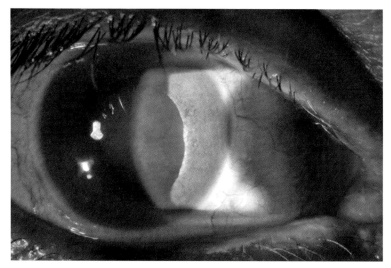

Fig. 11.6: Loss of pupillary ruff is an early sign of exfoliative syndrome.

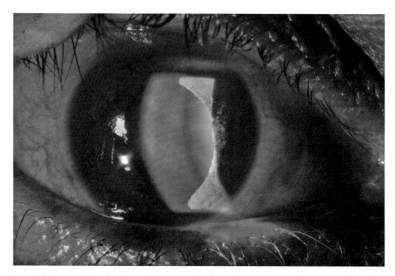

Fig. 11.7: Iris transillumination defects reflecting pigment loss from iris sphincter with consequent deposition on anterior chamber structures.

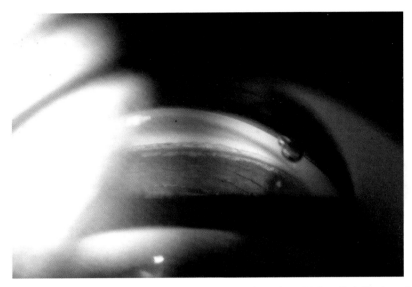

Fig. 11.8: Dense pigmentation of the trabecular meshwork and Schwalbe's line in exfoliation syndrome.

hypoperfusion, microneovascularization, reduced number of vessels associated with diffuse or patchy leakage of fluorescein, especially in the pupillary area. These observations account for atrophy of the iris musculature and rigid pupil resistant to dilatation, increased incidence of breakdown of blood aqueous barrier and inflammation following ocular surgery and incidence of iris new vessels and hyphema.

Pupil

Eyes with exfoliation dilate poorly. In unilateral, untreated exfoliation, the pupil in the involved eye is always observed to be smaller than the normal, uninvolved fellow eye. Histologic studies of the involved iris sphincter and dilator muscles[12] have revealed fibrotic, disorganized and degenerative muscle tissue. Pigment dispersion is also common and considerably profuse after dilatation. This pigment is released from the posterior pigment epithelium of the iris as the pupil dilates and is more common and marked in eyes with exfoliation[13] than in normal or in persons with POAG. Pigment in the anterior chamber is observed to be maximal at 1–2 h after mydriasis and lasts 12–24 h. Marked IOP rises can occur in these eyes after pharmacologic dilation with a positive correlation between the extent of IOP rise and the amount of pigment liberated. IOP rises usually reach a maximum after 2 h in eyes following pupillary dilatation. Ritch et al.[14] have observed that IOP may begin to rise only after 3–4 h after dilation. Since IOP is rarely measured at this hour, further possible glaucomatous damage in compromised eyes may occur. Postdilation IOPs should be checked routinely in all patients with exfoliation receiving mydriatics.

Cornea

Scattered or isolated deposits of exfoliation may be noticed on the corneal endothelium (Fig. 11.9) and is often mistaken for inflammatory precipitates. Diffuse, nonspecific pigmentation of the central endothelium, not amounting to typical Krukenberg spindle, is often seen. Decreased endothelial cell density with morphologic changes in shape and size of endothelial cells is noticed. Central corneal thickness is also increased[15] in eyes with exfoliation, reflecting corneal dysfunction. A true keratopathy[16] typical of exfoliation have been described, which predisposes these eyes to early corneal decompensation after uneventful cataract surgery or only with moderate elevation of IOP. The exfoliative keratopathy is characterized by diffuse and irregular thickening of Descemet's membrane, focal accumulation of exfoliation within or on the Descemet's membrane and melanin phagocytosis by the endothelial cells. Endotheliopathy of XFG significantly differs from Fuchs' endotheliopathy, aphakic or pseudophakic bullous keratopathy in that guttata are less in number and more diffusely distributed. In the tropical climates like India, there is a significant association of exfoliation with spheroidal degeneration and climatic droplet keratopathy.

Zonules and Ciliary Body

Exfoliation may be detected on the ciliary body and the zonules prior to observation on the anterior surface of the crystalline lens. Cycloscopy in patients with clinically unilateral exfoliation revealed exfoliative material on the ciliary processes and zonules of all the involved eyes and in approximately 80% of contralateral eyes,[17] without clinical evidence of exfoliation on the anterior segment. Abnormal zonular attachment from deposits of exfoliation may

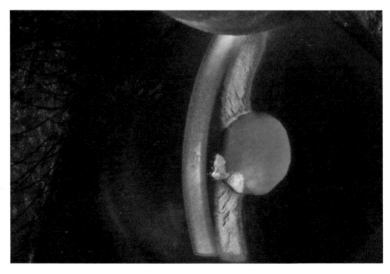

Fig. 11.9: Exfoliation on the endothelium.

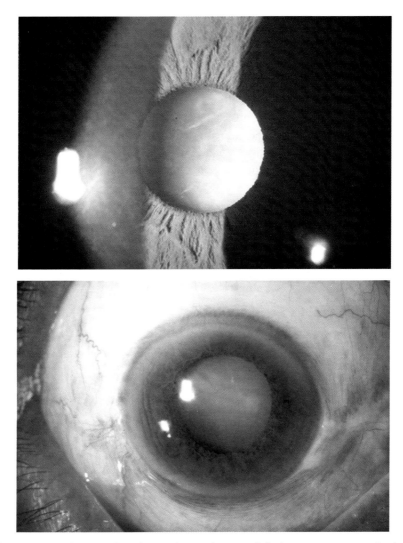

Figs. 11.10 and 11.11: Zonular weakness due to exfoliation can cause anterior lens subluxation, shallow chambers and phacodonesis. Exfoliation is often associated with pupillary block and angle-closure glaucoma.

account for increased incidence of lens subluxation (Figs. 11.10 and 11.11) and spontaneous dislocation (Fig. 11.12). Phacoemulsification in patients with exfoliation requires more skill since the zonules are fragile. Occasionally, the implanted IOL may be dislocated in the vitreous (Fig. 11.13) or may cause only a decentration of the intraocular lens in the pupillary axis.

Anterior Chamber Angle

Increased trabecular pigmentation is an early diagnostic sign in glaucoma and may precede the appearance of exfoliation on the anterior lens capsule or the

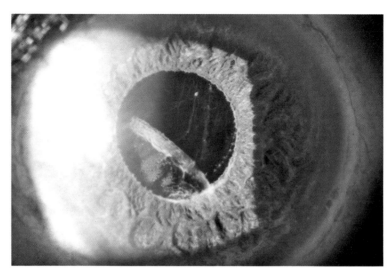

Fig. 11.12: Spontaneous dislocation of crystalline lens in exfoliation with deposits of exfoliative material on the vitreous and the lens capsule.

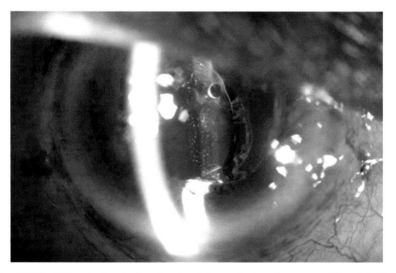

Fig. 11.13: Dislocated posterior chamber intraocular lens in an eye with exfoliation.

pupillary margin. The distribution tends to be patchy and less well defined. In unilateral exfoliation, trabecular pigmentation is more marked and denser in the involved eye (Fig. 11.8). Eyes with exfoliation and glaucoma have greater pigment deposition in the trabecular meshwork than in eyes with exfoliation without glaucoma. Exfoliative glaucoma also has greater pigment in the angle than POAG. There is a significant correlation between the magnitude of IOP elevation and the degree of trabecular pigmentation.[18] Severity of glaucoma is also related to the amount of exfoliation material present with in trabecular meshwork nearest to the Schlemm's canal (juxtacanalicular tissue). Pigment

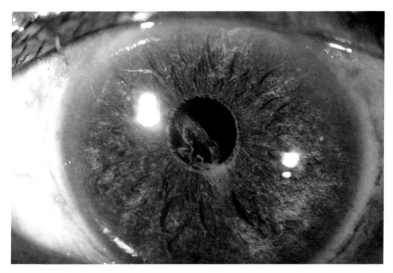

Fig. 11.14: Presence of exfoliative deposits on iris and lens capsule in aphakia.

is characteristically deposited on the Schwalbe's line or anteriorly (referred to as the Sampaolesi's line) and is an early sign of exfoliation. Occasionally flecks of exfoliation may be seen on posterior trabecular meshwork on gonioscopic evaluation.

Vitreous, Retina and Optic Disks

Exfoliation may be detected on the iris, vitreous, and posterior capsule (Fig. 11.14) following cataract surgery, proving incorrect the earlier hypothesis that crystalline lens was the source of exfoliation. Optic disk morphometric features in exfoliative eyes are not different than normal controls or eyes with POAG, although smaller disks may be found more frequently in eyes with XFG. Histologic and immunohistochemical studies of the lamina cribrosa in eyes with exfoliation have revealed extensive elastosis of the tissues comprising the lamina, which predisposes the optic nerve to typical glaucomatous damage even at lower IOP.

PATHOPHYSIOLOGY OF EXFOLIATION

Composition of Exfoliation Material

Exfoliation represents elastotic material arising from abnormal aggregation of elastic microfibril components. Immunohistochemical studies have shown exfoliation to represent a complex glycoprotein/proteoglycan structure. The characteristic fibrils are composed of microfibrillar subunits surrounded by an amorphous matrix comprising glycoconjugates. Amino-acid analysis of exfoliation[19] reveals a composition compatible with amyloid, noncollagen basement membrane components and elastic microfibrils. Recent studies with liquid chromatography coupled with mass spectrometry revealed that exfoliative material is composed of elastic microfibril components fibrillin 1, fibulin 2 and vitronectin, the proteoglycans syndecan and versican, clusterin and cross-linking enzyme lysyl oxidase and some proteins (Ovodento B, abstract presented in ARVO 2005). Differential gene expression analysis identified[20] more than 20 differentially expressed genes, mainly involved in extracellular matrix metabolism and in cellular stress. Several antioxidant defense enzymes and DNA repair proteins are down regulated in exfoliative tissues.

In summary the underlying pathophysiology of exfoliation seems to be associated with an excessive production of elastic microfibril components, enzyme cross-linking processes, over expression of TGF-1 (tissue growth factor-1), proteolytic imbalance between matrix metalloproteinase (MMP) and tissue inhibitor of metalloproteinases (TIMPs), low-grade inflammatory process, increased cellular and oxidative stress, and an impaired cellular stress response as reflected by downregulation of antoxidative enzymes and DNA repair proteins.

PATHOGENETIC FACTORS AND KEY MOLECULES AND THEIR ROLE IN EXFOLIATION PATHOPHYSIOLOGY

Aqueous humor studies in eyes with exfoliation showed increased concentration of growth factors,[21] a dysbalance of MMP and TIMP[22] (tissue inhibitor of MMP), an increase in oxidative stress markers (like 8-Isoprostaglandin F_2),[23] concomitant decrease in antioxidative protective factors such as ascorbic acid and an increase of vasoactive peptide,[24] Endothelin-1. The growth factor TGF-1, a major modulator for matrix formation in many fibrotic diseases, is a key moderator in fibrotic exfoliation process. It is markedly increased in aqueous humor of patients with exfoliation. TGF-1 is upregulated and synthesized by many anterior segment tissues, promotes exfoliation material formation in vitro and is known to regulate most genes differentially expressed in exfoliation tissues (e.g., Fibrillin-1, LTBP-1 and 2 and Clusterin).[25] Oxidative stress and hypoxia constitute major mechanisms involved in pathobiology of exfoliative syndrome. Decreased levels of ascorbic acid, the most effective free radical scavenger as well as increased levels of oxidative stress markers suggest faulty antioxidative process defense system.[26]

Exfoliative syndrome is also associated with ocular ischemia, especially iris hypoperfusion and anterior chamber hypoxia as well as reduced ocular and retrobulbar micro- and macrovascular blood flow.[27] Higher incidence of central retinal vein occlusion[28] is reported in patients with exfoliation. Increased levels of endothelin-1[29] (a potent vasoconstrictor) and decreased levels of nitric oxide[30] (a vasodilator) in the aqueous humor of patients with exfoliation play a key role in obliterative vasculopathy of the iris causing local ischemia. Increased homocysteine[31] levels in aqueous humor of patients with exfoliative syndrome further contribute to ischemic alterations such as endothelial dysfunction, oxidative stress, enhanced platelet aggregation, reduction of nitric oxide bioavailability, and abnormal perivascular matrix metabolism.

PATHOGENETIC CONCEPT OF EXFOLIATION SYNDROME

Immunohistochemical, biochemical and molecular biologic data provide strong support to the elastic microfibril[32] theory of pathogenesis, on the basis of histochemical similarities between exfoliation and zonular fibers and explain exfoliation as a type of elastosis affecting elastic microfibrils. Most recent evidence suggests exfoliation as a fibrillopathy. Fibrillin-1, a main component of elastic microfibrils and presumably of exfoliation fibrils as well, is a large glycoprotein with predominantly a cysteine component and a mosaic composition of several molecules like epidermal growth factor like motifs.

Current pathogenesis describes exfoliation as a specific type of stress-induced elastosis, an elastic microfibrillopathy, associated with excessive production of elastic microfibrils and their aggregation into typical, mature exfoliative fibrils by potentially elastogenic cells. Growth factors, especially TGF-1, increased cellular and oxidative stress, an impaired cellular protective system and stable aggregation of misfolded, stressed proteins appear to be involved in the fibrotic process. Due to imbalance between MMP and TIMP and extensive cross-linking processes involved in fiber formation, the pathologic material is not properly degraded, but progressively accumulates within tissues.

MECHANISMS OF DEVELOPMENT OF GLAUCOMA

Chronic Open-angle Glaucoma

The pathogenesis of elevated IOP in eyes with exfoliation remains controversial, although glaucoma with exfoliation is associated with increase in aqueous outflow resistance.[33] Aqueous outflow is reduced by 20% in eyes with XFG and in eyes with exfoliation without glaucoma; there was no significant variation in aqueous outflow in control eyes without exfoliation. Potential mechanisms of glaucoma in eyes with exfoliation include trabecular cell dysfunction, blockage of the trabecular meshwork by iris pigments and exfoliative material and coexisting POAG. Concomitant POAG appears unlikely since histological differences have been observed between eyes with these two major forms of glaucoma: there is a significant increase in juxtacanalicular plaque material and decrease in trabecular cellularity in eyes with POAG, while the plaque material concentration and trabecular cellularity in eyes with XFG is not significantly different from normal controls.

Obstruction of trabecular meshwork by pigments or exfoliation is generally accepted to be the cause of elevated IOP, although most patients with exfoliation do not develop elevated IOP or glaucoma. The presence of glaucoma, rise in IOP and optic nerve damage has been correlated with the amount of exfoliation observed histologically in juxtacanalicular tissue and other filtering portions of the anterior chamber angle.[34] In addition to mechanical obstruction of aqueous outflow pathways, active involvement of trabecular cells in the production of abnormal extracellular material and exfoliation has also been suggested as a contributing factor to outflow obstruction. Disorganization of juxtacanalicular tissue and Schlemm's canal has been observed in eyes with advanced glaucoma with exfoliation. In addition to these changes, immunohistochemistry has also revealed excessive deposition of albumin[35] in the trabecular meshwork of eyes with exfoliation which is likely to contribute to outflow obstruction.

Acute Elevation of IOP in Exfoliative Syndrome and Glaucoma

Patients with exfoliation and open-angle glaucoma may present with clinical features simulating acute angle-closure glaucoma with ciliary congestion, corneal edema and IOP exceeding 50 mm Hg.[36] Although a few of these may actually represent concomitant primary angle-closure glaucoma with classic pupillary block, or angle-closure glaucoma predisposed by exfoliation, a considerable number of eyes with acute glaucoma have open angles and is perhaps explained by pigment dispersion associated with pharmacological dilatation of pupils. A careful clinical examination with gonioscopy, and anterior segment imaging can differentiate between the exfoliation syndrome glaucoma and acute-angle closure glaucoma.

Angle-closure Glaucoma in Exfoliation

Associations between true angle-closure and exfoliation with glaucoma are not uncommon. Two series have reported a high incidence of narrow or occludable angles in eyes with exfoliation,[37,38] although some reports have mentioned exfoliation to be unusual or rare in angle-closure glaucoma. Ritch[39] had reported a third of patients with primary angle-closure glaucoma or occludable angles with evidence of exfoliation either clinically or on conjunctival biopsy. A number of characteristics in eyes with exfoliation predispose to angle-closure glaucoma. Pupillary block may be caused by a combination of posterior synechiae, increased iris thickness or rigidity, or anterior lens movement owing to zonular weakness or dialysis. Aqueous misdirection with angle-closure glaucoma following cataract or combined trabeculectomy and cataract surgery in eyes with open-angles and XFG have been observed in the authors' practice with an increased frequency as compared to POAG (unpublished data). Slackness of zonules cause forward shift in the position of the crystalline lens as soon as anterior chamber entry in eyes with exfoliation, predisposing to aqueous misdirection. Wound leak in the immediate postoperative phase can also increase risk of aqueous misdirection following filtering surgery, cataract extraction with or without intraocular lens implantation and combined glaucoma-cataract surgeries. Patients with exfoliation and occludable angles or angle-closure glaucoma tend to be more myopic,[40] reflecting cataract progression or a forward shift in the position of the crystalline lens contribution to narrow angles and angle closure.

Several characteristics in eyes with exfoliative syndrome predispose to angle-closure glaucoma. The iris pigment epithelium and the anterior lens surface, both coated with exfoliation, tend to adhere, especially when pupillary movement is inhibited by miotic therapy, a phenomenon referred to as iridocapsular block.[41] Development of posterior synechiae and angle-closure glaucoma is further stimulated by zonular weakness and forward movement of the lens. Owing to iridocapsular block at the pupil, aqueous pressure in the posterior chamber builds up, causing billowing of the iris at its weakest point, the iris root with consequent angle-closure glaucoma. Laser iridotomy can eliminate iridocapsular pupil block and prevent progressive angle-closure. Ciliary block glaucoma is precipitated in eyes with exfoliation following intraocular surgery, especially extracapsular cataract surgery with large incisions. Sudden collapse of the anterior chamber in these eyes after entering the anterior chamber causes forward shift in position of the crystalline lens and anterior vitreous, which contribute to cilio-lenticular-vitreal block and angle-closure glaucoma. Aqueous misdirection in these instances can be hastened or precipitated by poor wound apposition or wound leak in the postoperative phase. Since miotics like pilocarpine can cause forward shift of the lens aggravated by zonular laxity, miotic-induced angle-closure is more common in eyes with exfoliation as opposed to normal eyes.

Differential Diagnosis of Exfoliation Glaucoma

1. *Pigmentary glaucoma:* Pigmentary glaucoma is seen bilaterally at the time of presentation in young, myopic males most commonly in their third to fourth decade of life unlike XFG, which is unilateral, asymmetric, affecting elderly individuals after the age of 50 years. On gonioscopy, pigmentation of trabecular meshwork is patchy and segmental in XFG in contrast to diffuse dark brown or black pigmentation in pigmentary glaucoma. Iris transillumination defects also differ in these two situations: pigmentary glaucoma has elongated radial spokes in midperiphery of iris whereas XFG has moth eaten, patchy peripupillary transillumination defects often with some loss of pupillary ruff.

2. *True exfoliation or capsular delamination:* It is seen in glass blowers and people exposed to heat, trauma, irradiation or inflammation. A split occurs in anterior lens capsule without deposition of cross-linked polyethylene (PEX) material and the lens capsule has characteristic frosty appearance.

3. *Primary angle-closure glaucoma:* Eyes with exfoliation and angle-closure glaucoma tend to be myopic because of nuclear sclerosis and chambers

may appear deeper in the center. Eyes with primary angle-closure glaucoma tend to be hyperopic with convex iris configuration and features of classical pupillary block. Pupillary block and angle-closure in exfoliation is accentuated by zonular weakness and anterior lens movement and may be associated with diffusely shallow anterior chamber and lens tremulousness. The differentiation between primary angle-closure and angle-closure glaucoma due to exfoliation may be difficult to confirm clinically, although anterior segment imaging by optical coherence tomography (OCT) or ultrasonography may be of some significant assistance. Pupillary block in both conditions may be treated by laser iridotomy. Postdilatation IOP elevation in XFG is sometimes mistaken for acute angle-closure glaucoma, but gonioscopy reveals open iridocorneal angles.

4. *Inflammatory glaucoma:* Exfoliation glaucoma is occasionally characterized by small pupils and posterior synechiae especially if miotics are used to control elevated IOP. Pigmentation on the endothelium and exfoliative deposits may be mistaken for old keratic precipitates from past inflammation.

5. *Neovascular glaucoma:* Exfoliation is associated occasionally with iris neovascularization due to iris sector ischemia. Careful posterior segment evaluation reveals no primary retinal disease or retinal neovascularization.

MANAGEMENT

The sequential approach to management of glaucoma associated with exfoliation in general resembles that of POAG, although response to treatment is variable in individuals with XFG. The treatment includes beta-adrenergic antagonists, alpha-adrenergic agonists, miotics, carbonic anhydrase inhibitors, prostaglandin analogues, laser, and surgery.

Medical Therapy

Glaucoma associated with exfoliation in general tend to be less responsive to medical therapy with an increase in requirement for surgical option[37] more often than in POAG. Variable response to timolol has been reported in treatment of XFG and in spite of favorable initial reduction in IOP, eyes with XFG tended to have a sustained higher IOP and larger fluctuation in IOP as compared to POAG. Latanoprost has been studied to be effective in lowering IOP, and dorzolamide is as effective and additive to timolol in treatment of XFG. Prostaglandin analogs effectively reduce IOP in XFG by enhancing uveoscleral outflow. These drugs also decrease/antagonize growth factors like TGF-β1 and TIMP and favorably influence pathogenesis of exfoliation fibrils. Cholinergic agents like pilocarpine are effective and have been observed to have a greater additive effect with timolol in XFG than in primary-open angle glaucoma. Miotics seem to have multiple beneficial effects on lowering IOP in eyes with exfoliation. Apart from lowering IOP effectively by increasing trabecular out-flow of aqueous, they enable the trabecular meshwork to effectively clear the exfoliation and pigment clumps in the aqueous outflow pathways. Pigment liberation and further resistance to outflow facility is also reduced by miosis induced reduction in pupillary movement. Aqueous suppressants decrease aqueous inflow, and sluggish aqueous flow tends to increase the deposition of pigments and exfoliative material in the trabecular outflow pathways rather than their clearance. Suggestive evidence has been presented by Becker that long-term management of XFG with aqueous suppressants results in worsen-ing of glaucoma due to increase in trabecular dysfunction. In the light of these facts, miotics seem to be the first line of therapy in XFG. However, exfoliation is a disease of the aging and is often associated with nuclear sclerosis and senile cataracts and use of miotics may further worsen the vision. Long-term use of miotics results in posterior synechiae and worsening miosis, and renders subsequent cataract surgery difficult. It must be reemphasized that miotics in general increase posterior synechiae, causes smaller pupils, anterior lens movement with increased tendency for pupillary block or ciliary block glau-coma and worsening of angle-closure associated with exfoliation.

Laser Trabeculoplasty

Argon laser trabeculoplasty may particularly prove effective in XFG. The ini-tial IOP being higher than in POAG; the fall in IOP is likely to be greater fol-lowing argon laser trabeucloplasty in XFG.[41] The increased effectiveness of laser treatment in exfoliation is attributed to denser pigmentation observed in the trabecular meshwork of eyes with XFG. Initial laser trabeculoplasty controlled IOP better than treatment with pilocarpine in a 2-year prospective trial[42] though, there is, however, gradual reduction in effectiveness of laser treatment over time. Pretreatment with pilocarpine and apraclonidine may reduce postlaser IOP rise. Continued liberation of pigment following laser may result in late failure and increase in IOP, which can partly be counter-acted by treatment with miotics.

Laser Iridotomy

Laser iridotomy is indicated in eyes with angle-closure glaucoma and pupil-lary block mechanism. Angle-closure due to lens subluxation or anterior lens movement may not be relieved with laser iridotomy and may require supple-mentation with laser iridoplasty[43] to open the angles.

Surgery

Patients with XFG progress less after successful glaucoma filtering surgery than POAG, though surgical complications are reportedly more common. Markedly elevated IOP prior to surgery, if not adequately reduced preoperatively, may predispose to choroidal hemorrhage or effusions. Weakened zonular support with marked anterior lens movement during surgery predisposes to lens damage, vitreous loss, flat chamber and aqueous misdirection syndrome. Progression of cataracts following trabeculectomy is reportedly more common in XFG. Trabeculectomy tends to bypass the mechanical blockage in trabecular meshwork in XFG; it has also been reported to be effective in XFG, with 64% success rate with adjunctive medications at 5 years follow-up. Trabecular aspiration (with the objective of improvement in outflow facility) with or without phacoemulsification for concomitant cataracts also causes significant IOP lowering[44,45] with reduced need for glaucoma medications in eyes with exfoliation glaucoma, when compared to cataract extraction alone. Trabecular aspiration and cataract extraction, however, has been observed to be less efficacious than trabeculectomy combined with phacoemulsification[46] in IOP lowering.

REFERENCES

1. Ritch R. Exfoliation syndrome: the most common identifiable cause of open angle glaucoma. J Glaucoma. 1994;3(2):176-7.
2. Aasved H. Prevalence of fibrillopathia epitheliocapsularis (pseudoexfoliation) and capsular glaucoma. Trans Ophthalmol Soc UK. 1975;99(2): 293-5.
3. Forsius H. Exfoliation syndrome in various ethnic populations. Acta Ophthalmol. 1988;184(Suppl):71-85.
4. Krishnadas R, Praveen K, Nirmalan, et al. Pseudoexfoliation in a rural population of South India: The Aravind Comprehensive Eye Survey. Am J Ophthalmol. 2003;135(6):830-7.
5. Arvind H, Raju P, Paul PG. Pseudoexfoliaiton in South India. Br J Ophthalmol. 2003;87(11):1321-23.
6. Damji K. Is pseudoexfoliation syndrome inherited? A review of genetic and nongenetic factors and a new observation. Ophthal Genet. 1998;19(4): 175-85.
7. Thorlifesson G, Magnusson KP, Sulem P, et al. Common sequence variants in LOXL1 gene confer susceptibility to exfoliation glaucoma. Science. 2007; 317(5843):1397-400.
8. Kozart DM, Yanoff M. Intraocular pressure status in 100 consecutive patients with exfoliation syndrome. Ophthalmology. 1982;89(3):214-8.
9. Aasved H. Intraocular pressure in eyes with and without fibrillopathia epitheliocapsularis (senile exfoliation or pseudoexfoliation). Acta Ophthalmol (Copenh). 1971;49(4):601-10.
10. Henry JC, Krupin T, Schmitt M, et al. Long term follow up of pseudoexfoliation and the development of elevated intraocular pressure. Ophthalmology. 1987;94(5):545-52.
11. Prince AM, Ritch R. Clinical signs of the pseudoexfoliation syndrome. Ophthalmology. 1986;93(6):803-7.

12. Repo LP, Naukkarinen A, Paljarvi L, et al. Pseudoexfoliation syndrome with poorly dilating pupil (a light and electron microscopic study of the sphincter area). Graefes Arch Clin Exp Ophthalmol. 1996;234(3):171-6.

13. Krause U, Helve J, Forsius H. Pseudoexfoliation of the lens capsule and liberation of iris pigment. Acta Ophthalmol (Copenh). 1973;51(1): 39-46.

14. Ritch R, Schlötzer-Schrehardt U. Exfoliation syndrome. Surv Ophthalmol. 2001;45(4):265-315.

15. Puska P, Vasara K, Harju M, et al. Corneal thickness and corneal endothelium in normotensive subjects with unilateral exfoliation syndrome. Graefes Arch Clin Exp Ophthalmol. 2000;238(8):659-63.

16. Naumann GOH, Schlötzer-Schrehardt U. Keratopathy in pseudoexfoliation syndrome as a cause of corneal endothelial decompensation. A clinicopathologic study. Ophthalmology. 2000;107(6):1111-24.

17. Mizuno K, Muroi S. Cycloscopy of pseudoexfoliation. Am J Ophthalmol. 1979;87(4):513-8.

18. Moreno-Montañés J, Quinteiro Alonso A, Alvarez Serna A, et al. [Exfoliation syndrome: clinical study of the irido-corneal angle]. J Fr Ophtalmol. 1990;13(4): 183-8.

19. Ringvold A. A preliminary report on the amino acid composition of pseudo exfoliation material. Exp Eye Res. 1973;15(1):37-42.

20. Zentel M, Posch E, Von der Mark K, et al. Differential gene expression in pseudoexfoliation syndrome. Invest Ophthalmol Vis Sci. 2005;46(10): 3742-52.

21. Gartaganus SP, Georgapoulos CD, Exarchou AM, et al. Increased aqueous humor, basic fibroblast growth factor and hyaluronon levels in relation to exfoliation syndrome and exfoliation glaucoma. Acta Ophthalmol Scand. 2001;79(6):572-5.

22. Schlötzer-Schrehardt U, Lommatzsch J, Küchle M, et al. Matrix metalloproteinases and their inhibitors in aqueous humor of patients with pseudoexfoliation syndrome, pseudoexfoliation glaucoma, and primary open-angle glaucoma. Invest Ophthalmol Vis Sci. 2003;44(3):1117-25.

23. Koliakos GG, Konstas AGP, Schlötzer-Schrehardt U, et al. 8-Isoprostaglandin F2A and ascorbic acid concentration in the aqueous humor of patients with exfoliation syndrome. Br J Ophthalmol. 2003;87(3):353-6.

24. Koliakos GG, Konstas AGP, Schlötzer-Schrehardt U, et al. Endothelin-1 concentration is increased in the aqueous humor of patients with exfoliation syndrome. Br J Ophthalmol. 2004;88(4):523-7.

25. Schlötzer-Schrehardt U, Zenkel M, Küchle M, et al. Role of transforming growth factor-1 and its latent form binding protein in pseudoexfoliation syndrome. Exp Eye Res. 2001;73(6):765-80.

26. Koliakos GG, Konstas AGP, Schlötzer-Schrehardt U, et al. 8-Isoprostaglandin F2A and ascorbic acid concentration in the aqueous humor of patients with exfoliation syndrome. Br J Ophthalmol. 2003;87(3): 353-6.

27. Yüksel N, Karabas VL, Arslan A, et al. Ocular hemodynamics in pseudoexfoliation syndrome and pseudoexfoliation glaucoma. Ophthalmology. 2001; 108(6):1043-9.

28. Gillies WE, Brooks AM. Central retinal vein occlusion in pseudoexfoliation of the lens capsule. Clin Exp Ophthalmol. 2002;30(3):176-87.

29. Koliakos GG, Konstas AGP, Schlötzer-Schrehardt U, et al. Endothelin-1 concentration is increased in the aqueous humor of patients with exfoliation syndrome. Br J Ophthalmol. 2004;88(4):523-7.

30. Kotikoski H, Moilanen E, Vapaatalo H, et al. Biochemical markers of the L-arginine-nitric oxide pathway in the aqueous humor in glaucoma patients. Acta Ophthalmol Scand. 2002;80(2):191-5.

31. Bleich S, Roedl J, von Ahsen N, et al. Elevated homocysteine levels in aqueous humor of patients with pseudoexfoliation glaucoma. Am J Ophthalmol. 2004;138(1):162-4.

32. Streeten BW, Gibson SA, Dark AJ. Pseudoexfoliative material contains an elastic microfibrillar-associated glycoprotein. Trans Am Ophthalmol Soc. 1986; 84:304-20.

33. Johnson DH, Brubaker RF. Dynamics of aqueous humor in the syndrome of exfoliation with glaucoma. Am J Ophthalmol. 1982;93(5):629-34.

34. Gottanka J, Flügel-Koch C, Martus P, et al. Correlation of pseudoexfoliation material and optic nerve damage in pseudoexfoliation syndrome. Invest Ophthalmol Vis Sci. 1997;38(12):2435-46.

35. Schlötzer-Schrehardt U, Küchle M, Naumann GOH. Mechanisms of glaucoma development in pseudoexfoliation syndrome. In: Gramer E, Grehn F (Eds). Pathogenesis and Risk Factors of Glaucoma. Heidleberg: Springer; 1999. pp. 34-49.

36. Brooks AM, Gillies WE. The presentation and prognosis of glaucoma in pseudoexfoliation of the lens capsule. Ophthalmology. 1988;95(2):271-6.

37. Layden WE, Shaffer RN. Exfoliation syndrome. Am J Ophthalmol. 1974; 78(5):835-41.

38. Wishart PK, Spaeth GL, Poryzees EM. Anterior chamber angle in the exfoliation syndrome. Br J Ophthalmol. 1985;69(2):103-7.

39. Ritch R. Exfoliation syndrome and occludable angles. Trans Am Ophthalmol Soc. 1994;92:845-944.

40. Bartholomew RS. Pseudoexfoliation and angle-closure glaucoma. Glaucoma. 1981;3:213-6.

41. Tuulonen A, Airaksinen PJ. Laser trabeculoplasty in simple and capsular glaucoma. Acta Ophthalmol (Copenh). 1983;61(6):1009-15.

42. Bergeå B, Bodin L, Svedbergh B. Primary ALT vs pilocarpine. Acta Ophthalmol (Copenh). 1995;73(3):216-21.

43. Ritch R. Techniques of Argon Laser Iridectomy and Iridoplasty. Palo Alto, CA: Coherent Medical Press; 1983.

44. Jacobi PC, Dietlein TS, Krieglstein GK. Comparative study of trabecular aspiration versus trabeculectomy in glaucoma triple procedure to treat pseudoexfoliation glaucoma. Arch Ophthalmol. 1999;117(10):1311-8.

45. Georgopoulos GT, Chalkiadakis J, Livir-Rallatos G, et al. Combined clear cornea phacoemulsification and trabecular aspiration in the treatment of pseudoexfoliative glaucoma associated with cataract. Graefes Arch Clin Exp Ophthalmol 2000;238(10):816-21.
46. Jacobi PC, Dietlein TS, Krieglstein GK. The risk profile of trabecular aspiration versus trabeculectomy in glaucoma triple procedure. Graefes Arch Clin Exp Ophthalmol. 2000;238(7):545-51.

12

Traumatic Glaucoma

Moorthy LP, Ramakrishnan R

INTRODUCTION

Traumatic glaucoma is a secondary glaucoma that occurs as a consequence to an injury to the globe. Ocular trauma is a leading cause of morbidity with early and late onset complications that eventually affect the final visual outcome. Traumatic glaucoma is a condition in which there is raised intraocular pressure (IOP) as a result of ocular trauma; eventual optic neuropathy may likely develop in the long term if IOP is not controlled. Glaucoma associated with trauma is a multifactorial disease process. It usually occurs following a blunt injury that causes anterior segment deformation during the impact. It can also occur following penetrating injuries. Transient or prolonged elevations in IOP and damage to trabecular meshwork (TM) and other structures predispose traumatized eyes to the development of glaucomatous optic nerve atrophy. Also the treatment to trauma—like steroid therapy or scleral buckling can cause increase in IOP.

Patients with ocular trauma must be counseled for lifelong risk of glaucoma. Close follow-up is recommended with specific attention paid to any early signs of glaucomatous changes in the injured eye.

PREVALENCE AWND INCIDENCE

Most ocular trauma patients are young, with an average age less than 30 years. Trauma is an important cause of ocular morbidity among children. Two peak incidences of traumatic glaucoma have been reported; one is within a year and another at least 10 years posttrauma. The lifetime prevalence of ocular trauma is estimated to be 19.8%.[1] Children represent 27–48% of total number of patients affected; males are more susceptible with the ratio being 3.4:1.

About 3.4% cases develop raised IOP within 6 months after ocular trauma and this percentage increases to 10% within 10 years.

The incidence of traumatic hyphema is 17 per 100,000 people. About 30–94% of these patients have angle recession[2,3] and 20–30% of the reported patients had IOP more than 21 mm Hg. A 10 years prospective study of 31 patients with traumatic glaucoma and angle recession revealed a 9% incidence of traumatic glaucoma with 6% of the cases being late onset.[3] Late-onset glaucoma from blunt trauma ranges from 1.3% to 20% in other studies.

A gross impairment of vision, hyphema, elevated mean IOP at presentation, angle recession > 180°, lenticular subluxation/dislocation and heavily pigmented TM are considered significant risk factors. On other hand, presence of a cyclodialysis cleft has been seen to be a protective mechanism.[4] Occupational injuries are more likely to be of penetrating mechanism when compared to blunt rupture in non-work related open globe injury.[5]

MECHANISM OF GLAUCOMA FOLLOWING TRAUMA

1. Glaucoma following blunt injury
    - Early onset
        - Iritis
        - Hyphema
        - Traumatic lens subluxation or dislocation
        - Traumatic intumescence of lens
    - Delayed onset
        - Angle recession
        - Ghost cell glaucoma
2. Glaucoma following penetrating injury
    - Epithelial/stromal down growth
    - Siderosis
    - Peripheral anterior synechiae (PAS)
3. Chemical injury
4. Glaucoma following ocular surgery
    - Cataract surgery
    - Penetrating keratoplasty
    - Vitreoretinal procedures

PATHOGENESIS OF CLOSED GLOBE INJURY

The closed globe injuries are more likely to be affected by long term sequelae because blunt trauma initially compresses the globe in an antero-posterior axis, resulting in a distortion of anterior segment anatomy. At initial impact of an object to the eye, the cornea and anterior sclera are rapidly displaced posteriorly with a compensatory expansion at the equator of the eye. The expansion causes tears in various parts of anterior segment that are affected by hemorrhage, inflammation and scarring and referred to as seven anterior rings of tissue by Campbell.[6,7]

1. Iris sphincter tear—causing traumatic mydriasis
2. Iridodialysis—tear at the iris base
3. Angle recession—tear of anterior ciliary body
4. Cyclodialysis—tear at the attachment of ciliary body with scleral spur
5. Trabecular meshwork tear
6. Zonulodialysis—tear of the zonules
7. Retinal dialysis—detachment of the retina at the ora serrata

EARLY-ONSET GLAUCOMA

Acute rise in IOP without hemorrhage may occur because of the presence of inflammatory cells and pigment in the anterior chamber (AC), which clog the TM. Iritis/iridocyclitis occurring soon after trauma leads to low IOP due to decreased aqueous production: hypotony phase. There is leakage of proteins and cells due to vascular permeability accompanied by osmotic influx of water leading to increased IOP. The cellular debris, hemorrhage, platelets, ghost cells, fibrous growth or scar tissue also block the TM.

Other causes of raised IOP following blunt trauma are the following:

- Blockage of the angle by vitreous, iris, free lens matter or macrophages from phacolysis
- Secondary angle closure may occur with subluxation or dislocation of lens causing pupillary block
- Angle recession or edema of iris root with formation of PAS
- Trabecular damage
- Choroidal hemorrhage

LATE-ONSET GLAUCOMA

The causes of late onset glaucoma are the following.

- Angle recession
- Peripheral anterior synechiae
- Ghost cell glaucoma
- Lens-induced glaucoma
- Intumescent cataract
- Phaco-antigenic uveitis. Lens particle glaucoma (retained lens fragments)

Symptoms

In case of an acute rise in IOP, patient complains of headache, nausea, blurring of vision or photophobia whereas in late-onset glaucoma due to gradual rise in IOP, the patient is usually asymptomatic. Therefore, a detailed history of events should be taken.

Signs

- *Hyphema:* Blood in the AC (Fig. 12.1) results from torn anterior ciliary or iris stromal arteries. It is described later.
- *Rebleeding:* Obvious or subtle rebleeding appears as bright red blood layered over the old blood. This is easily confused with the bright red color of dissolving clot at the periphery. Rebleeding is associated with a poor prognosis related to the increased risk of IOP rise and corneal blood staining.[8]
- *Microhyphema:* Circulating pigmented red blood cells should be differentiated from inflammatory cells because of the 7% rebleeding rate noted in children with no frank hyphema.[9]
- *Vossius ring:* Presence of pigments on the anterior lens capsule indicates impression of the pupillary margin onto the anterior capsule during blunt trauma (Fig. 12.2).
- *Sphincter tears:* Fine radial tears at the pupillary margin or sphincter dysfunction with traumatic mydriasis are not rare (Fig. 12.3).
- *Iridodialysis:* A tear at the iris base is seen as a separation of the iris at the limbus exposing zonular fibers below.
- *Anterior displaced lens:* It causes a relative pupillary block and narrow angle.
- *Cyclodialysis cleft:* The internal scleral wall is seen because the ciliary body is torn from the scleral spur. Intraocular pressure may be low. Cyclodialysis cleft usually affects less than 90° of the angle (Fig. 12.4).

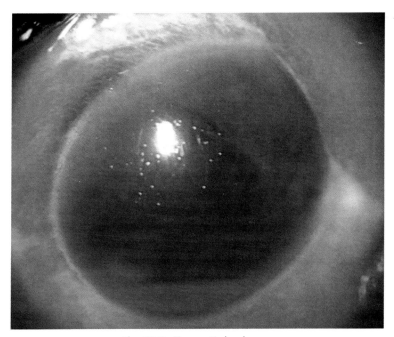

Fig. 12.1: Traumatic hyphema.

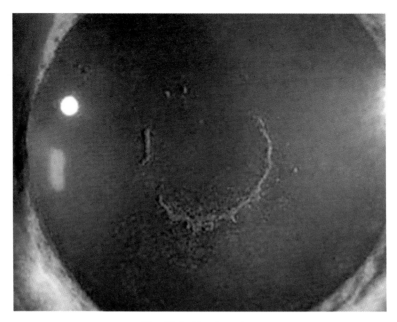

Fig. 12.2: Vossious ring.

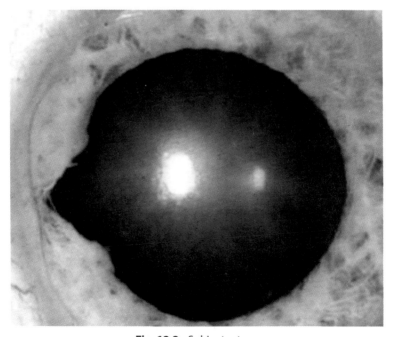

Fig. 12.3: Sphincter tear.

- *Angle recession:* A tear between the longitudinal and circular muscles of the ciliary body causes angle recession.
- *Trabecular meshwork damage:* These findings are subtle. Torn iris processes at the angle, prominent white scleral spur, and the glistening back

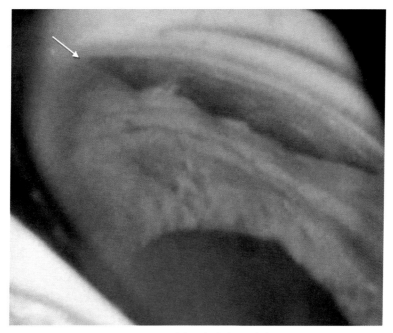

Fig. 12.4: Old cyclodialysis cleft.

wall of the canal may be apparent if the tear extends through the corneo-scleral meshwork.[7] In addition debris, pigment, PAS and blood can be present in the angle.

TRAUMATIC IRITIS/IRIDOCYCLITIS

Iridocyclitis occurring immediately following trauma leads to low IOP (hypotony phase). Later the IOP is increased (hypertony phase). The IOP elevation is mild and can be easily controlled.[10] Recommended treatment for traumatic iridocyclitis includes cycloplegia and topical steroids. These alone can reduce IOP to acceptable range. If hypotensive agents are used, β-blockers and carbonic anhydrase inhibitors (CAIs) are usually the first choice. Prostaglandin analogs and pilocarpine are usually avoided as they can exacerbate inflammation and risk for posterior synechiae.

HYPHEMA

The anterior segment is the most commonly injured after ocular trauma, with hyphema being the most frequent complication. Bleeding from the highly vascularized ciliary body and iris leads to a hyphema. It eventually stops due to acute rise in IOP, vasospasm of the ciliary body vessels and clot formation. Clot lysis and retraction occurs usually 2–5 days after the trauma when there is maximal risk of rebleeding. The rebleed is often more severe than the initial episode and can lead to total hyphema (Fig. 12.5). Usually total hyphema is

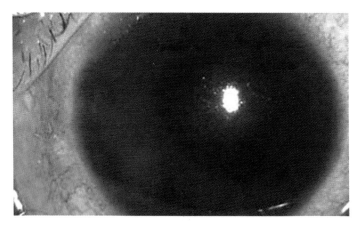

Fig. 12.5: Total hyphema.

associated with sudden visual loss, high IOP, severe pain and nausea as well as other symptoms of acute glaucoma. The mechanism for the rise of IOP is mechanical obstruction of the TM by red blood cells and sometimes pupillary block from clot.

If hyphema persists longer (more than a week), there is a risk of damage to the trabecular meshwork, uveitis and possible rebleeding. The hyphema can be graded by the volume of the AC filled with blood after layering of the red blood cells. They may also be graded on the basis of actual height in millimeter of blood layering in the AC. An evidence of suspended red blood cells on slit-lamp examination in a small AC without layering is termed as microcopic hyphema.

Grading of Hyphema

Grade 1: Less than one-third of the AC
Grade 2: One-third to one-half of the AC
Grade 3: One-half to nearly total
Grade 4: Total ('eight ball')

Two subgroups of hyphema patients warrant special attention: sickle cell patients and those with rebleed. The rate of rebleed after a traumatic hyphema has been variably reported at anywhere from 3.5 to 3.8%.[11] Rebleed is usually more severe and more damaging than initial hyphema. Sickle cell patients are not only at higher risk for rebleed but also more likely to develop glaucomatous nerve damage even with moderate IOP elevations.[12] Hyphema patients need to be followed daily for 3–5 days to monitor for rebleed and for IOP check-up. Eye rest and shielding throughout this period is important. IOP more than 25 mm Hg should always be treated. Surgical washout of AC is usually reserved for cases with elevated IOP uncontrolled by medical therapy or evidence of corneal blood staining.

A careful gonioscopic examination of both eyes is typically performed 3-6 weeks after injury to see changes of angle recession.[13] Baseline visual fields and disk photographs should be obtained.

LENS-INDUCED GLAUCOMA

The lens-induced glaucomas are a group of secondary glaucomas that share the lens as a common pathogenic cause. Traumatic changes to the integrity or position of the lens may result in glaucoma through several distinct mechanisms. Lens subluxation and phacomorphic glaucoma lead to secondary angle-closure, whereas phacolytic, lens particle and lens-induced uveitic glaucomas present secondary open angle mechanism.

Lens Dislocation

The lens may be dislocated or subluxated as a direct result of trauma that disrupts the zonules (Figs. 12.6A and B). Once mobilized, the lens may advance forward, producing pupillary block with angle closure. With a complete dislocation of the lens posteriorly, the pupil may become blocked with vitreous, which can also produce a pupillary block angle-closure glaucoma.

Phacomorphic Glaucoma

Occasionally, a cataractous lens following trauma becomes intumescent. Subsequently, swollen lenses can cause angle-closure glaucoma as a result of pupillary block or direct angle compromise by mass effect.

Phacolytic Glaucoma

Phacolytic glaucoma is seen in the setting of a hypermature cataract. Open-angle glaucoma occurs as a result of leakage of high-molecular-weight proteins through an intact lens capsule. These high-molecular-weight proteins are engulfed by macrophages and together they obstruct the TM.[14]

Lens Particle Glaucoma

Lens particle glaucoma is characterized by the presence of a frankly disrupted lens capsule following trauma with obvious fragments of lens material in the AC causing phacoanaphylactic uveitis, leading to uveitic glaucoma. This inflam-

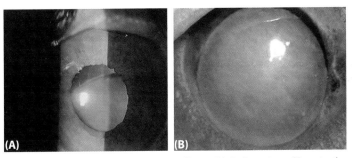

Figs. 12.6A and B: (A) Subluxation of lens. (B) Dislocation of lens in the anterior chamber.

mation can also cause PAS closing the angle. Relative pupil block can occur with posterior synechiae, anterior subluxated lens or traumatic lens swelling.[15]

ANGLE RECESSION

Blunt trauma causes shearing forces upon the globe with tearing of angle structures, the commonest being recession of the angle (Fig. 12.7),[16] one of the most devastating form of trauma related glaucoma. On gonioscopy, a wide dark ciliary body band is seen, which may not be uniform across the entire angle. Always compare with the other normal eye. Angle recession seen by gonioscopy is not responsible for outflow obstruction but it is a visible marker of invisible damage sustained by TM. Usually the IOP rises a few months after the initial injury. The AC is deep or of irregular depth. Sphincter tears at the pupillary margin, rosette-shaped cataract (Fig. 12.8), TM pigmentation, iridodialysis, sometimes dark-clotted blood in the angle on gonioscopy indicate trauma in the past.

Usually 5–20% of cases of ocular trauma may develop glaucoma.[17] Patients who have 180° or more angle recession have more chances of glaucoma.[18] Up to 50% will eventually develop glaucoma in fellow eye, which suggests that these patients have a predisposition to glaucoma and that trauma can predispose to the initiation of the cascade of glaucomatous damage. Angle recession is reported to occur in 60–90% cases of traumatic hyphema.

Initial treatment of angle recession glaucoma is medical. If it fails, filtering surgery is recommended. Trabeculectomy with antimetabolites results in the greatest reduction of IOP and fewest postoperative glaucoma medications. Laser trabeculoplasty tends to be relatively ineffective.[19] Cyclodestructive procedures are reserved for patients with limited visual potential but can offer effective and long lasting IOP control in refractory cases.

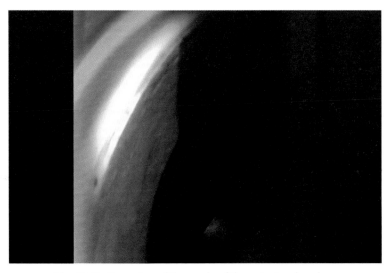

Fig. 12.7: Recession of the angle of the anterior chamber.

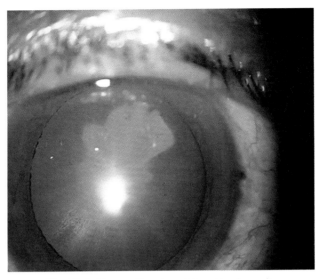

Fig. 12.8: Traumatic cataract (rosette-shaped).

GHOST CELL GLAUCOMA

Fresh red blood cells present in hyphema are pliable and percolate through TM but not the degenerated ghost cell erythrocytes. These cells are rigid, khaki colored over the course of several weeks can raise IOP, obstructing the meshwork.[20] It occurs 2–3 weeks after vitreous hemorrhage with rupture of the anterior hyaloid face. The ghost cells are seen wandering freely in the AC or as a tan stripe against a back ground of red cells, giving so-called candy stripe sign.

Diagnosis is made by microscopic examination of an AC specimen.[21] On light-microscopy, the ghost cells appear as rigid spheres with small dense adherent spots on their surface called 'Heinz bodies'. Medical treatment mostly is sufficient to control IOP. Certain cases where IOP is not adequately controlled by medical therapy may require AC wash or vitrectomy procedures to aid in pressure control.

GLAUCOMA FOLLOWING PENETRATING INJURY

Any penetrating injury can initiate inflammation that eventually leads to uveitic glaucoma. Mechanisms associated with blunt trauma such as hyphema, angle recession and ghost cell glaucoma can also coexist. Thus, inflammation should be carefully controlled; cycloplegia is usually recommended during acute postinjury phase. Long-term use of corticosteroids is common and can lead to elevated IOP. The rise in IOP tends to occur 2–3 weeks after initiation of therapy and is dose-dependent.[22] Even after cessation of steroid treatment patients require lifelong IOP control due to irreversible changes in the TM.

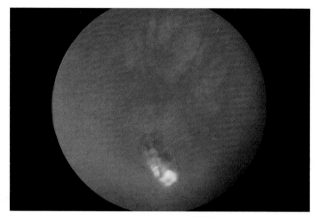

Fig. 12.9: Retained IOFB.

Retained Intraocular Foreign Body

Penetrating trauma will always be associated with a high degree of suspicion of retained intraocular foreign body (RIOFB; Fig. 12.9). Approximately, 40% of patients with open-globe injuries retain intraocular foreign body.[23] All patients with open-globe injury should undergo radiological imaging to confirm RIOFB. Glaucoma may develop due to the complication of RIOFB. Iron and copper foreign bodies are most likely to cause damage due to toxic discharge. Iron released will clog and damage the TM. Iron is toxic to the epithelial tissues of the eye. Excess iron either from retained foreign body or from chronic intraocular hemorrhage (hemosiderosis) can lead to a pattern of tissue damage in the eye termed *siderosis*. Copper is oxidized within the eye and will damage the TM.

Clinical findings of the retained IOFB include iris heterochromia with darkening of iris in the affected eye, a dilated and poorly reactive pupil, rust-like deposits on the corneal endothelium and anterior lens surface, optic nerve head edema, raised IOP and pigmentary retinopathy. Degenerative changes in TM include sclerosis and loss of intertrabecular spaces. Any eye with retained metallic foreign body or long-standing intraocular hemorrhage must be followed closely for glaucoma and record electroretinogram changes.[24]

Management of all foreign bodies is prompt removal, except in some cases of encapsulated RIOFB, which is difficult to extract. Visual prognosis is also limited due to retinal toxicity of the metallic foreign bodies. Treatment should be administered with steroids and cycloplegics to avoid cyclitic membranes and antibiotics to prevent endophthalmitis. Raised IOP is controlled medically.

CHEMICAL INJURIES

Both acid and alkali burns can acutely raise the IOP. Alkali agents penetrate into the AC within seconds, causing severe anatomical deformity.

Prostaglandin is released and causes an acute rise in IOP. If there is severe ciliary body damage, hypotony will follow permanently. Usually there is rise in IOP due to inflammatory reaction. After a period of months, there is intense scarring, leading to irreversible trabecular damage as well as formation of PAS (Fig. 12.10). The mechanism is poorly understood and thought to be due to contraction of anterior tissues of the eye.[25] Topical steroids and aqueous suppressants can be helpful in managing the pressure. Cases that progress to sterile corneal ulceration typically have most extensive anterior segment damage (Fig. 12.11) and more likely to develop glaucoma and eventful phthisis.[26]

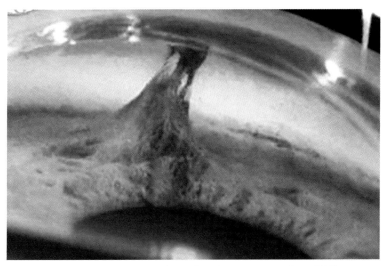

Fig. 12.10: Formation of Peripheral anterior synechiae (PAS).

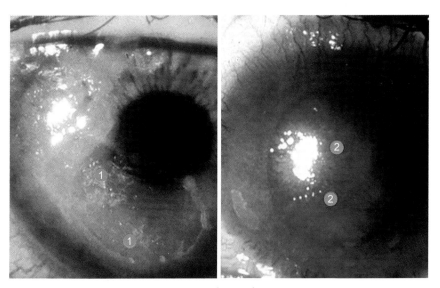

Fig. 12.11: Chemical injury.

ORBITAL INJURIES

Orbital disorders, particularly carotid cavernous fistulas, and embolization treatments have been associated with acute rise in IOP. The mechanism involves venous thrombosis and stasis, concomitant exudative retinal detachment and choroidal detachment, intraorbital engorgement, raised episcleral venous pressure and blood in Schlemm's canal on gonioscopy. Embolization results in increased superior ophthalmic venous pressure, choroidal transudation, anterior displacement of the iris-lens diaphragm and nonpupillary block glaucoma.

GLAUCOMA FOLLOWING OCULAR SURGERY

Glaucoma can develop in the postoperative period in following conditions:
- Malignant glaucoma (aqueous misdirection syndrome)
- Glaucoma in aphakia and pseudophakia
- Glaucoma following penetrating keratoplasty
- Glaucoma following vitreoretinal surgery

The diagnosis of traumatic glaucoma is mainly clinical and includes a detailed history of the mechanism of injury, slit-lamp examination, IOP measurements, gonioscopy, optic nerve head and nerve fiber analysis. Most importantly, patients with a history of blunt trauma (especially in those with documented angle recession or hyphema) should have yearly examination for life to look for any development of late-onset glaucoma.

Black patients have as 8% risk for sickle cell and in the presence of hyphema, they produce sickled cells that may not easily pass through the TM and lead to rapid increases in IOP. Laboratory tests in patients with a history of a bleeding disorder should also be considered: platelet counts, liver function tests, prothrombin time and partial thromboplastin time.[9]

MANAGEMENT

Treatment of traumatic glaucoma involves lowering IOP or precluding its rise to prevent optic nerve damage. It depends on the cause of the unstable IOP and the amount of time after the traumatic event.

Medical Management

Usually, the increase in IOP is usually caused by blockage of the angle with hyphema, debris, and inflammatory cells. Because these patients are usually young, they can tolerate acute increase in IOP without nerve damage. Therefore, most ophthalmologists advocate treatment with aqueous suppressants such as beta-blockers, alpha-2 agonists and CAIs when IOP is more than 30 mm Hg. CAIs should not be used in patients with sickle-cell disease or trait. Parasympathomimetics and prostaglandin analogs are associated with increased inflammation and should be avoided. Topical steroid should also be used for up to 6 weeks to decrease inflammation and cellular infiltration of the damaged angle.

Rebleeding

Rebleeding in the acute phase (usually in the first 2–5 days after trauma) increases IOP. Use of anticoagulants or nonsteroidal anti-inflammatory drugs such as aspirin, and heavy physical activities should be avoided. The head of the patient is elevated 30°, and an eye shield is used for all times. Hospital admission is recommended for hyperactive children with a large hyphema, high IOP and sickle cell disease.

Antifibrinolytic agents: Tranexamic acid and aminocaproic acid have been shown in numerous studies to significantly reduce the incidence of rebleeding by stabilizing the fibrin clot. More recent studies do not show an improvement in visual outcome and thus these drugs have fallen out of favor. The patients have to be monitored closely for the many side effects of these drugs such as dizziness, hypotension, and vomiting. They are contraindicated in patients with renal or hepatic insufficiency or hemophilia.

Topical and oral steroids commonly used in eye trauma, also help to prevent rebleeding by inhibiting fibrinolysis and stabilizing the blood ocular barrier.[8] If rebleeding occurs, an IOP check will help evaluate further treatment options, which may include the use of an antifibrinolytic drug.

Surgical Management

Indications for surgical intervention are:
- Intraocular pressure >50 mm Hg for 5 days
- Intraocular pressure >30 mm Hg for 7 days
- Total hyphema unresolved for 10 days on maximal medical therapy
- Early signs of corneal blood staining

Surgical intervention is done to decrease the rate of optic nerve damage, PAS formation and corneal blood staining. Patients with sickle cell and IOP more than 30 mm Hg (for more than 24 h)[8] and AC washout should be considered.

Hyphema

Different techniques for hyphema evacuation include the following:
- Creating two paracentesis incisions with saline irrigation through one incision and a depression of the posterior lip of the second paracentesis for a thorough AC washout.
- Clot expression and limbal delivery. Eight-ball hyphema can be removed by the conventional limbal clot delivery method.

- Bimanual cutting/aspiration of clotted blood using the vitrectomy probe. Occasionally, a larger organized hyphema will require a vitrector. Vitrectomy will actually debulk the clot without shearing the anatomical structures and causing a rebleed. Anterior chamber stability is important and hypotony should be prevented otherwise a rebleed can occur. In case there is a bleed, inject viscoelastic to tamponade the AC.

Late-onset Glaucoma

Numerous studies report different treatment options for late-onset glaucoma. Many patients may need lifelong treatment with topical medications. In those refractory to medical therapy, argon laser trabeculoplasty and trabeculectomy without antimetabolite have shown failure.[23] This may be due to increased fibroblast proliferation in younger patients or a change in their aqueous humor after trauma. The use of mitomycin C or 5-fluorouracil has decreased the rate of trabeculectomy failure. Also, glaucoma drainage implants (except Molteno implants) in eyes with past failed filtering procedures have been shown to control IOP.[7,27]

SUMMARY

Both open and closed globe injuries can cause elevated IOP and glaucoma due to a number of mechanisms. In most cases, the rise in IOP is temporary and can be effectively managed with topical medication. In the more severe cases, surgical intervention is often necessary. Despite the presence of normal IOP, patients with severe ocular injury should understand that their lifetime risk of glaucoma is increased and they therefore require regular periodic monitoring of IOP on long-term basis for preservation of vision.

REFERENCES

1. Wong T, Klein B, Klein R. The prevalence and 5-year incidence of ocular trauma—The Beaver Dam Eye Study. Ophthalmology. 2000;107(12): 2196-202.
2. Sihota R, Sood NN, Agarwal HC. Traumatic glaucoma. Acta Ophthalmol Scand. 1995;73(3):252-4.
3. Kaufman JH, Tolpin DW. Glaucoma after traumatic angle recession. A ten-year prospective study. Am J Ophthalmol. 1974:78(4):648-54.
4. Macewen CJ. Eye injuries: a prospective survey of 5671 cases. Br J Ophthalmol. 1989;73(11):888-94.
5. Canavan YM, Archer DB. Anterior segment consequences of blunt ocular injury. Br J Ophthalmol. 1982;66(9):549-55.
6. Campbell, DG. Traumatic glaucoma. In: Shingleton BG, Hersh PS, Kenyon KR (Eds). Eye Trauma. St. Louis, MO: Mosby Year Book; 1991. pp. 117-25.

7. Chi TS, Netland PA. Angle-recession glaucoma. Int Ophthalmol Clin. 1995; 35:117-24.

8. Walton W, Von Hagen S, Grigorian R, et al. Management of traumatic hyphema. Surv Ophthalmol. 2002;47(4):297-334.

9. Shingleton BJ, Hersh PS. Traumatic hyphema. In: Shingleton BG, Hersh PS, Kenyon KR (Eds). Eye Trauma. St. Louis, MO: Mosby Year Book; 1991. Wp. 107.

10. De Leon-Ortega JE, Girkin C. Ocular trauma-related glaucoma. Ophthalmol Clin N Am. 2002;15(2):215-23.

11. Volpe NJ, Larrison WI, Hersh PS, et al. Secondary hemorrhage in traumatic hyphema. Am J Ophthalmol. 1991;112(5):507-13.

12. Goldberg MF. Sickled erythrocytes, hyphema, and secondary glaucoma: I. The diagnosis and treatment of sickled erythrocytes in human hyphemas. Ophthal Surg. 1979;10(4):17-31.

13. Filipe JA, Barros H, Castro-Correia J. Sports-related ocular injuries: a three year follow up study. Ophthalmology. 1997;104:313-8.

14. Zimmerman LE. Lens induced inflammation in human eyes. In: Maumenee AE, Silverstein AM (Eds). Immunopathology of Uveitis. Baltimore, MD: Williams & Wilkins; 1964. pp. 221-32.

15. Irvin JA, Smith RE. Lens injuries. In: Shingleton BG, Hersh PS, Kenyon KR (Eds). Eye Trauma. St. Louis, MO: Mosby Year Book; 1991. pp.127-8.

16. Sihota R, Kumar S, Gupta V, et al. Early predictors of traumatic glaucoma after closed globe injury—trabecular pigmentation, widened angles and a higher baseline intra ocular pressure. Arch Ophthalmol. 2008:126(7);921-6.

17. Salmon JF, Mermoud A, Ivey A, et al. The detection of post-traumatic angle recession by gonioscopy in a population-based glaucoma survey. Ophthalmology. 1994;101(11):1844-50.

18. Alper M. Contusion angle deformity and glaucoma. Arch Ophthalmol. 1963; 69:77-89.

19. Goldberg I. Argon laser trabeculoplasty and the open angle glaucomas. Aust N Z J Ophthalmol. 1985;13(3):243-8.

20. Campbell DG. Ghost cell glaucoma following trauma. Ophthalmology 1981; 88(11):1151-8.

21. Cameron J, Havener VR. Histologic confirmation of ghost cell glaucoma by routine light microscopy. Am J Ophthalmol. 1983;96(2):251-2.

22. Polansky JR, Weinreb RN. Steroids as anti-inflammatory agents. In: Sears ML (Ed). Pharmacology of the Eye. Handbook of Experimental Pharmacology. Vol. 69. Berlin: Springer-Verlag; 1984. pp. 538-40.

23. De Juan E, Sternberg P Jr, Michels R. Penetrating ocular injuries. Ophthalmology. 1983;90(11):1318-22.

24. Schechner R, Miller B, Merksamer E, et al. A long term follow-up of ocular siderosis: quantitative assessment of the electroretinogram. Doc Ophthalmol. 1990;76(3):231-40.

25. Paerson CA, Eakins EA, Paterson E, et al. The ocular hypertensive response following experimental acid burns in the rabbit eye. Invest Ophthalmol Vis Sci. 1979;18(1):67-74.

26. Kuckelkorn R, Kottek A, Reim M. Intraocular complications after severe chemical burns—incidence and surgical treatment. Klin Monatsbl Augenheilkd. 1994;205(2):86-92.

27. Mermoud A, Salmon JF, Barron A, et al. Surgical management of post-traumatic angle recession glaucoma. Ophthalmology. 1993;100(5):634-42.

13

Neovascular Glaucoma

David R, George RJ

HISTORY

Rubeosis iridis was first described by Coats[1] in 1906 in association with central retinal vein occlusion (CRVO). Since his original description, neovascularization of the iris and angle has been identified in many diseases and 97% of which are proceeded by retinal ischemia.[2] Rubeosis iridis is often associated with a severe form of glaucoma. On the basis of their varied clinical presentations, this condition was historically called by different names, namely, hemorrhagic glaucoma, congestive glaucoma, thrombotic glaucoma and robotic glaucoma. However, the term 'neovascular glaucoma (NVG)' proposed by Weiss et al.[3] has become the most accepted one.

RISK FACTORS OF RUBEOSIS IRIDIS

Rubeosis is not a rare entity, it may be predisposed by a number of risk factors[4] such as ischemic retinal diseases, ocular inflammatory diseases and neoplasm. It can be induced surgically or following radiation therapy. They are tabulated in Table 13.1.

Table 13.1: Risk factors of rubeosis iridis.

1. *Retinal ischemic diseases*
Diabetes
Central retinal vein occlusion
Ocular ischemic syndrome/carotid occlusive disease
Central retinal artery occlusion
Retinal detachment

(Contd.)

(Contd.)

Lebers congenital amaurosis
Coats' disease
Eales disease
Sickle cell retinopathy
Retinal hemangioma
Persistent hyperplastic primary vitreous
Norrie's disease
Wyburn Mason syndrome
Carotid-cavernous fistula
Dural shunt
Stickler's syndrome
X-linked retinoschisis
Takayasu's aortitis
Juxtafoveal telangiectasis
2. Surgically induced
Carotid endarterectomy
Cataract extraction
Pars plana vitrectomy/lensectomy
Silicone oil injection
Scleral buckle
Neodymium: yttrium–aluminium–garnet capsulotomy
3. Tumors
Iris: melanoma, hemangioma, metastatic lesion
Ciliary body: ring melanoma
Retina: retinoblastoma, large cell lymphoma
Choroid: melanoma
Conjunctiva: squamous cell carcinoma
4. Radiation
External beam
Charged particle: proton, helium
Plaques
Photoradiation
5. Inflammatory diseases
Uveitis: chronic iridocyclitis, Behçet's disease
Vogt-Koyanagi-Harada syndrome, Syphilitic
Retinitis, Sympathetic ophthalmia, endophthalmitis
6. Miscellaneous
Vitreous-wick syndrome
Interferon alpha

Source: Sivak-Callcott JA, O'Day DM, Gass JD, et al. Evidence-based recommendations for the diagnosis and treatment of neovascular glaucoma. Ophthalmology. 2001;108(10):1767-76.

PATHOGENESIS

Retinal ischemia stimulates the production of vascular endothelial growth factor (VEGF),[5] a key molecule in ocular neovascularization. Elevated levels of VEGF have been identified in the aqueous humor of patients with NVG.[6] The VEGF is primarily produced by the Muller cells of the retina and it reaches the iris tissue and angles. The removal of the lens or a breach in the posterior capsule is associated with a higher incidence of rubeosis.

Although VEGF is the most studied factor, a multitude of other endogenous growth factors[7] have also been implicated for the cause of angiogenesis, namely insulin-like growth factor Iand II, insulin-like growth factor binding protein 2 and 3, transforming growth factor-alpha, beta (TGF-β, TGF-α), fibroblast growth factors, tumor necrosis factor–alpha (TNF-α), angiogenin , platelet-derived endothelial cell growth factor (PD- ECGF) and interleukin-8 (IL-8).[8,9]

CLINCOPATHOLOGIC COURSE

Rubeosis or Preglaucoma Stage

Rubeosis or preglaucoma stage is characterized by normal intraocular pressure (IOP). Careful slit-lamp biomicroscopy using bright light and high magnification reveals tufts of new vessels randomly oriented at the pupillary margin (Figs. 13.1A and B). Occasionally, angle neovascularization precedes neovascularization of the iris. These vessels should not be confused with normal iris stromal vessels, which have a more radial orientation and are intrastromal unlike the new vessels, which are on the surface of the iris and a have a random course. Gonioscopy reveals either normal angles or variable levels

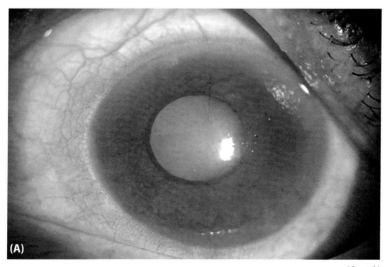

(A)

(Contd.)

(Contd.)

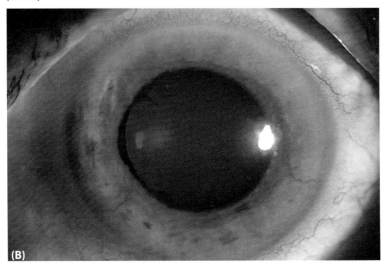

Figs. 13.1A and B: Rubeosis iridis.

of neovascularization of the angles. The IOP may remain normal until a significant portion of the trabecular meshwork is left uncovered.

Neovascularization begins as endothelial buds from the capillaries of the minor arterial circle at the pupil; however, they may appear from anywhere on the iris. The endothelial buds progress to become glomerulus-like vascular tufts. These peripupillary tufts extend over the iris in an irregular, meandering manner growing toward the collarette to reach the angle; in the angle the vessels cross the ciliary body band and scleral spur to arborize on the trabecular meshwork. The old axiom that an abnormal vessel crosses the scleral spur still holds good till date.

Neovascularization may first be seen at the site of a peripheral iridotomy or iridectomy since circulating angiogenic factors invoke neovascularization in areas where aqueous flow is high such as the pupil or iridotomies.

Stage of Open-angle Glaucoma

In this stage, IOP is elevated and florid rubeosis iridis is observed. On gonioscopy the angles may be open but the neovascularization is intense (Fig. 13.2). Angle neovascularization gives rise to fibrovascular tissue, which covers the trabecular meshwork and causes rise in IOP.

Stage of Angle-closure Glaucoma

At the stage of angle-closure glaucoma, fibrovascular membrane, composed of myofibroblasts, proliferates and contracts tenting the iris toward trabecular meshwork, forming peripheral anterior synechiae (PAS) (Fig. 13.3). When these PAS coalesce, permanent synechial angle closure occurs (Fig. 13.4) and

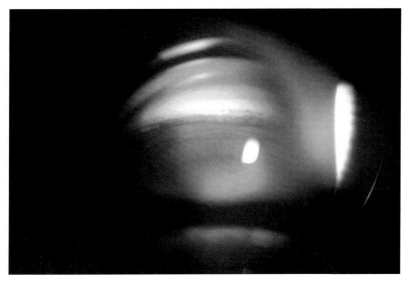

Fig. 13.2: Neovascularization of angle.

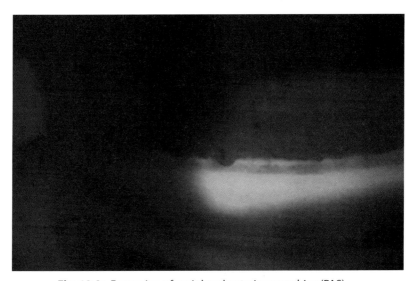

Fig. 13.3: Formation of peripheral anterior synechiae (PAS).

IOP rises. As angle closure progresses it becomes a total smooth zippered-up line of iridocorneal adhesion, which is pathognomic of NVG.

The contraction on the membrane over the iris pulls the posterior pigment epithelium of the iris around the pupillary margin onto the anterior surface known as ectropion uveae (Fig. 13.5).

COMMON CAUSES OF NEOVASCULAR GLAUCOMA

The commonest conditions associated with NVG related to the retinal hypoxia are diabetic retinopathy, retinal vessel occlusion and ocular ischemic syndrome.

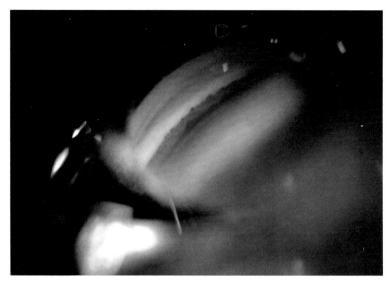

Fig. 13.4: Stage of angle-closure.

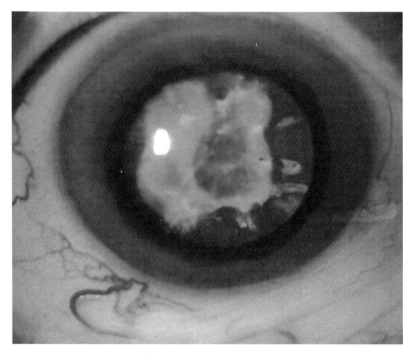

Fig. 13.5: Ectropion uveae.

Diabetic Retinopathy

Diabetes is one of the most common causes of NVG, accounting for approximately one-thirds of cases. It is most often seen in patients with proliferative diabetic retinopathy (PDR). Rubeosis occurs in 33–64% of those with PDR.[10]

The incidence of NVG increases after vitrectomy[11] and lensectomy.[12] A breach in the posterior capsule and removal of the lens allows the angiogenic factors to gain easy access to the iris and angles accelerating angiogenesis.

Central Retinal Vein Occlusion

Central retinal vein occlusion accounts for 30% of those with NVG. About 40% of those with ischemic CRVO develop NVG.[13] The central vein occlusion study (CVOS)[14] demonstrated that the percentage of conversion of nonischemic to ischemic CRVO is 30%. Hence a careful undilated slit lamp evaluation and gonioscopy is vital for detecting early signs of anterior segment neovascularization. The CVOS also found that 10% of eyes with nonischemic CRVO and 6% of eyes with ischemic CRVO had neovascularization of the angle without iris new vessels. Neovascularization is less frequently associated with branch retinal vein occlusion.

Ocular Ischemic Syndrome

Ocular ischemic syndrome is the third most common cause of NVG. Neovascularization secondary to ocular ischemic syndrome has the most variable course as it can present with mere neovascularization with normal IOP, which may be attributable to ischemia of the ciliary body.

Central Retinal Artery Occlusion

Central retinal artery occlusion (CRAO) has also been associated with neovascularization in 15% of patients. However, panretinal photocoagulation (PRP) does not prevent formation of new vessels.[15]

Miscellaneous Causes

The chances of developing NVG increases post vitrectomy. In a recent study done Akiko Gotta et al.[16] they reported that the incidence of NVG in PDR eyes postvitrectomy was 5.3% and increases to 7.1% at 1 year. The risk factors are male gender, younger age, NVG in the fellow eye, high baseline IOP and presence of NVA. Neovascularization, a sequela of chronic retinal ischemia, occurs in 10% of those with retinal vasculitis. NVG can also develop postradiation, probably owing to radiation induced damage to the posterior segment.[17]

CLINICAL PRESENTATION

Early in the course of the disease a high index of suspicion and careful examination of iris and angle of anterior chamber are essential to detect early neovascularization. Anterior chamber flare may be present due to leakage of proteins from the new vessels.

In a fully developed NVG, the clinical picture may be dramatically different; the condition becomes painful and the IOP increases as high as 60 mm Hg or more. There is usually corneal epithelial edema, which can make identification of iris and angle neovascularization difficult. The visual acuity may be grossly reduced, either due to the corneal edema or due to the associated retinal pathology.

Gonioscopy reveals new vessels crossing the scleral spur and in the end stages synechial closure, which is anterior to the Schwalbe's line, classically appearing as a zippered-up line of iridocorneal adhesion. Neovascularization of the iris and the angle of the anterior chamber is graded on the basis of extent of involvement (Table 13.2).[18]

Fluorescein angiography allows early detection of iris neovascularization before the development of clinically visible new vessels. In a study by Ehrenberg et al.,[19] 54% of the eyes despite leakage on the angiogram did not show clinically visible any new blood vessels. Stromal leakage is considered a risk for severe forms of rubeosis. Grading of iris neovascularization on fluorescein angiography is shown in Table 13.3.

MANAGEMENT OF NEOVASCULAR GLAUCOMA

The management of NVG is targeted toward treating the underlying disease process responsible for the neovascular stimulus and treatment of the increased IOP.[4]

Table 13.2: Grading of neovascularization of iris and the angle of the anterior chamber.

Grade	Neovascularization of iris	Neovascularization of the angle of anterior chamber
I	Fine surface neovascularization of the pupillary zone of the iris involving less than two quadrants	Fine neovascular twigs cross the scleral spur and branch on the trabecular meshwork involving less than 2 quadrants
II	Surface neovascularization of the pupillary zone of the iris involving more than two quadrants	Fine neovascular twigs cross scleral spur branching on the trabecular meshwork involving more than 2 quadrants
III	In addition to neovascularization of the pupillary zone, neovascularization of the ciliary zone of the iris or ectropion uveae involving one to three quadrants	In addition to neovascularization of the trabecular meshwork peripheral anterior synechiae (PAS) involving one to three quadrants
IV	Neovascularization of the ciliary zone of the iris or ectropion uveae involving three or more quadrants	PAS involving three or more quadrants

Table 13.3: Grading of iris neovascularization on fluorescein angiography.

Grade	Signs
0	No iris neovascularization
1	Neovascular tufts, one- to two-sphincter quadrants
2	Neovascular tufts, three- to four-sphincter quadrants
3	Diffuse stromal iris neovascularization, one to two quadrants
4	Diffuse stromal iris neovascularization, three to four quadrants
5	Diffuse stromal neovascularization, three to four quadrants with neovascular glaucoma

Panretinal Photocoagulation

Panretinal photocoagulation is considered the standard treatment for retinal ischemic diseases. Since retinal ischemia is critical to the development of NVI, PRP eliminates the source of the angiogenesis factor by selectively ablating the outer photoreceptor retinal pigment epithelium, which is a high oxygen-consuming layer. This allows the choroidal oxygen to diffuse into inner retinal layer and decrease inner retinal hypoxia. Vascular endothelial growth factor levels in patients with ischemic retinal pathologic features are reduced indirectly after laser photocoagulation.[6]

With the appearance of rubeosis, PRP is indicated in all the cases. Although not all patients with rubeosis progress to NVG, it is justified in performing PRP on all of them as the frequency of developing NVG is very high. Ohnishi and colleagues[20] documented regression of rubeosis in 68% of patients and normalization of IOP in 42% of patients treated with PRP. In 1993, Striga and Ivanisevic[21] demonstrated the importance of applying an adequate treatment dose of PRP. They reported that application of 1,200 to 1,600 spots produced regression of rubeosis in 70.4% of diabetic patients.

According to the CVOS, PRP should be done when the NVI/NVA appears. Prophylactic PRP makes it less effective when done before the appearance of new vessels. In PDR and non-PDR with extensive capillary nonperfusion areas, PRP helps the regression of rubeosis and prevents NVG. In carotid diseases where hypoxia may not be limited to the retina alone, PRP has been shown to cause regression of NVI until definitive treatment can be instituted. However, PRP has not shown very promising results in CRAO.

In the end stage, even when the angles are completely closed synechially, PRP improves the success of the filtering surgery eliminating the angiogenic stimulus.[22] Regression of NVI occurs within 3–4 weeks following PRP.

Endophotocoaguation

When adequate PRP cannot be done due to a poor view of the fundus, another option is to surgically improve the view. Pars plana vitrectomy and lensectomy (if necessary) along with endolaser application can be performed.

Anterior Retinal Cryotherapy

Whenever PRP is indicated but the media are too hazy due to diseases of the cornea, lens or vitreous to allow adequate visualization, pan retinal cryotherapy can be performed. A total of 32 spots are applied 8 mm away from the limbus and extending just outside the major arterial circle. The probe tip is kept in contact with the sclera until –70°C has been maintained for 5–10 s. In a prospective study done by Sihota et al.[23] more than 90% of the patients achieved symptomatic relief and regression of neovascularization. Panretinal cryotherapy can be combined with cyclodestructive procedures in order to reduce the IOP, in eyes with poor visual potential.

Goniophotocoagulation

Goniophotocoagulation involves direct application of argon laser to the new vessels in the angle in the early stages of the disease thereby preventing irreversible changes in the angle. Low-energy argon laser (0.2 s, 50–100 μm, 100–200 mW) are applied to the neovascular tufts as they cross the scleral spur. It is a useful adjunct to PRP.

Medical Management of NVG

Medical management of NVG includes IOP-lowering agents, including topical β-adrenergic antagonists, α-2 agonists, and topical and oral carbonic anhydrase inhibitors. Prostaglandin analogs should be used with caution as their use may cause permanent synechial closure. Miotic should also be avoided as they increase the inflammation and synechiae formation. Topical steroids can be given for reduction of inflammation and providing symptomatic relief. Topical atropine is used for its cycloplegic effect. Medical treatment is effective to control the IOP in the open-angle stage of the disease. In the later stages the role of medical treatment is limited.

ANTI-VASCULAR ENDOTHELIAL GROWTH FACTOR

The pathogenesis of NVG is linked to locally produced angiogenic growth factor: VEGF. Therefore, directly targeting the VEGF is a logical therapeutic strategy to treat NVG.

Bevacizumab (Avastin, Genentech, South San Francisco, CA) is a full-length humanized monoclonal antibody that binds all isoforms of VEGF. It is proven beneficial for the short-term regression of NVI and considered safe for the management of NVG when injected into the anterior chamber or vitreous cavity.[24] The dose of intracameral[25] bevacizumab and intravitreal[26] bevacizumab is 1.25 mg/0.05 mL. NVI usually regress within 1 week after the injection but however its duration of action is short, lasting for 4 weeks. Repeated injections may be required for recurrence of NVI.[27]

Injection of Avastin is a useful alternative when PRP does not work or when media opacities preclude visualization. Intravitreal injection is a more logical choice as it bypasses the blood ocular barrier and provides high local concentrations of the agent. Intravitreal injections of bevacizumab accentuate the effect of PRP, reduces NVI and IOP in NVG and may be considered as an adjunct to more definitive surgical procedures for NVG.[28]

Ehlers et al.[29] reported that intravitreal bevacizumab when given on the same day as PRP in comparison to PRP alone had a significantly higher frequency and rapid regression of NVI at around 4 months follow-up.

In a retrospective study done by Wasabayashi et al.,[30] patients were divided into three subgroups: NVI without elevated IOP, NVG with an open angle and NVG with angle closure. Intravitreal bevacizumab effectively stabilized NVI, and controlled IOP in patients with NVI alone and early-stage NVG without angle closure. In advanced NVG, IV bevacizumab could not control IOP. It may be used as an adjunct to improve results of subsequent surgical results.

A recent Cochrane review assessed available evidence on anti-VEGF agents in NVG and concluded that there was a lack of well-designed controlled trials comparing different treatment options leading to inadequate evidence that justified its use in NVG.[31]

SURGICAL MANAGEMENT

Several factors influence the choice of surgical technique for the control of the NVG. The surgeries most commonly performed are trabeculectomy combined with antifibrotic agent, glaucoma drainage devices and cyclodestructive procedures. The glaucoma drainage implant is preferred when the inflammation is severe and the disease is advanced.

When the visual potential is poor, less invasive method like cyclodestructive procedure is preferred.

Trabeculectomy

Trabeculectomy in NVG patients is associated with frequent intraoperative complications and poor surgical outcomes. The prior pan retinal photocoagulation and use of adjunctive antimetabolite like Mitomycin C increase the success of the surgery to a certain extent. Kuchi et al.[32] reported a success of 61.8%, 2–3 years after trabeculectomy with Mitomycin C in patients with NVG. However, they found extensive PAS and previous vitrectomy as negative predictors for surgical outcome.

The use of intravitreal anti-VEGF before trabeculectomy improves the surgical outcome by reducing the chances of hyphema and reduces the IOP in the early postoperative period. Trabeculectomy with intraoperative Mitomycin C after an adjunctive treatment with intravitreal bevacizumab and PRP is a good treatment modality in the management of NVG.[33]

Takihara et al.,[34] in a retrospective study, compared the surgical success between intravitreal bevacizumab before trabeculectomy and trabeculectomy with mitomycin C. The results confirmed the previous statement but the long-term outcome was the same 63% in the intravitreal bevacizumab group and mitomycin C group. This may be explained by the transient nature of the molecule, which gets eliminated in 4 weeks.[35]

The prognostic factors for failure of filtering surgery were studied in detail by Takihara et al.[36] They were younger age, history of previous vitrectomy, fellow eye with NVG and persistent proliferative membrane and/or retinal detachment after vitrectomy.

Glaucoma Drainage Devices

Considering the poor prognosis for success of trabeculectomy, glaucoma drainage implants have been auseful alternative in the treatment of intractable elevation of IOP in NVG. The initial description of the use of glaucoma drainage implants in NVG was by Molteno et al.,[37] who described the technique for implantation and reported on the IOP in 12 patients with an average of 13 months follow-up. Mermoud et al.[38] analyzed 60 eyes with NVG who underwent Molteno implantation with a mean follow-up of 24.7 months. They achieved a success rate of 62% and 10.3% at 1 and 5 years follow-up intervals, respectively. A similar study with a larger series of cases by Every et al.[39] achieved more or less similar results.

The Bareveldt implant is also effective in controlling the IOP associated with NVG. According to Sodoti et al.,[40] preoperative visual acuity and increased age were positively correlated to the surgical outcome with the Bareveldt implant. They also reported that the implant size did not affect success of surgery.

Netland et al.[41] compared 38 eyes with NVG to controls without NVG undergoing Ahmed glaucoma valve implant (AGV), they found that the surgical success rates at 1 year, 2 years and 5 years in the NVG group were 73.1%, 81.8% and 20.6% respectively while in the control group corresponding rates were 89.2%, 81.8% and 73.1%. It was concluded that AGV implantation was less successful in eyes with NVG.

The levels of VEGF in NVG affect fibrosis and so conceivably affect the success of glaucoma drainage surgery. In a study done by Kim et al.,[42] in subjects with a lower level of VEGF had a better success rate than those who had a higher level.

In a retrospective case series done by Kyong Tak et al.[43] 52 eyes with NVG who had intraoperative intravitreal bevacizumab (1.25 mg/mL) prior to AGV were compared to a control group who underwent only AGV. Although the success rate in the IVB group (70%) was higher than the controls (62.5%) the difference was not statistically significant at 1 year follow up.

In a long-term study done by Yalvac et al.[44] AGV and single-plate Molteno were found effective for lowering IOP in NVG patients. However, both procedures were poor for maintaining the long-term success of the surgery due to the progression of the disease.

Cyclodestructive Procedures

Partial destruction of the ciliary body is a safe and effective procedure for lowering IOP in patients with poor visual potential. Bloom and colleagues[45] reported a mean IOP reduction of 53% (from a preoperative mean IOP of 45 mm Hg) in 25 patients treated with the diode laser for refractory NVG. Uram et al.[46] directly treated the ciliary processes with the endoscopic diode laser and achieved a mean IOP-lowering effect of 65% in 10 eyes with NVG. Nine eyes had a pressure of less than 21 mm Hg at 11 months.

Cyclodestructive procedures have been combined with anti-VEGF injection with variable results.

Fong et al.[47] observed no statistical difference in the IOP-lowering effect between the transcleral cyclophotocoagulation group and the transscleral cyclophotocoagulation combined with intravitreal bevacizumab group. Ghosh et al.[48] reported that transscleral cyclophotocoagulation with intravitreal bevacizumab dramatically reduced the IOP and caused regression of new vessels in 14 eyes followed up for 6 months.

REFERENCES

1. Coats G. Further cases of thrombosis of central retinal vein. Roy London Ophthal Hosp Rep. 1906;16:516.
2. Brown GC, Magargal LE, Schachat A, et al. Neovascular glaucoma: etiologic considerations. Ophthalmology. 1984;91(4):315-20.
3. Weiss DI, Shaffer RN, Neherenberg TR. Neovascular glaucoma complicating carotid-cavernous fistula. Arch Ophthalmol. 1963;69:304-7.
4. Sivak-Callcott JA, O'Day DM, Gass JD, et al. Evidence-based recommendations for the diagnosis and treatment of neovascular glaucoma. Ophthalmology. 2001;108(10):1767-77.
5. Aiello LP, Avery RL, Arrigg PG, et al. Vascular endothelial growth factor in ocular fluid of patients with diabetic retinopathy and other retinal disorders. N Engl J Med. 1994;331(22):1480-7.
6. Tripathi RC, Li J, Tripathi BJ, et al. Increased level of vascular endothelial growth factor in aqueous humor of patients with neovascular glaucoma. Ophthalmology. 1998;105(2):232-7.
7. Casey R, Li WW. Factors controlling ocular angiogenesis. Am J Ophthalmol. 1997;124(4):521-9.
8. Meyer-Schwickerath R, Pfeiffer A, Blum WF, et al. Vitreous levels of the insulin-like growth factors I and II, and the insulin-like growth factor binding proteins 2 and 3, increase in neovascular eye diseases. Studies in nondiabetic and diabetic subjects. J Clin Invest. 1993;92(6):2620-5.
9. Chen KH, Wu CC, Roy S, et al. Increased interleukin-6 in aqueous humor of neovascular glaucoma. Invest Ophthalmol Vis Sci. 1999;40(11):2627-32.

10. Ohrt V. Glaucoma due to rubeosis iridis diabetic. Ophthalmologica. 1961; 142:356-64.
11. Wand M, Madigan JC, Gaudio AR, et al. Neovascular glaucoma following pars plana vitrectomy for complications of diabetic retinopathy.Ophthalmic Surg. 1990;21(2):113-8.
12. Rice TA, Micheals RG, Maguire MG, et al. The effect of lensectomy on the incidence of iris neovascularization. Am J Ophthalmol. 1983;95(1):1-11.
13. Hayreh SS, Rojas P, Podhajsky P, et al. Ocular neovascularization with retinal vascular occlusion-III. Incidence of ocular neovascularization with retinal vein occlusion. Ophthalmology.1983;90(5):488-506.
14. Natural history and clinical management of central retinal vein occlusion. The Central Vein Occlusion Study Group. Arch Ophthalmol. 1997;115(4):486-91.
15. Duker JS, Brown GC. Efficacy of panretinal photocoagulation for neovascularization of iris after central retinal artery obstruction. Ophthalmology. 1989;96(1):92.
16. Goto A, Inatani M, Awai-Kasaoka N, et al. Frequency and risk factors for neovascular glaucoma after vitrectomy in eyes with proliferative diabetic retinopathy. J Glaucoma. 2013;22(7):572-6.
17. Fernandes BF, Weisbrod D, Yücel YH, et al. Neovascular glaucoma after stereotactic radiotherapy for juxtapapillary choroidal melanoma: histopathologic and dosimetric findings. Int J Radiat Oncol BiolPhys. 2011;80(2):377-84.
18. Weiss DI, Gold D. Neofibrovascularization of iris and anterior chamber angle: a clinical classification. Ann Ophthalmol. 1978;10(4):488-91.
19. Ehrenberg M, Brooks W, McCuen II, et al. Rubeois iridis. Ophthalmology. 1984;91(4):321-5.
20. Ohnishi Y, Ishibashi T, Sagawa T. Fluorescein gonioangiography in diabetic neovascularization. Graefes Arch Clin ExpOphthalmol. 1994;232(4):199-204.
21. Striga M, Ivanisevic M. Comparison between efficacy of full and mild scatter (pan retinal photocoagulation) on the course of diabetic rubeosis iridis. Ophthalmologica. 1993;207:144-7.
22. Wolbarst ML, Landers MB III. A rational for photocoagulation therapy for proliferative diabetic retinopathy a review and model. Ophthalmic Surg. 1980; 11(4):235-45.
23. Sihota R, Sandramouli S, Sood NN. A prospective evaluation of anterior retinal cryoablation in neovascular glaucoma. Ophthal Surg.1991;22(50):256-9.
24. Chilov MN, Grigg JR, Playfair TJ. Bevacizumab (Avastin) for the treatment of neovascular glaucoma. Clin ExpOphthalmol. 2007;35:494-6.
25. Iliev ME, Domig D, Wolf-Schnurrbursch U, et al. Intravitreal bevacizumab (avastin) in the treatment of neovascular glaucoma. Am J Ophthalmol. 2006; 142(6):1054-6.
26. Grisanti S, Biester S, Peters S, et al. Intracameral bevcizumab for iris rubeosis. Am J Ophthalmol. 2006;142(1):158-60.
27. Oshima Y, Sakaguchi H, Gomi F, et al. Regression of iris neovascularization after intravitreal injection of bevacizumab in patients with proliferative diabetic retinopathy. Am J Ophthalmol. 2006;142(1):155-7.
28. Yazdani S, Hendi K, Pakravan M, et al. Intravitreal bevacizumab for neovascular glaucoma, a randomized control trial. J Glaucoma. 2009;18(8):632-7.

29. Ehlers JP, Sprin MJ, Lam A, et al. Combination of intravitreal bevacizumab/panretinal photocoagulation versus pan retinal photocoagulation alone in the treatment of neovascular glaucoma. Retina. 2008;28(5):696-702.

30. Wakabayashi T, Oshima Y, Sakaguchi H, et al. Intravitreal bevacizumab to treat iris neovascularization and neovascular glaucoma secondary to ischemic retinal diseases in 41consecutive cases. Ophthalmology. 2008;115(9):1571-80.

31. Simha A, Braganza A, Abraham L, et al. Anti-vascular endothelial growth factor for neovascular glaucoma. Cochrane Database Syst Rev. 2013;2(10): CD007920.

32. Kuchi Y, Sugimoto R, Nakae K, et al. Trabeculectomy with mitomycin C for treatment of neovascular glaucoma in diabetic patients. Ophthalmologica. 2006;220(6):383-8.

33. Alkawas AA, Shahien EA, Hussein AM. Management of neovascular glaucoma with pan retinal photocoagulation, intravitreal bevcizumab, and subsequent trabeculectomy with mitomycin C. J Glaucoma. 2010;19(9):622-6.

34. Takihara Y, Inatani M, Fukushima M, et al. Combined intravitreal bevacizumab and trabeculectomy with mitomycin C versus Trabeculectomy with miotmycin C alone. J Glaucoma. 2011;20(3):196-201.

35. Iliev ME, Domig D, Wolf-Schnurrbursch U.Intravitreal bevacizumab (Avastin) in the treatment of neovascular glaucoma. Am J Ophthalmol. 2006;142(6):1054-6.

36. Masaruinatani T, Fukushima M, Iwao K, et al. Trabeculectomy with Mitomycin C for neovascular glaucoma: prognostic factors for surgical failure. Am J Ophthalmol. 2009;147(5):912-8.

37. Molteno AC, Van Rooyen MM, Bartholomew RS. Implants for draining neovascular glaucoma. Br J Ophthalmol. 1977;61(2):120-5.

38. Salmon MA, Alexander JF, et al. Tube implantation for neovascular glaucoma: long-term results and factors influencing outcome. Ophthalmology. 1993;100:892-902.

39. Every SG, Molteno ACB, Bevin TH, et al. Long-term results of Molteno implant insertionin cases of neovascular glaucoma. Arch Ophthlamol. 2006;124(3): 355-60.

40. Sidoti PA, Dunphy TR, Baerveldt G. Experience with the Baerveldt glaucoma implant in treating neovascular glaucoma. Ophthalmology. 1995; 102(7):1107-18.

41. Netland PA, Ishida K, Boyle JW. Ahmed glaucoma valve in patients with and without neovascular glaucoma. J Glaucoma. 2010;19:851-6.

42. Kim YG, Hong S, Lee CS. Level of vascular endothelial growth factor in aqueous humor and surgical results of Ahmed glaucoma valve implantation in patients with neovascular glaucoma. J Glaucoma. 2009;18(6):443-7.

43. Ma KT, Yang JY, Kim JH, et al. Surgical results of Ahmed valve implantation with intraoperative bevacizumab injection in patients with neovascular glaucoma. J Glaucoma. 2012;21(5):331-6.

44. Yalvac IS, Eksioglu U, Satana B, et al. Long-term results of Ahmed valve and Molteno implant in neovascular glaucoma. Eye (Lond). 2007;21(1):65-70.

45. Bloom PA, Tsai JC, Sharma K et al. "Cyclodiode." Transscleral diode laser cyclophotocoagulation in the treatment of advanced refractory glaucoma. Ophthalmology. 1997;104(9):1508-19, discussion 1519-20.

46. Uram M. Ophthalmic laser microendoscope ciliary process ablation in the management of neovascular glaucoma. Ophthalmology. 1992;99(12):1823-8.
47. Fong AW, Lee GA, O'Rourke P, et al. Management of neovascular glaucoma with transscleral cyclophotocoagulation with diode laser alone versus combination transscleral cyclophotocoagulation with diode laser and intravitreal bevacizumab. Clin Exp Ophthalmol. 2011;39(4):318-23.
48. Ghosh S, Singh D, Ruddle JB, et al. Combined diode laser cyclophotocoagulation and intravitreal bevacizumab (Avastin) in neovascular glaucoma. Clin Exp Ophthalmol. 2010;38(4):353-7.

14

Epidemic Dropsy Glaucoma

Chandravanshi SL

INTRODUCTION

Epidemic dropsy glaucoma is an ocular manifestation of epidemic dropsy. Epidemic dropsy is an acute toxic state resulting from consumption of cooking media (edible oil) mixed with *Argemone mexicana* (Mexican prickly poppy) seed oil. It is characterized by massive pitting edema of the legs, gastrointestinal tract disturbances, dyspnea, cardiac insufficiency, renal failure and open angle glaucoma. Epidemic dropsy has been seen in many countries such as India, Australia, Fiji Islands, Myanmar, Pakistan, South Africa, Mauritius, Madagascar and Nepal.[1] Lyon reported the first case series of four cases of argemone seed oil toxicity from Calcutta, West Bengal, in 1877. Since then, many epidemics have been reported from different states of India namely West Bengal (1878, 1879, 1907, 1908, 1909), Assam (1893), Orissa (1928), Bihar (1950), Maharashtra (1968, 1969, 1972), Andhra Pradesh (1972), New Delhi (1975, 1994, 1998), Rajasthan (1985), Uttar Pradesh (1994, 2002, 2005, 2013), Jammu and Kashmir (1998), Madhya Pradesh (2000), Gujarat (2012), Haryana (2013), and Punjab (2013).

Epidemic dropsy has both systemic and ocular manifestations. In epidemic dropsy, massive edema of the lower extremities is the most consistent clinical sign, hence the name of the disease.

ETIOLOGY

Argemone oil contains two toxic alkaloids called sanguinarine and dihydrsanguinarine. They are responsible for epidemic dropsy. These toxic compounds interfere in pyruvic acid metabolism, which results in an accmulation of pyruvate in blood. The contamination of mustard oil or other edible oils

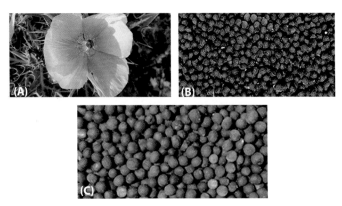

Figs. 14.1A to C: Flower and seeds of argemone plant (A and B), seeds of mustard (C).

with argemone oil may be deliberate or accidental. The 'argemone' plant is a common weed in India. It has spiky leaves and bright orange-yellow flowers. Hence it is also called prickly poppy (Fig. 14.1A). Seeds of *Argemone mexicana* (*Satyanashi*) are very similar to mustard (*Brassica nigra*) seeds in terms of color, size, shape and appearance (Figs. 14.1B and C).

The seeds of argemone mature in March and during the same period, the crops of mustards are also harvested and likely to be gathered along with mustard seeds. This mixup of seeds may lead to accidental contamination of mustard seeds. Sometimes unscrupulous dealers deliberately mix argemone oil in edible oils such as mustard oil, rapeseed oil, linseed oil, groundnut oil and other cooking media. Epidemic dropsy has also been reported secondary to consumption of argemone adulterated wheat flour in South Africa.[1]

CLINICAL PRESENTATIONS

Systemic Features

Affected Organs

Epidemic dropsy affects many organs of our body mainly skin, lungs, gastrointestine, heart, liver, kidney and eye. No age group is immune to epidemic dropsy except breast-fed infants. However, infants may be affected due to skin massage with adulterated oils. Epidemic dropsy affects males and females equally. Majority of the epidemics of dropsy reported from India have taken place during rainy season (July–August months). Onset of the disease may be subacute or insidious in nature with gastrointestinal disturbances such as watery diarrhea and vomiting.

Fever is usually mild, ranging from 99 to 100.5°F, which may be intermittent or continuous in nature.[1]

Cutaneous Manifestations

Cutaneous features are pitting edema of the lower extremities, erythema, tenderness, alopecia and pigmentary changes. Bilateral symmetrical pitting

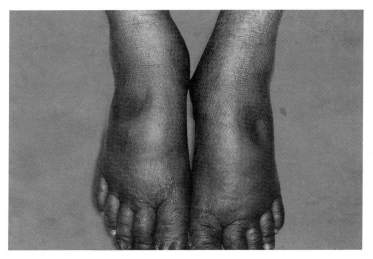

Fig. 14.2: Pitting edema of feet.

edema involving the lower extremities (Fig. 14.2), scrotum and abdominal wall is the hallmark feature of epidemic dropsy. Widespread profuse capillary dilatation develops due to the toxic effect of alkaloids resulting in extravasation of protein-rich plasma into the interstitial (extravascular) compartment causing edema.[1]

Raised local temperature and tingling sensations in the edematous area help in differentiating epidemic dropsy edema from other causes of edema. The edema may persist for up to 2 months in most of the cases. Erythema may be resolved earlier, leaving pigmentary changes.[2]

Gastrointestinal Manifestations

Main gastrointestinal manifestations of epidemic dropsy are seen in 90% of cases and these include diarrhea, vomiting, abdominal pain, tenesmus, melena and hepatomegaly. Acute stage of disease is characterized by abdominal pain, watery diarrhea and vomiting due to the direct toxic effect of sanguinarine to the enterocytes of small intestine. Intestinal mucosal congestion develops due to vascular leakage. Hepatomegaly is congestive and non-tender. It is seen in 25% of cases and thought to be due to congestive cardiac failure. However, it has also been reported without congestive cardiac failure. Direct toxic liver injury by alkaloids present in argemone oil may be the other possibility in such cases.[1,3]

Cardiac Manifestations

Pericardial effusion, tachycardia, and high output cardiac failure are major cardiac manifestations of epidemic dropsy.[4] Sanguinarine blocks cardiac Na^+/K^+-ATPase enzyme function by interacting with the cardiac glycoside receptor site of the enzyme, which probably causes degenerative changes in cardiac muscle fibers and cardiac failure.[5]

Pulmonary Manifestations

Cough, breathlessness, respiratory alkalosis with mild hypoxia, ortho-pnea, pulmonary edema, decreased vital capacity, patchy pneumonitis and pleural effusions are its pulmonary manifestations. Sanguinarine causes increase in blood pyruvate levels due to activation of glycogenolysis. In the animal model, it has been seen that sanguinarine causes thickening of interalveolar septa and structural disorganization of alveolar spaces in lungs. Accumulation of interstitial fluid in alveoli of lung leads to ventila-tory dysfunction and right-sided cardiac failure with normal activities of left ventricle.

Renal Manifestations

Renal manifestations of epidemic dropsy are uncommon. Kidney function test may show bland urinary sediments, decreased glomerular filtration rate, renal azotemia (mild to moderate) and proteinuria. Timely management of these manifestations is necessary to prevent acute renal failure. Sanguinarine induces extensive capillary dilatation and increased permeability, caus-ing extravasation of protein-rich plasma component of the blood into the interstitial tissues, which causes rise in its oncotic pressure relative to cap-illary network. The raised oncotic pressure causes movement of fluid from the intravascular compartment to extravascular compartment and leads to a hypovolemic state, causing renal hypoperfusion, which may progress to acute tubular necrosis and acute renal failure.[6,7]

Neurological Manifestations

Neurological manifestations are rare. Electrophysiological testing of retina, peripheral nerves and muscles have been observed normal in epidemic dropsy. Brachial neuritis and palatal palsy are rarely seen in epidemic dropsy patients.[9]

Pregnancy and Epidemic Dropsy

Pregnancy is usually unaffected by epidemic dropsy. Rarely, it may cause spontaneous abortion and still birth secondary to hemangiomatous changes in the endometrium of uterus and placenta.[10]

Ocular Features

Ocular manifestations include open-angle glaucoma and subconjunctival hemorrhages. A number of retinal changes are found in epidemic dropsy. Superficial retinal hemorrhages and retinal venous dilatation and tortuos-ity were most commonly observed fundus findings (Fig. 14.3). Liberation of histamine and prostaglandin E were thought to be responsible for these ret-

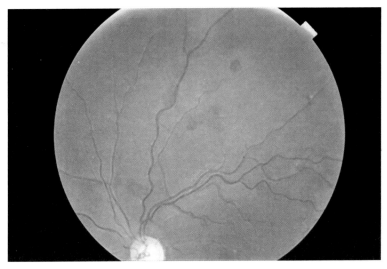

Fig. 14.3: Fundus showing retinal hemorrhages and venous tortuosity in a patient with epidemic dropsy.

inal manifestations. Microaneuryms, papillophlebitis and optic disc edema may also be found. Very few cases of epidemic dropsy have been reported with central retinal vein occlusion.[11,12]

Fundus fluorescein angiography may show dilatation and tortuosity of retinal vessels, prominent and prolonged staining of vessels, microaneuryms, optic disc edema, blocked fluorescence in area of retinal hemorrhages and leakage of dye around the optic disk head.[12] These fundus fluorescein angiography findings are well correlated with the systemic severity of epidemic dropsy. Ocular electrophysiological studies have been reported to be normal.[8]

Special Features of Epidemic Dropsy Glaucoma

- Ocular manifestations of epidemic dropsy have been reported in various epidemics in 0–12% of cases[11,13]
- Patients usually complain of irritation and burning eyes, sensations in diminution of vision and colored haloes
- It is usually bilateral as a rule, though one eye is more severely involved than the fellow one
- The rise in intraocular pressure often develops 1–2 months after appearance of dropsy[1,15]
- The eye has normal depth of anterior chamber and no signs of ocular inflammations[1,14]
- Gonioscopic examination shows open angle of the anterior chamber
- Normal outflow also demonstrated on tonography
- Variable pattern of IOP is recorded[15]
- It is a hypersecretion open-angle glaucoma

- Sachdev et al.[14] suggested that high level of prostaglandin E_2 and histamine activity in the aqueous humor is probably responsible for development of epidemic dropsy glaucoma
- Development of acute visual field defects does not depend on rise of intraocular pressure especially in the early stage of the disease[16]

DIAGNOSIS

Diagnosis of epidemic dropsy glaucoma requires a high degree of clinical suspicion. It should be suspected if patients have:
- Bilateral raised intraocular pressure with normal drainage angle
- Bilateral pitting edema of the legs
- Cutaneous manifestations such as erythema, flushing, raised local temperature in edematous area and tenderness
- Family history of similar illness along with history of intake of loose cooking oil and
- Detection of sanguinarine in serum or urine by appropriate test is confirmatory[1]

DIFFERENTIAL DIAGNOSIS

The differential diagnosis of epidemic dropsy includes congestive cardiac failure, beriberi, hypoproteinemia, myxedema, nephrotic syndrome, and anemia.

Epidemic dropsy glaucoma should be differentiated from primary as well as secondary open-angle glaucoma.

INVESTIGATIONS

No specific hematological or biochemical changes have been described in literature.[1]

Hematology

- Anemia is quite common, but sometimes it may be severe. Microcytic hypochromic or normocytic normochromic anemia is usually seen in epidemic dropsy. Anemia in epidemic dropsy is multifactorial in origin. Bleeding from gastrointestinal tract, suppression of bone marrow and decreased red blood cell life span are common factors behind development of anemia.

Kidney Function Test

- Impairment of renal function may result in raised blood urea and serum creatinine.
- Serum protein derangement such as raised alpha-2 globulin, hypoalbuminemia and reversal of albumin/globulin ratio have been documented.
- Elevated plasma pyruvate level has been seen occasionally.

Liver Function Test

- Serum bilirubin and hepatic enzymes are usually normal.

Electrocardiography

- Electrocardiography may show non-specific ST segment and T-wave changes, or atrial and/or ventricular extrasystoles.[1]

X-ray Chest

X-ray chest may reveal cardiomegaly, pulmonary edema or pneumonia.

Chemical Test for Detection of Argemone Oil

- Nitric acid test or thin-layer chromatography is usually applied for detection of argemone oil in adulterated cooking oil.
- Thin-layer paper chromatography is a gold standard technique because it is the most sensitive and more specific technique to detect argemone. It can detect 0.0001% of argemone oil in edible oil.

TREATMENT

Although epidemic dropsy is known for more than 135 years, still there is no established treatment.[17] Complete cessation of consumption of adulterated cooking oil along with symptomatic therapy is the mainstay of epidemic dropsy management.[1]

Systemic Treatment

Diuretics, calcium, multi-vitamins, antihistaminic, antioxidants and protein-rich diet are given as supportive therapy.[1] Multivitamins and antioxidants are helpful in recovering from antioxidant depletion.[17] Complete bed rest with leg elevation and protein-rich diet are useful in relieving edema of legs. Corticosteroids have been also recommended for relieving edema. However, its efficacy is yet to be proved. Oral antihistamine, promethazine, is helpful in relieving itching caused by histamine and related substance.

Diuretics are used universally in patients with epidemic dropsy, especially if congestive cardiac failure occurs. Diuretics are not helpful in relieving leg edema because the pathogenesis behind the leg edema is increased capillary permeability. Diuretics should be used judiciously; otherwise depletion of intravascular volume may occur.

Cardiac failure may be managed by complete bed rest, restriction of salt intake, digitalization and administration of diuretics. Treatment of pneumonia include appropriate antibiotics according to culture and sensitivity report. Acute renal failure may require dialysis in some patients.

Ophthalmic Treatment

- Epidemic dropsy glaucoma is a self-limiting entity but if left untreated, it may lead to glaucomatous optic atrophy
- Intraocular pressure usually became normal within 3 months once affected individual stopped consuming adulterated cooking oils
- Intraocular pressure generally responds very well to topical anti-glaucoma medicines; however, glaucoma filtration surgery is required in rare circumstances.[14] Therefore, in some cases, topical anti-glaucoma medicines may be needed to be tailored on a weekly basis.[15]
- Aqueous humor suppressants are more effective and pilocarpine has no role in the treatment of epidemic dropsy glaucoma

Prognosis

- Mortality is reported in 5% of cases and most frequently due to cardiopulmonary/renal complications such as cardiac failure, pneumonia, respiratory distress syndrome or renal failure[1]
- Most of the patients completely recover within 3 months after withdrawal of toxic cooking oil
- Intraocular pressure also normalizes within 3 months

Prevention

- The accidental contamination of mustard seeds can be prevented at fields by removing the argemone weeds growing among mustard crops.[1]
- Intentional mixing of edible oil with argemone oil should be dealt under the Prevention of Food Adulteration Act, 1954

REFERENCES

1. Sharma BD, Malhotra S, Bhatia V, et al. Epidemic dropsy in India. Postgrad Med J. 1999;75(889):657-61.
2. Kar HK, Jain RK, Sharma PK, et al. Epidemic dropsy: a study of cutaneous manifestations with histopathological correlation. Indian J Dermatol Venereol Leprol. 2001;67:178-9.
3. Tandon RK, Tandon HD, Nayak NC, et al. Liver in epidemic dropsy. Indian J Med Res. 1976;64:1064-9.
4. Sanghvi LM, Misra SN, Bose TK, et al. Cardiovascular manifestations in argemone mexicana poisoning (epidemic dropsy). Circulation. 1960;21:1096-106.
5. Seifen E, Adams RJ, Riemer RK. Sanguinarine: a positive inotropic alkaloid which inhibits cardiac Na$^+$,K$^+$-ATPase. Eur J Pharmacol. 1979;60(4):373-7.
6. Sharma BD, Bhatia V, Rahtee M, et al. Epidemic dropsy: observations on pathophysiology and clinical features during the Delhi epidemic of 1998. Trop Doct. 2002;32(2):70-5.
7. Das M, Khanna SK. Clinicoepidemiological, toxicological, and safety evaluation studies on argemone oil. Crit Rev Toxicol. 1997;27(3):273-97.

8. Sachdev HP, Sachdev MS, Verma L, et al. Electrophysiological studies of the eye, peripheral nerves and muscles in epidemic dropsy. J Trop Med Hyg. 1989;92(6):412-5.

9 Sahoo S, Bandyopadhyay A, Mahapatra NC. Unusual association of epidemic dropsy with brachial neuritis and palatal palsy. Indian J Pediatr. 2013; 80(5):428-9.

10. Bhadury KP. Epidemic dropsy complicating pregnancy. Ind Med Gaz. 1950;85(3):98-9.

11. Rathore MK. Ophthalmological study of epidemic dropsy. Br J Ophthalmol. 1982;66(9):573-5.

12. Sachdev MS, Sood NN, Mohan M, et al. Optic disc vasculitis in epidemic dropsy. Jpn J Ophthalmol. 1987;31(3):467-74.

13. Mohan M, Sood NN, Dayal Y, et al. Ocular and clinico-epidemiological study of epidemic dropsy. Indian J Med Res. 1984;80:449-56.

14. Sachdev MS, Sood NN, Verma LK, et al. Pathogenesis of epidemic dropsy glaucoma. Arch Ophthalmol. 1988;106(9):1221-3.

15. Malik KP, Dadeya S, Gupta VS, et al. Pattern of intraocular pressure in epidemic dropsy in India. Trop Doct. 2004;34(3):161-2.

16. Singh K, Singh MJ, Das JC. Visual field defects in epidemic dropsy. Clin Toxicol (Phila). 2006;44(2):159-63.

17. Kumar A, Husain F, Das M, et al. An out-break of epidemic dropsy in the Barabanki District of Uttar Pradesh, India: a limited trial for the scope of antioxidants in the management of symptoms. Biomed Environ Sci. 1992;5(3):251-6.

Current Role of Imaging in Glaucoma Management

Palani M, Rajagopal S, Madhivanan N, Murali A

INTRODUCTION

Glaucoma is a progressive optic neuropathy with characteristic optic disk changes and corresponding visual field loss, for which elevated intraocular pressure (IOP) is one of the main risk factor.[1] In glaucoma the structural damage usually precedes the functional deterioration and by the time white on white perimetry shows defect, about 40–45% of retinal ganglion cells (RGC) are lost. This is attributed to the fact that even if some RGC are lost, the surrounding ganglion cells subserving the same area would signal the presence of the target and there would be no functional visual field loss. Hence structural evaluations of the optic nerve head (ONH) and retina are the key for the early diagnosis and follow-up of glaucoma patients. There are three predominant imaging technologies currently in use for the detection and progression of glaucoma, namely:

1. Scanning laser polarimetry—GDx
2. Confocal scanning laser ophthalmoscopy—Heidelberg retina tomograph (HRT)
3. Optical coherence tomography (OCT)

These imaging technologies provide objective quantitative measurements of the posterior segment structures that are involved in glaucoma.

SCANNING LASER POLARIMETRY

Scanning laser polarimetry is an objective imaging technique of the retinal nerve fiber layer (RNFL), based on retardation of the polarized light.

Evolution

The earlier versions of the instrument were equipped with a fixed corneal compensator. This was not able to adjust for the variability of the corneal thickness among different individuals. Hence with the goal of providing more reliable and reproducible measurements of the RNFL thickness, the initial versions of the device have been upgraded several times. The new generation instrument has the GDx VCC (variable corneal compensation) and the latest has the GDx ECC (enhanced corneal compensation) both from Carl Zeiss Meditec, Dublin, CA, USA.[2]

Principle

The principle used in GDx is birefringence. The birefringent intraocular tissues are cornea, lens and retina. The variable corneal compensator in GDx VCC individually corrects for the polarization induced by the cornea and lens, improving the ability of GDx to discriminate between glaucomatous and healthy eyes. GDx ECC performs significantly better than GDx VCC in glaucoma detection in patients with more severe atypical retardation patterns as seen in eyes with high myopia.[3,4]

Interpretation of the GDx VCC Report

Patient data: This contains the name, date of birth, gender, ethnicity of the patient with the ID number and date of examination (Figs. 15.1 to 15. 3).

Quality score: The image quality is shown in a box above the fundus image that ranges from scale 1 to 10. An ideal image quality score is from 7 to 10.

Fundus image: The fundus image is used to check the quality of the image, focus, illumination and proper centration of the black ring around the ONH. The calculation circle is a fixed circle centered on the ONH. The band is 0.4 mm wide and has an outer diameter of 3.2 mm and an inner diameter of 2.4 mm, which measures the temporal-superior-nasal-inferior-temporal (TSNIT) and nerve fibre indicator (NFI) parameters.

RNFL thickness map: This is a color-coded representation of the peripapillary RNFL thickness. Thick RNFLs are colored yellow, orange and red, while thinner areas are colored blue and green. A typical normal scan of vertical bow-tie pattern is the one with brighter colors in the superior and inferior quadrants corresponding to the thicker RNFL superiorly and inferiorly.

Deviation map: This map compares patient's RNFL thickness with the values derived from normative database. The map is averaged into a grid 32×32 squares, where each square is compared with age-matched normative database.

TSNIT graph: This graph demonstrates the patient's RNFL thickness as a black line drawn over a green and purple shaded area of normality for the right and left eye respectively.

TSNIT symmetry graph: The graph overlays the individual TSNIT graphs of the right and left eye.

TSNIT comparison graph and serial analysis graph: These graphs compare two or more scans of the same eye obtained on different visits. They do not appear on regular printouts.

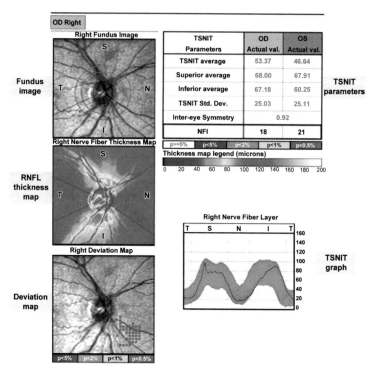

Fig. 15.1: Normal GDx VCC report—single eye.

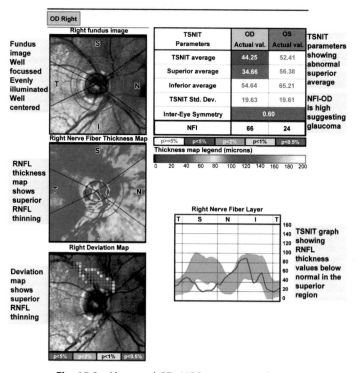

Fig. 15.2: Abnormal GDx VCC report—single eye.

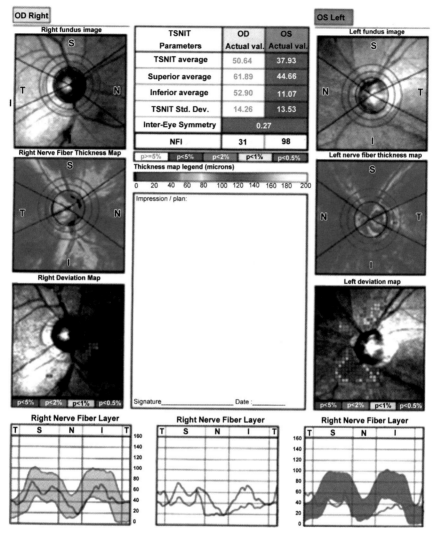

Fig. 15.3: Both eyes GDx VCC report: OD shows normal report. OS shows thinning of RNFL in the superior & inferior region, abnormal TSNIT (total, superior & inferior) average RNFL values, NFI < 50, TSNIT graph below the normal suggesting glaucoma.

TSNIT Parameters

TSNIT average: The average RNFL thickness around the entire circle.

Superior average: The average RNFL thickness in the superior 120° region of the calculation circle.

Inferior average: The average RNFL thickness in the inferior 120° region of the calculation circle.

TSNIT standard deviation: It represents the standard deviation of the overall measurements, bigger the number healthier the eye.

Intereye symmetry: It is a correlation coefficient of the total measurement from both eyes. A value close to 1 indicates high symmetry between the eyes.

Nerve fiber indicator (NFI): It is a global measure based on the entire RNFL thickness map. It is calculated using an advanced form of neural network called a support vector machine. It ranges from 0 to 100. The higher NFI reflects toward patient being glaucomatous. GDx offers the following guidelines on the NFI interpretation:

- 1 to 30: Normal
- 31 to 50: Borderline
- 51+: Abnormal

Diagnostic Accuracy

Sensitivity, specificity of GDx VCC in the early diagnosis of glaucoma ranges from 72 to 78% and 56 to 92% respectively.[5-8] The sensitivity of GDx VCC in the detection of glaucoma increased with the severity of glaucoma.

Strengths and Limitations

- GDx is easy, rapid and simple to operate
- Does not require pupillary dilatation
- Good reproducibility
- This device can only provide RNFL data
- The technique does not measure the actual RNFL value, but an inferred value
- Measures RNFL at different locations for each patient
- GDx VCC does not differentiate true biological change from variability
- It has limited use in moderate/advanced glaucoma
- It is affected by anterior and posterior segment pathology, ocular surface disorder, macular pathology, large peripapillary atrophy,[9] cataract and refractive surgery

CONFOCAL SCANNING LASER OPHTHALMOSCOPE

The confocal scanning laser ophthalmoscope (CSLO) is an imaging technology that is based on the principle of spot illumination and spot detection. HRT (Heidelberg Retinal Tomograph, Heidelberg Engineering, Germany) is the major commercially available instrument based on the principle of confocality. It gives a rapid and reproducible quantitative analysis of the optic disk parameters and RNFL.

Evolution

Confocal imaging procedures were initially developed over 30 years ago as a technique to provide optical sectioning of biologic and industrial specimens. Modified techniques have been used in ophthalmology for in-vivo corneal, retinal, and optic disk imaging. Since 1992, CSLO has been used for glaucoma diagnosis. The first commercially available instrument was the HRT, which was studied extensively in the Ocular Hypertension Treatment Study (OHTS). However, it was highly operator dependant and required fine tuning of several manual settings. The current glaucoma practice uses the HRT II and HRT III, which are designed to be more user-friendly with high precision.

Principle

HRT and HRT II use a rapid scanning 670 nm diode laser based on the principle of confocality. The emitted beam is redirected in the x-axis and y-axis along a plane of focus perpendicular to the optic axis (z-axis) using two oscillating mirrors to obtain a $15° \cdot 15°$, two-dimensional image reflected from the surface of the retina and optic disk.

In the confocal optical system, a small diaphragm placed in front of the detector at a location that is optically conjugate to focal plane of illuminating system. A luminance detector measures the light reflected from each point in the image after passing through a confocal imaging aperture. This reflected light from the focal plane, is detected only if it focuses at the level of diaphragm.

The HRT II utilizes a higher resolution of 384×384 pixels and measures a 15° scan area with higher resolution than original HRT. A typical imaging session with HRT II is done in less than 7 s, including the pre-scan and three confocal scans. It has automatic quality control measures to detect scans that are interrupted by blinks and saccades and obtains three high-quality scans. The software automatically aligns and averages the images to obtain a matrix of maximum height measurement.

Interpretation

The stepwise analysis of HRT is done in the following way (Figs. 15.4 and 15.5):
- *Patient data:* This contains the name, date of birth, gender, ethnicity of the patient with the ID number and date of examination.
- *Image quality:* If the standard deviation is equal to or less than 30 μm, it is acceptable, else the scan has to be repeated.
- *Optic disk size:* The position of the contour line in both the topographic image and in the reflectance image should be carefully evaluated. It should be placed at the inner margin of the disk margin, as the HRT parameters are calculated based on the location of the contour line. The optic disk is evaluated as small, average and large disks. The Moorfield's regression analysis (MRA) is valid only for disk size within a range of 1.2–2.8 mm². Disk size outside this range may not be represented in database, and in such cases the interpretation must be done with caution.
- *Structure of optic disk:* HRT gives a color-coded topography map of the optic disk. The cup (red) and the rim (blue and green) are represented as an overlay on the topographic image. This facilitates a quick qualitative

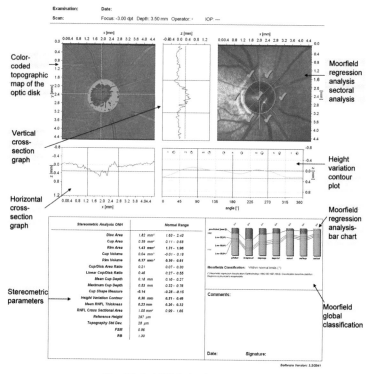

Fig. 15.4: HRT II single eye report.

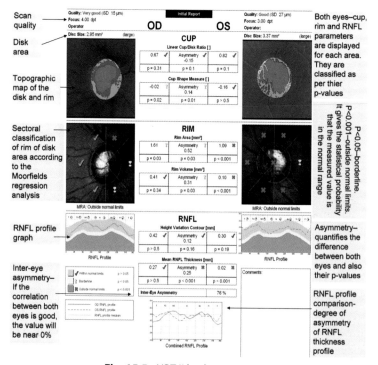

Fig. 15.5: HRT II both eyes report.

assessment of the relation of rim tissue and cup and detection of localized area of rim thinning.

- *Stereometric parameters:* The disk area, rim area and C/D ratio are more
  useful at follow-up visits to monitor progression.
- *Moorfield's regression analysis:* It is able to identify the structural damage
  by comparing the patient's data to a normative database of Caucasian eyes
  (refractive error less than 6 diopters and disk size between 1.2 and 2.8 mm^2).
  - The analysis results for each sector are indicated as overlay on the
    reflectivity image.
  - A bar diagram representing global as well as six sectors analysis of
    neuro-retinal rim to disk area ratio is also given.
    Individual values are classified as within normal limits if they are inside
    the 95% confidence interval for normality (green check), borderline
    if between 95% and 99.9% (yellow exclamation mark) and outside
    normal limits if outside the 99.9% confidence interval (red cross).
- *Height variation contour plot:* It provides useful information about status
  of RNFL. In normal subjects, the plot usually has a double hump appearance, but has wide variability. When the RNFL is lost, the nerve fiber layer
  contour line represented in green line flattens and reaches the red reference plane.

Sensitivity and Specificity

HRT is found to be sensitive and specific for glaucoma detection[10] and progression. This imaging technology has been evaluated extensively in various
studies. HRT has been used in CSLO study as an ancillary project of OHTS.[11,12]

Sensitivity and specificity of HRT in the diagnosis of healthy eyes and
glaucomatous visual field defects ranges from 77 to 92% and 81 to 97%,
respectively.[13-16]

Strengths and Limitations

- Does not need pupillary dilatation though image quality is often improved
  with dilatation in dense cataracts
- Needs only low level of illumination improving patient comfort during
  the scan
- Normative database includes a large, race-specific normal subjects
- Sophisticated analysis software for glaucoma detection and progression
- Ability to monitor quality control during image acquisition
- Most of the measurement relies on the user-defined contour line for the
  reference plane. However, in the recent HRT III, the contour line and the
  reference plane are not user defined
- The data are not reliable in disk sizes that are outside the normal range
- The stereometric measurements may be influenced by moderate changes
  in IOP[17]

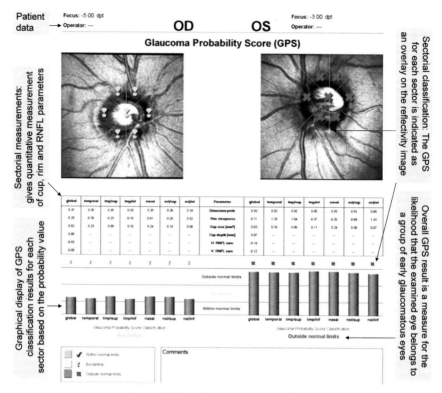

Fig. 15.6: HRT III—Glaucoma probability score.
Courtesy: www.heidelbergengineering.com

HRT III

This is the latest software version of HRT (Fig. 15. 6). This is operator independent for contour line placement as it automatically fits the ONH and the RNFL to that of a model optic disk. The technique provides stereometric data by applying an automatic model of the ONH shape.[18] These data are analyzed by a machine learning classifier and yields the glaucoma probability score (GPS). This version uses GPS for analysis instead of MRA (Table 15.1).

GPS is more advantageous in detecting early-stage glaucoma, but does not differentiate normal and ocular hypertensive eyes. It is more sensitive but less specific than MRA. The agreement between MRA and GPS was low.[20]

OPTICAL COHERENCE TOMOGRAPHY

Optical coherence tomography is a non-invasive optical imaging technology that provides high-resolution, cross sectional in-vivo images of the retina. Optical coherence tomography has the ability to scan the following three distinctive ocular structures for the detection and progression of glaucoma.
1. The peripapillary RNFL
2. The ONH and
3. The macular region

Table 15.1: Glaucoma probability score and Moorfield regression analysis.

Glaucoma probability score	Moorfield regression analysis
Operator independent	Operator dependent
Normative database—733 patients of Caucasian descent, 215 patients of African descent, and 100 Indian participants	Normative database—112 normal Caucasian eyes
Analyzes the topographic image of the optic disk, including the cup size, cup depth, rim steepness and horizontal/vertical RNFL curvature	Analyzes the logarithmic relationship between the neuro-retinal rim and optic disk areas
Reproducibility is not affected by refraction, disk size, disk characteristics like paripapillary atrophy or tilting or the severity of the glaucoma[19]	Affected by refraction and disk size

Evolution

Optical coherence tomography was first described by Huang and his associates in the year 1991.[21] Optical coherence tomography became popular in 2002 with the release of Stratus OCT, a time-domain technology (TD-OCT). Four years later, several companies started to release the next generation technology, spectral-domain OCT (SD-OCT). Currently, the most common commercially available SD-OCT devices are: Cirrus HD-OCT (Carl Zeiss Meditec, Dublin, CA, USA), RTVue-100 (Optovue Inc., Fremont, CA, USA), Spectralis OCT (Heidelberg Engineering, Heidelberg, Germany) and Topcon 3D-OCT 2000 (Topcon Corporation, Tokyo, Japan), Nidek RS-3000. The older time domain OCT machines are now being replaced by the spectral domain OCT for increased axial resolution, faster scanning speeds and improved reproducibility.[22,23] Ultrahigh-speed swept source OCT, ultrahigh-resolution OCT, adaptive optics OCT and polarization sensitive OCT are all on the horizon.

Principle of Optical Coherence Tomography

Optical coherence tomography is based on the principle of low-coherence interferometry.[24] It uses non-contact transpupillary approach to capture the images. The TD-OCT is based on the ability to discriminate the retinal layers depending on the difference in the time delay of their reflections. In SD-OCT, a dispersive detector is used to break the optical beam into light beam of different wavelengths and the scan is obtained by analyzing the interference signal based on the wavelength of light.

This section will review the practical approach towards the role of OCT in glaucoma.

Normative Database

Each machine has different glaucoma scan patterns, proprietary software segmentation algorithms and display outputs. The normative database, which is utilized for comparison of the subject's measurement to that of the normal values, varies from machine to machine. Thus the size, age limit, refractive error, ethnicity of a particular OCT machine's normative database can influence the interpretation of OCT results and the subsequent management by the clinician. Sometimes the results obtained may be statistically flagged abnormal who are not represented in the normative database. Review of literature revealed various studies conducted in different centers in India using the various spectral domain OCT machines. It revealed maximum RNFL thickness is in the inferior quadrant followed by superior, nasal and temporal quadrants supporting the ISNT (inferior ≥ superior ≥ nasal ≥ temporal) rule. The mean nerve fiber layer thickness along the circumference was also comparable.[25-28]

Patient Data

Identification of the patient data including name, sex and in particular age is vital. The results are interpreted in comparison to the age-matched controls.

Scan Quality

Particular attention to the signal strength (SS) or the scan quality index (SQI) should be given. A poor SS or SQI may make the interpretation less reliable. A simple comparison of SS between different OCT machines may not be possible as each OCT machine and their versions might vary in their image processing strategy and data analysis.

Scan quality may be influenced by age, visual acuity and extent of media opacity. The SS can range from 1 to 10, with 10 being the maximum. Signal strength of more than 5 is considered desirable.

Scan Quality Index—Optovue iVue: The good SQI is indicated in green and the poor quality in red. The scan is said to be of poor quality when they are below 40 in retina scan; below 27 in ONH scan and below 32 in ganglion cell complex (GCC) scan.

Retinal Nerve Fiber Layer Analysis

Spectral-domain OCTs are capable of segmenting the RNFL layer around the ONH and measure the area between the internal limiting membrane and the RNFL border.

The RNFL thickness map is represented in a false color scale with thickness value in reference to the normative database progressing from blue to red.

The normal pattern is a symmetrical hourglass shape of bright colors in superior and inferior quadrants corresponding to thicker RNFL in superior

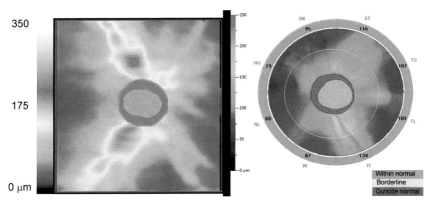

Figs. 15.7A and B: (A) Zeiss Cirrus OCT—RNFL thickness map showing nomal vertical hourglass pattern of RNFL thickness with bright colors in the superior and inferior quadrant. (B) Optovue—iVue OCT showing normal RNFL thickness map depicting the average thickness of RNFL in clock hour distribution.

and inferior quadrant and thinner RNFL in nasal and temporal quadrant (Figs. 15.7A and B).

The analysis of RNFL should include the following steps:

- Focal defects of RNFL corresponding to fundus image
- Diffuse loss
- Superior–inferior asymmetry
- Intereye asymmetry

Deviation Map

The deviation map is an estimate of deviation of the subject's RNFL thickness profile compared to the age-matched normative database. The thickness that falls below the normal range is color coded based on the probability of normality (Fig. 15.8).

TSNIT RNFL Thickness Profile

The TSNIT RNFL thickness profile is the linear representation of the RNFL thickness along the scan circle that starts temporally and then superiorly, nasally, inferiorly and ends temporally. As the RNFL is thicker in superior and inferior quadrants than nasally and temporally, the TSNIT thickness profile in a normal eye has a 'double hump' pattern. When the subject's RNFL thickness follows the pattern of normal eye it falls in the green area (representing >95 % of normal eyes), borderline loss if falling in yellow area (1–5% of normal eyes), and severe loss if falling in red (<1% of normal eyes) (Fig. 15.9).

The numerical data values of the RNFL parameters are given in the analysis. All the values are color coded according to the probability levels that are given in the print out (Fig. 15.10).

Healthy eye
RNFL deviation map

Glaucomatous eye
RNFL deviation map

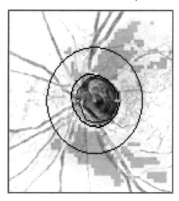

Disk center (0.21, 0.24) mm   Disk center (0.12, 0.06) mm

Fig. 15.8: Ziess Cirrus OCT—RNFL deviation map showing deviation of the subject's RNFL thickness profile compared to the age matched normative database. It is color coded based on the probability of normality when the values are less than normal range.

RNFL thickness on diameter 3.45 mm

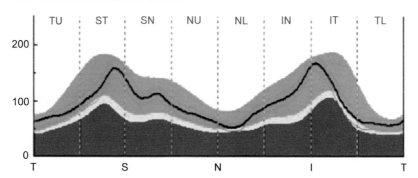

Fig. 15.9: Optovue—iVue OCT showing the TSNIT—RNFL thickness profile of a normal eye with the classic double-hump pattern.

- Average RNFL thickness—the average RNFL thickness around the entire RNFL calculation circle
- Average superior RNFL—the average RNFL thickness in the superior 120° of the scan circle
- Average inferior RNFL—the average RNFL thickness in the inferior 120° of the scan circle
- Superior–inferior difference calculates the difference between the average superior–inferior RNFL thickness
- RNFL symmetry—shows the percentage of RNFL symmetry between right and left eyes

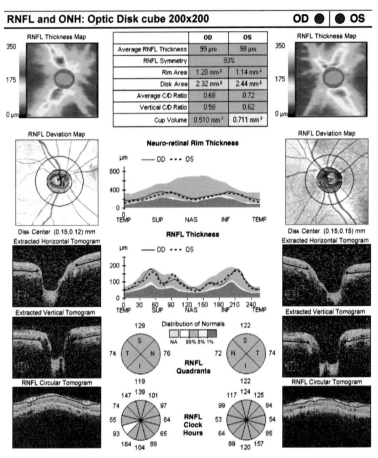

Fig. 15.10: Zeiss Cirrus OCT both eyes shows analysis of optic nerve head and peripapillary nerve fiber layers in a healthy patient.

- RNFL quadrants and RNFL clock hours—shows the average thickness along the four quadrants and 12 clock hours

   The sensitivity and specificity of various RNFL parameters in Cirrus OCT is comparable to Stratus OCT.

Optic Nerve Head Analysis

The Stratus-OCT defines the ONH margin automatically as the termination of the retinal pigment epithelium. A straight line is drawn connecting the edges of the RPE and a parallel line is constructed 150 μm anterior to this line. The neuro-retinal rim is identified as the area above this line, whereas the cup is the area located below this plane (Fig. 15.11A). A topographic image of the ONH is constructed with the optic disk borders, corresponding to the edges of the RPE, that shown in red and the cup shown in green (Fig. 15.11B).

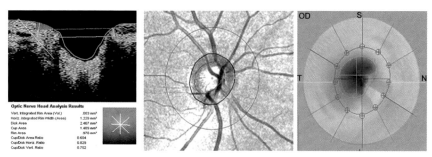

Figs. 15.11A and B: (A) Optic nerve head analysis by Stratus OCT showing a straight line drawn connecting the edges of the RPE and a parallel line is constructed 150 μm anterior to this line. The neuro-retinal rim is identified as the area above this line and the cup is the area located below this plane. (B) A topographic image of the optic nerve head is constructed with the optic disc borders, corresponding to the edges of the RPE, shown in red and the cup is shown in green.

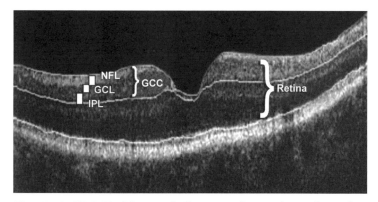

Fig. 15.12: SD-OCT of the macula illustrating the ganglion cell complex.

The SD-OCT produces high-resolution three-dimensional volume of the ONH, which can be automatically segmented to provide objective measurements of the optic cup, optic disk and the neuro-retinal rim. The optic disk is delineated as the termination of Bruch's membrane[29] and then finds the shortest perpendicular distance to the internal limiting membrane (minimum band distance) to define the inner cup margin. Each SD-OCT provides several built-in scan pattern options for imaging the ONH.

The ONH parameters that are analyzed by SD-OCT are: disk area, rim area, average CD ratio, cup volume, vertical and horizontal CD ratio.

Neuro-retinal (NRR) rim thickness profile: This is a graphical representation of the NRR thickness along the TSNIT circle. It is interpreted in the same way as RNFL thickness profile.

Ganglion Cell Complex Analysis

The GCC (Fig. 15.12) includes:
• Axons of RGC—nerve fiber layer

- The cell bodies of the RGC—inner nuclear layer
- The dendrite of RGC—inner plexiform layer Macula has the highest concentration of ganglion cells in the retina, approximately 50% of RGC of the entire retina.[30] Glaucoma affects the macular ganglion cells early in its course. The GCC becomes thinner as the ganglion cells die from glaucoma. Hence study of ganglion cell complex is very useful for the early detection and progression of glaucoma. GCC analysis directly measures the thickness of these three layers and provides an analysis of the percent loss of these layers compared to an extensive normative database. The results are presented as significant loss from normal, which makes clinical interpretation straightforward. The macular GCC parameters are able to identify early glaucoma eyes and this ability is comparable to that of the disk and RNFL parameters.[31]

In a normal eye, thickness map contains a bright 'doughnut-shaped' circular band surrounding the macula representing thick GCC from the healthy ganglion cells. It is false color coded with the color scale present in the printout. The center of the macula is thin due to absence of ganglion cells in fovea. The GCC deviation map or the GCC normative data base (NDB) reference map shows the amount of deviation of the subject's GCC thickness profile in macula from the normal values.

The Cirrus OCT (Fig. 15.13) gives the macular GCC thickness along six sectors (each 60° of the entire macular circle).

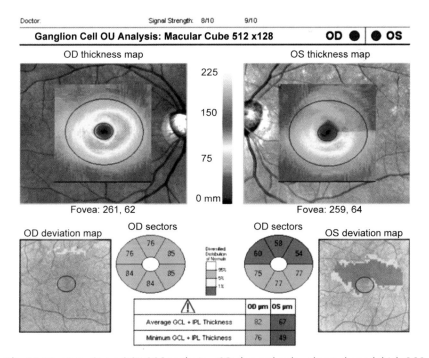

Fig. 15.13: Zeiss Cirrus OCT GCC analysis—OD shows the doughnut-shaped thick GCC around macula in a normal eye. OS shows loss of GCC in the superior quadrant in a glaucomatous eye with corresponding changes in the GCC deviation map.

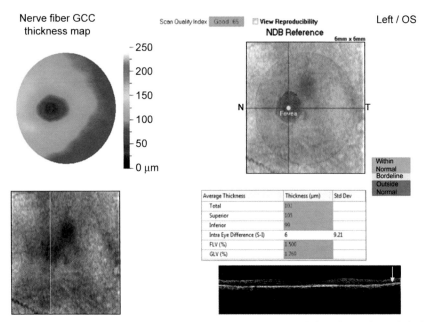

Fig. 15.14: Optovue—iVue GCC analysis showing the normal doughnut-shaped thick GCC around the macula in a normal eye.

The optovue iVue macular GCC analysis (Fig. 15.14) has the parameter table showing the total, superior and inferior average GCC thickness. Focal loss volume (FLV) percentage indicates the FLV indicating the amount of focal loss over the entire GCC map representing focal depressions. The FLV is the most accurate parameter to differentiate normal from glaucomatous eyes. Global loss volume (GLV) percentage indicates the average GCC loss over the entire GCC map representing overall depression of the GCC thickness. FLV and GLV are analog to the total and pattern deviation maps in visual field tests.

Limitations of Optical Coherence Tomography in the Diagnosis of Glaucoma

- Results are less reliable when the SS is poor[32,33]
- RNFL thickness values are affected by age,[34] axial length, disk size and tilt
- When the scan circle is not centered on the optic disk, it can lead to erroneous measurements
- During eye blinking or saccade when acquiring scan, the alignment of the scans is improper, leading to unreliable RNFL measurements
- Conditions that lead on to segmentation error should be ruled out[35] (e.g., ERM, disk edema)
- Age-related loss can confound with the identification of glaucoma progression

Floor Effect

Optical coherence tomography is a very useful tool for assessing early to moderate glaucoma but in advanced glaucomatous disease, SD-OCT is clinically less useful due to the 'floor-effect.' The RNFL is not only made up of retinal ganglion cells but also contains blood vessels and supporting cells like glial and Muller cells. Therefore, in advanced glaucomatous eye disease, the RNFL thickness levels off and rarely falls below 40–50 μm due to the assumed presence of the residual glial and non-neural tissue including the blood vessels.[36]

Role of Imaging in Follow-up

The detection of progression of glaucoma is critical as glaucoma is a slowly progressing optic neuropathy and thus identification of glaucomatous changes is essential for glaucoma management. These imaging instruments take multiple scans at baseline and at each follow-up, providing reproducible data of the ONH and RNFL changes, both globally and regionally. The GDx-GPA, HRT-topographic change analysis (TCA) and OCT-GPA are studied to be highly sensitive in detecting the glaucoma progression by the ONH and RNFL parameters, especially in eyes showing progression based on stereo-photographic images and visual field analysis than in non-progressing eyes.[37,38]

SCANNING LASER POLARIMETRY

Serial Analysis

The serial analysis printout has five elements (Fig. 15.15) that should be considered when assessing RNFL change over time.
* Thickness map
* Deviation map
* Deviation from reference maps
* Parameters
* TSNIT graphs

Serial analysis can compare upto four examinations. The first examination is the baseline or reference examination and follow-up examinations are compared to the baseline. The deviation from reference map displays the RNFL difference pixel by pixel of the follow-up examinations compared to the baseline examination. A colored rectangular box to the left side of the thickness map contains the date and quality score of each examination. The same color is used in the TSNIT graph to indicate the TSNIT curve of that examination.

The deviation from reference map shows the RNFL difference of the follow-up examination compared to the baseline examination. If the difference exceeds 20 μm, the pixel is color coded. The areas of RNFL change shown on the deviation from reference map will frequently correspond to the

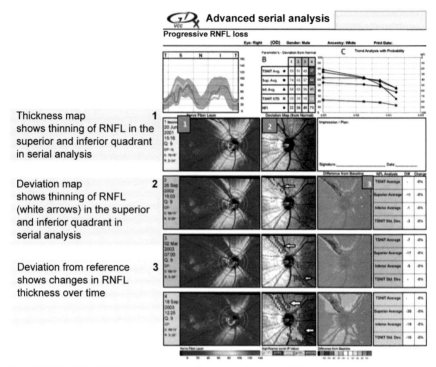

Fig. 15.15: GDx VCC Serial Analysis shows progressive RNFL loss as depicted in the Trend analysis and Nerve fiber layer analysis.
Courtesy: Carl Zeiss Meditec.

areas of loss detected by the deviation map. This is because the 'deviation map' shows loss compared to the normative database while the 'deviation from reference maps' shows RNFL change over time in the same eye. The TSNIT curves are overlaid on the shaded area representing the normal range for the patient's age. RNFL loss will result in a lower TSNIT curve on the follow-up examination compared to the baseline examination.

GDx-Guided Progression Analysis

The GDx VCC guided progression analysis (GPA) is a software that evaluates and compares progression over time and determines whether the difference is statistically significant. GDx GPA reports progression of glaucoma as:

- 'Possible progression' when significant change is detected once
- 'Likely progression' when significant reduction is detected in at least two consecutive examinations and
- 'Possible increase' if an increase in RNFL thickness is detected

Progression analysis has two modes: fast and extended mode. Fast mode is for analyzing data sets that include single measurements. It compares change to a predetermined average measurement variability derived from a

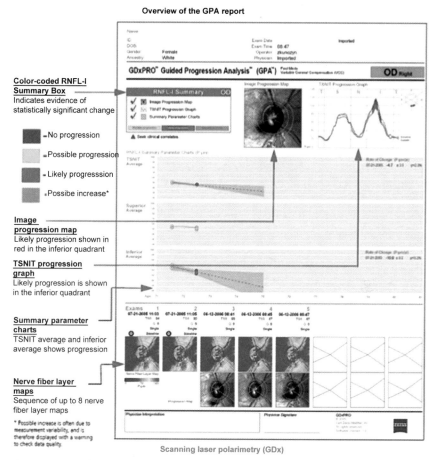

Fig. 15.16: Guided progression analysis for GDx shows Likely progression depicted in red in the inferior quadrant suggestive of glaucoma progression.

sample population. In contrast, extended mode requires the mean of three measurements and GPA calculates the individual measurement variability of each eye for a selected patient. It measures and detects the progression based on three different parts of the analysis (Fig. 15.16):

1. Image progression map
2. TSNIT progression graph
3. Summary parameters charts

Image progression map recognizes the change in the reflectance image. The minimal cluster size considered is 150 pixels, which is 2% of the image size. Possible progression areas are shown in yellow, likely progression areas in red and possible increase areas in purple. It can detect narrower and deeper defects.

TSNIT Progression Graph: The ring around the optic nerve is divided into 64 equal segments and compared on follow-up. If three adjacent segments show significant change on follow-up, the progression is indicated. Areas between current baseline set and current examination that report significant change are displayed with possible progression in yellow, likely progression in red and possible increase in purple. This detects shallower and broader defects.

Summary Parameter Charts: The TSNIT average, superior average and inferior average are compared. On the chart, regression line is drawn to show likely progression and $P < 5\%$. This can detect diffuse changes in the RNFL. This parameter can also compare the rate of progression before and after treatment, thus helpful for guiding the treatment protocol.

CONFOCAL SCANNING LASER OPHTHALMOSCOPE

The two progression algorithms available with HRT are:
1. Trend analysis
2. Topographical change analysis

HRT Trend Analysis

The trend analysis compares the global and stereometric summary indices from the baseline examination to that of the follow-up visits (Fig. 15.17A). The analysis is represented graphically as the normalized change from the baseline over time. The changes in volume (red line) and area (blue line) of the neuroretinal rim are displayed as two independent lines. The changes in volume are represented in red triangles and the changes in area are represented in blue squares along the y-axis. The examination date is represented along the x-axis.

HRT Topographic Change Analysis

Topographic change analysis (TCA) gives a quantitative change analysis within the disk margin contour and analyzes the changes in the topographical height of the HRT image at the super pixel level. The HRT images of at least three examinations (baseline and two or three follow-up exams) are compared. Before the analysis, these images are automatically aligned.

Change probability map: The statistical method estimates the probability of the difference in heights between the baseline and follow-up and generates a 'change probability map.' It shows significant and repeatable changes in picture elements over the topographic map, with red pixels representing height depression and green pixels representing significant elevation.

TCA change summary parameters can be used to describe size and location of regions of change. The color intensity reflects the extent of change measured.

Studies suggest that HRT-TCA analysis may be helpful in detecting more subtle change in glaucoma patients for assessing progression earlier than stereo-photographic assessment and visual field analysis.[39]

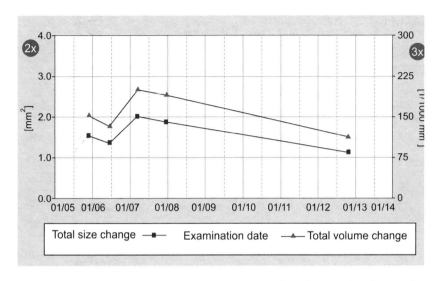

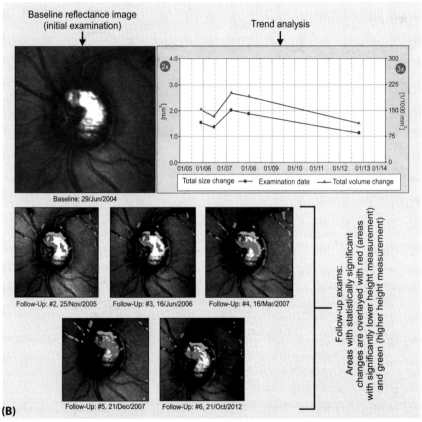

Figs. 15.17A and B: (A) HRT II—Trend analysis—shows the development of the entity of all red marked clusters over time. Changes in volume and area are displayed separately as two independent lines. (B) Topographic change analysis (TCA) shows statistically significant progression in the areas overlayed with red.

Limitation of HRT-TCA

The standard stereographic follow-up assessment of the optic disk examines nerve fiber layer defects, peripapillary hemorrhages and rim loss whereas the TCA analyzes the surface changes, which is not easily identified by disk stereophotograph. This suggests that visual fields, stereophotographs and the TCA should be used in complementary fashion.

OPTICAL COHERENCE TOMOGRAPHY

Guided Progression Analysis

Spectral-domain OCT[40-46] is more sensitive in identifying progression than TD-OCT.[47-49]

Among the SD-OCT devices that are manufactured by several companies, only Cirrus OCT and Optovue iVue currently offer progression analysis as part of their commercially available software. With guided progression analysis, Cirrus OCT can perform event analysis and trend analysis of RNFL thickness and ONH parameters. Event analysis assesses change from baseline compared to expected variability. If change is outside the range of expected variability, it is identified as progression. Trend analysis looks at the rate of change over time, using linear regression to determine rate of change. Figure 15.18 illustrates the interpretation of the Cirrus OCT guided progression analysis map.

The progression analysis offered by the Optovue–iVue (Fig. 15.19) includes side-by-side RNFL thickness measurements and overlay of the RNFL profiles for the consecutive scans. Similar reports are also provided for ganglion cell complex thickness (Fig. 15.20) along with thickness change plots. Changes are presented in a similar fashion for the ganglion cell complex of the macula. However, a formal statistical analysis of change over time is not currently included in the latest version of the software for this device (version 6.1).

Figures 15.21 to 15.31 illustrate clinical examples that depicting the structure–function correlation of the ONH and the retina in the diagnosis and follow-up of glaucoma.

Figure 15.21 depicts the structure–function correlation of a diabetic patient with pre-perimetric glaucoma. He presented with IOP of 26 mm Hg, central corneal thickness (CCT) of 501 μm, fundus examination showing vertical cup disk ratio (VCDR) of 0.7 with normal reliable visual fields by Humphrey visual field analyzer and thinning of RNFL at superotemporal quadrant by Optovue iVue SD OCT.

Figure 15.22 portrays the details of a patient with primary open angle glaucoma with IOP of 24 mm Hg, fundus showing VCDR 0.6 with disk hemorrhage, superior wedge-shaped RNFL defect and focal thinning of supero-temporal neuroretinal rim. Visual field shows early field defect. OCT-ONH analysis shows borderline changes in the supero-temporal quadrant with corresponding depression in the TSNIT graph and GCC thickness.

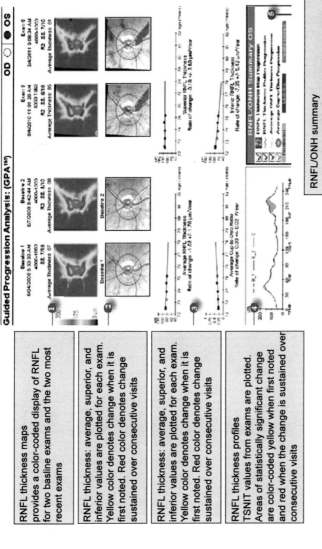

Fig. 15.18: Cirrus SD OCT—Guided Progression Analysis: RNFL thickness maps show gradual progression in the infero-temporal region (yellow and red sectors). The infero-temporal progression is also notable in the RNFL thickness profiles (red). Average RNFL thickness plots show statistically significant thinning in the overall, superior and inferior RNFL thickness.

Courtesy: www.zeiss.com.

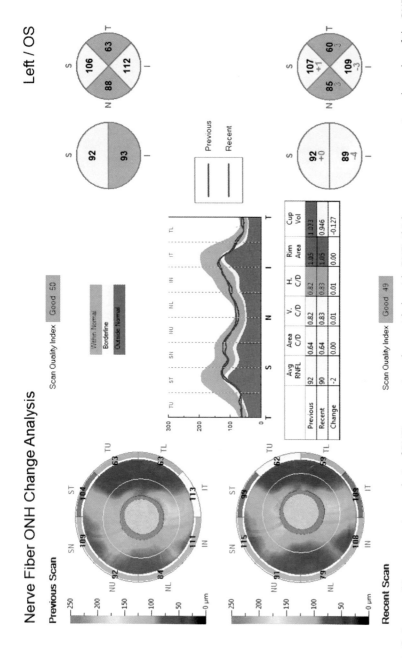

Fig. 15.19: Optovue—iVue progression analysis of RNFL parameters shows side by side RNFL thickness measurements and overlay of the RNFL profiles of the consecutive scans.

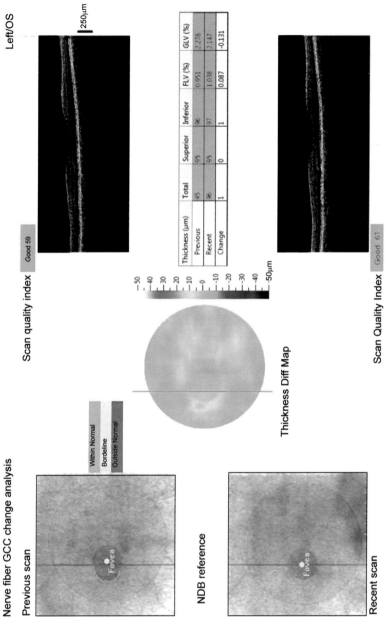

Fig. 15.20: Optovue—iVue progression analysis of ganglion cell complex.

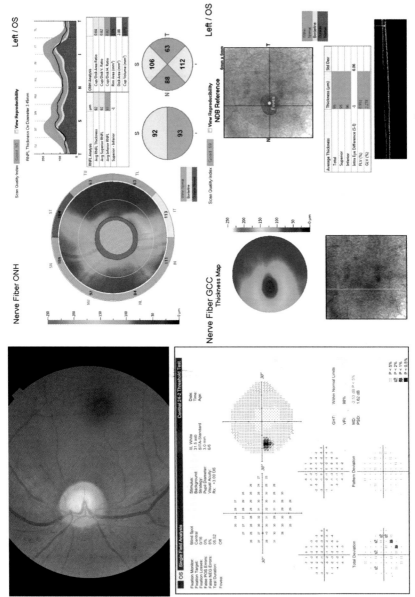

Fig. 15.21: Fundus photo, visual fields and OCT of a patient with pre-perimetric glaucoma.

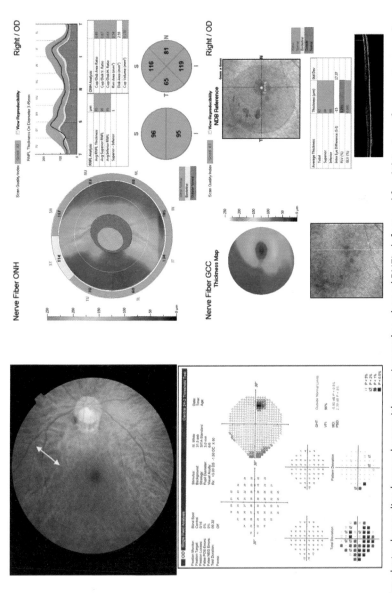

Fig. 15.22: Fundus photo shows disc hemorrhage with superior wedge-shaped RNFL defect and focal thinning of supero-temporal neuroretinal rim. Visual field shows early field defect. OCT-ONH analysis shows borderline changes in the supero-temporal quadrant with corresponding depression in the TSNIT graph and GCC thickness.

Figure 15.23 reveals fundus photograph showing myopic disk with thinning of inferior neuroretinal rim and early superior scotoma with borderline changes in OCT suggesting early glaucomatous damage.

Figure 15.24 shows the fundus photograph with increased VCDR, superior wedge-shaped RNFL defect with thinning of superior and inferior neuroretinal rim. Visual field shows inferior arcuate scotoma with areas of depressed sensitivity along the superior area. OCT ONH analysis shows reduction in superior and inferior RNFL thickness with depressed TSNIT graph and corresponding reduction of GCC thickness.

Figure 15.25 depicts the structure–function correlation details of a patient with normotensive glaucoma. Patient was a diabetic and hypertensive on treatment. Fundus photograph shows inferior notching with peripapillary atrophy more in the inferior quadrant. Visual field shows superior arcuate scotoma. Nidek RS 3000 OCT ONH analysis shows reduction in RNFL thickness in the inferotemporal clock hour with corresponding depressed TSNIT graph.

Figure 15.26 depicts the structure–function details of an 18-year-old patient with myopia and pigmentary glaucoma. Fundus photograph shows VCDR 0.7 with wedge-shaped inferior RNFL defect. Visual field shows superior scotoma. Optovue iVue OCT ONH analysis shows reduction in RNFL thickness in the inferior quadrant with corresponding depression in the TSNIT graph and reduction of GCC thickness.

Figure 15.27 shows the details of a diabetic patient who came to the glaucoma clinic with IOP of 28 mm Hg in both eyes, right eye fundus photograph shows thinning of inferior neuroretinal rim. Visual field shows corresponding scotoma in the superior quadrant. OCT ONH analysis depicts reduction of inferior RNFL thickness with corresponding depression in the TSNIT graph and NDB map.

Figure 15.28 reveals structure–function correlation of the same patient, left eye fundus photograph shows increased VCDR with thinning of inferior neuroretinal rim. Visual field shows superior arcuate scotoma. OCT ONH analysis depicts reduction of inferior RNFL thickness with corresponding depression in the TSNIT graph and reduction of GCC thickness.

Figure 15.29 shows a fundus photograph of a patient depicting enlarged VCDR of 0.7 with thinning of superior and inferior neuroretinal rim. Visual field shows a corresponding superior and inferior arcuate scotoma. OCT ONH analysis shows reduction in superior and inferior RNFL thickness with depressed TSNIT graph and corresponding reduction of GCC thickness is noted in the NDB map.

Figure 15.30 depicts the fundus photograph showing increased VCDR with thinning of superior and inferior neuroretinal rim. Visual field shows a corresponding superior arcuate scotoma with areas of depressed sensitivity along the inferior arcuate area. OCT ONH analysis shows reduction in superior and inferior RNFL thickness with depressed TSNIT graph and corresponding reduction of GCC thickness.

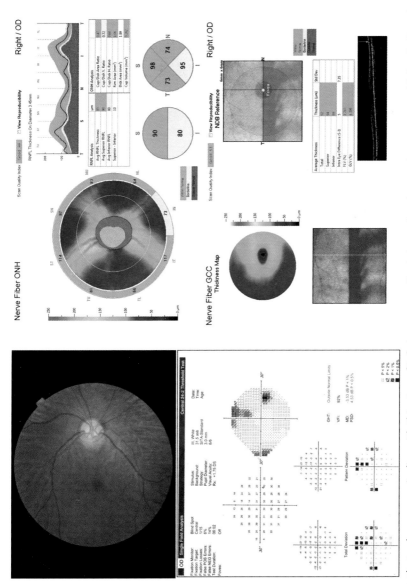

Fig. 15.23: Fundus photo shows myopic disc with thinning of inferior neuro-retinal rim and early superior scotoma with borderline changes in OCT suggesting early glaucomatous damage.

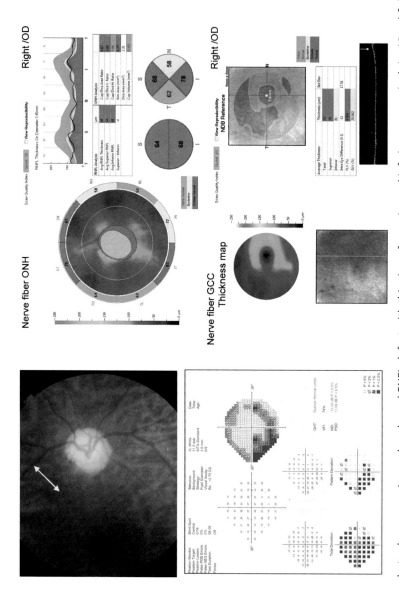

Fig. 15.24: Fundus photo shows superior wedge-shaped RNFL defect with thinning of superior and inferior neuro-retinal rim. Visual field shows inferior arcuate scotoma with areas of depressed sensitivity along the superior area. OCT ONH analysis shows reduction in superior and inferior RNFL thickness with depressed TSNIT graph and corresponding reduction of GCC thickness.

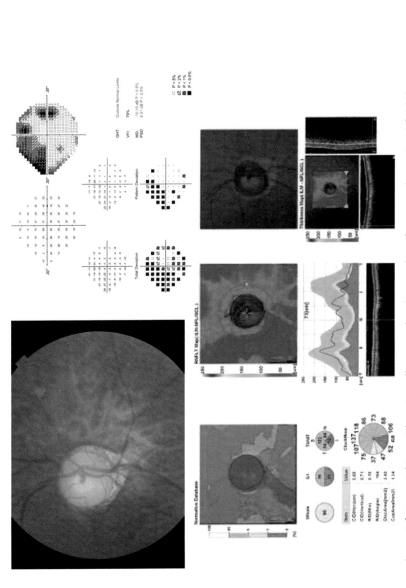

Fig. 15.25: Fundus photo shows inferior notching with peripapillary atrophy more in the inferior quadrant. Visual field shows superior arcuate scotoma. OCT ONH analysis shows reduction in RNFL thickness in the inferotemporal clock hour with corresponding depressed TSNIT graph.

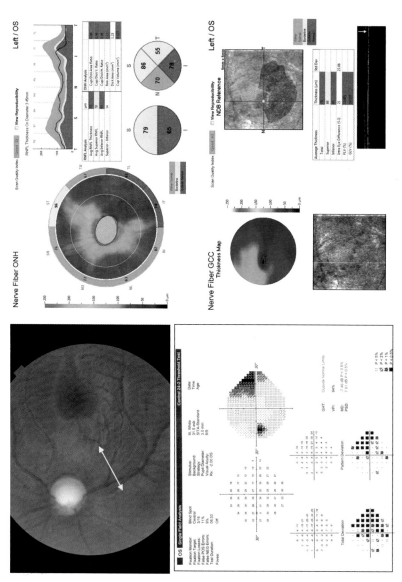

Fig. 15.26: Fundus photo shows VCD ratio 0.7 with wedge-shaped inferior RNFL defect. Visual field shows superior scotoma. OCT ONH analysis shows reduction in RNFL thickness in the inferior quadrant with corresponding depression in the TSNIT graph and reduction of GCC thickness.

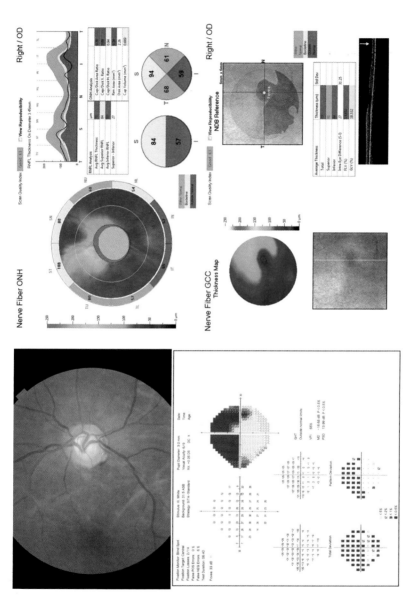

Fig. 15.27: Fundus photo shows thinning of inferior neuroretinal rim. Visual field shows scotoma in the superior quadrant. OCT ONH analysis depicts reduction of inferior RNFL thickness with corresponding depression in the TSNIT graph and NDB map.

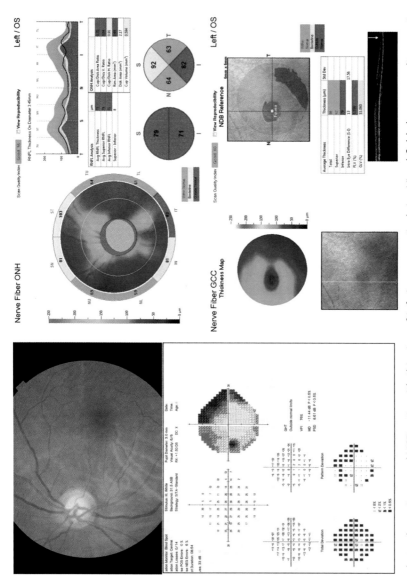

Fig. 15.28: Fundus photo shows increased VCD ratio with thinning of inferior neuroretinal rim. Visual field shows superior arcuate scotoma. OCT ONH analysis depicts reduction of inferior RNFL thickness with corresponding depression in the TSNIT graph & reduction of GCC thickness is noted in NDB map.

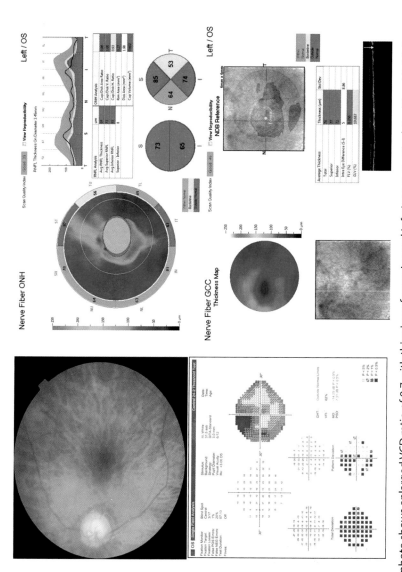

Fig. 15.29: Fundus photo shows enlarged VCD ratio of 0.7 with thinning of superior and inferior neuroretinal rim. Visual field shows a corresponding superior and inferior arcuate scotoma. OCT ONH analysis shows reduction in superior and inferior RNFL thickness with depressed TSNIT graph and corresponding reduction of GCC thickness is noted in NDB map.

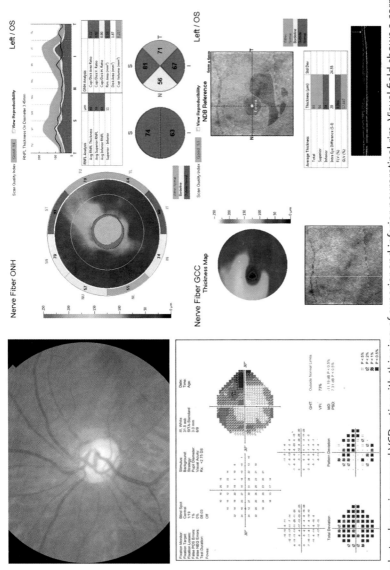

Fig. 15.30: Fundus photo shows increased VCD ratio with thinning of superior and inferior neuroretinal rim. Visual field shows a corresponding superior arcuate scotoma with areas of depressed sensitivity along the inferior arcuate area. OCT ONH analysis shows reduction in superior and inferior RNFL thickness with depressed TSNIT graph and corresponding reduction of GCC thickness.

Figure 15.31 portrays the details of a patient who underwent glaucoma surgery prior with controlled IOP. Fundus photograph shows enlarged VCDR of 0.8 with thinning of superior and inferior neuroretinal rim. Visual field shows severe visual field loss. OCT ONH analysis shows reduction in superior, nasal and inferior RNFL thickness with severely depressed TSNIT graph.

FUTURE DEVELOPMENTS IN GLAUCOMA IMAGING

Swept-source OCT (SS-OCT)

Swept-source OCT is the latest milestone in retina, choroid and ONH imaging. It differs from SD-OCT (Table 15.2).

The widefield scan of SS-OCT enables the view of macula and ONH simultaneously, helping to understand the relationship of macular damage and ONH damage in glaucoma. It displays the RNFL thickness data across 12×9 mm grid format. SS-OCT also gives in vivo study of the lamina cribrosa. The histological studies suggest that the lamina cribrosa can undergo morphological changes in glaucomatous eyes. Thinning and the posterior displacement of lamina have been observed and are thought to be a result of raised intraocular pressure.[50] The three-dimensional SS-OCT imaging allows visualization of the lamina cribrosa defects, which may be more prevalent in eyes with longer axial length and related to disk hemorrhages.[51]

Longer Wavelength OCT

Currently, clinical OCT imaging of the retina mainly occurs at wavelengths in the 800–870 nm range; however, the melanin contained in the retinal pigment epithelial (RPE) is highly scattering and absorbing in this range of wavelength,[52] making it difficult to image structures below this tissue layer, such as the choroid and choriocapillaris. Additionally, due to the rapid signal drop off, the penetration of light into the ONH is limited. Current research is focused on exploring OCT imaging at wavelengths of 1000–1100 nm to achieve deeper imaging capabilities, and allow penetration below the RPE. Long-wavelength imaging may also improve OCT signal quality in patients with media opacity.[53,54] High-speed retinal OCT in the 1000–1100 nm wavelength range has been shown to allow the imaging of choroidal layers. Therefore, it is helpful in the evaluation of glaucoma and age-related macular degeneration.[55]

Adaptive Optic OCT (AO-OCT)

Early detection of axonal tissue loss is critical for managing diseases that destroy the RNFL such as glaucoma. Adaptive optic-OCT systems have been used to capture volume images of retinal structures that were previously visible only with histology. Examples include the bundles within the RNFL; retinal microvasculature such as the capillaries that form the rim of the foveal avascular

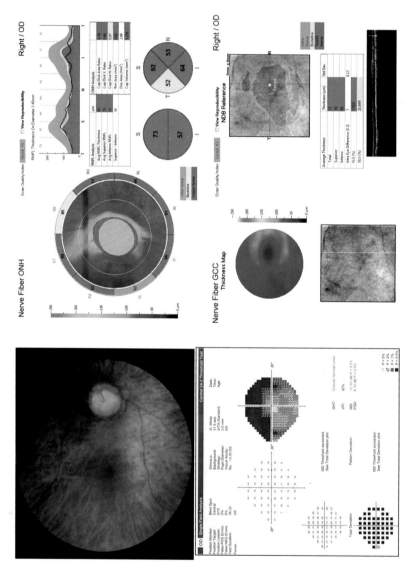

Fig. 15.31: Fundus photo shows enlarged VCD ratio of 0.8 with thinning of superior and inferior neuroretinal rim. Visual field shows severe visual field loss. OCT ONH analysis shows reduction in superior, nasal and inferior RNFL thickness with severely depressed TSNIT graph.

Table15.2: Difference between Swept-source OCT and SD-OCT.

	Swept source OCT	**Spectral domain OCT**
Wavelength	1050 nm	840 nm
Laser source	Short-cavity swept laser	Superluminescent diode laser
Scan speed	100000 A-scans/sec	50000 A-scans/sec
Field of scan	12 mm	6–9 mm
Field of view	Optic nerve and macula on the same scan	Optic and macula not possible on the same scan
Depth of image	Deeper choroidal layers and lamina cribrosa visible	Only till RPE layer

zone (FAZ); microstructures in the ganglion cell layer and Henle's fiber layer; the 3D photoreceptor mosaic; retinal pigment epithelium; and the tiny pores of the lamina cribrosa of the optical nerve. Adaptive optic–OCT represents a potential means to measure cross-sectional retinal nerve fiber bundles (RNFB) dimensions, owing to its micron-level 3D resolution.[56] The technical benefits of adding AO to OCT are increased lateral resolution, smaller speckle and enhanced sensitivity there by increasing the imaging capability of the OCT.

The volume of retinal tissue visualized by AO-OCT is shown as a composite that is made by reimaging the same retinal patch, with focus systematically shifted to different depths. In this way, it preserves the high image quality provided by AO for the retinal layer of interest. Extracted en face slices are shown of individual RNFBs, microstructures in the ganglion cell layer, retinal capillaries, and outer segments of cone photoreceptors.

Polarization-sensitive OCT (PS-OCT)

Polarization-sensitive OCT extends the concept of OCT and utilizes the information that is carried by polarized light to obtain additional information on the tissue. Several structures in the eye like cornea, RNFL and retinal pigment epithelium alter the polarization state of the light and therefore show a tissue-specific contrast in PS-OCT images. In PS-OCT images of the eye, birefringent structures like the RNFL, depolarizing tissues like the retinal pigment epithelium and polarization preserving structures like the photoreceptor layer, can be distinguished.[57]

OCT Angiography: ANGIO-VUE

It is a noninvasive technique that acquires volumetric angiographic information without the use of dye. The en-face images (OCT angiograms) images are obtained and they can be analyzed layerwise from internal limiting membrane to the choroid along with the vascular plexus. It employs motion contrast imaging to high-resolution volumetric blood flow information generating angiographic images.

In patients with glaucoma, it is useful in evaluating the optic disk perfusion, which shows attenuation in both superficial disk vasculature as well as the microvascular network along the lamina cribrosa. In eyes with glaucoma, the flow index is reduced, which is obtained by averaging the de correlation signal and the area of microvasculature. The flow index has been shown to have both a very high sensitivity and specificity in differentiating glaucomatous eyes from normal eyes.[58,59]

REFERENCES

1. Simmons ST. American Academy of Ophthalmology. Basic and clinical science course, Glaucoma Section 10, 2005-2006.
2. Vizzeri G, Kjaergaard SM, Rao HL, et al. Role of imaging in glaucoma diagnosis and follow-up. Indian J Ophthalmol. 2011;59(Suppl S1):59-68.
3. Medeiros FA, Bowd C, Zangwill LM, et al. Detection of glaucoma using scanning laser polarimetry with enhanced corneal compensation. Invest Ophthalmol Vis Sci. 2007;48(7):3146–53.
4. Reus NJ, Zhou Q, Lemij HG. Enhanced imaging algorithm for scanning laser polarimetry with variable corneal compensation. Invest Ophthalmol Vis Sci. 2006;47(9):3870-7.
5. Bowd C, Zangwill LM, Berry CC, et al. Detecting early glaucoma by assessment of retinal nerve fiber layer thickness and visual function. Invest Ophthalmol Vis Sci. 2001;42(9):1993-2003.
6. Da Pozzo S, Fuser M, Vattovani O, et al. GDx-VCC performance in discriminating normal from glaucomatous eyes with early visual field loss. Graefes Arch clin Exp Ophthalmol. 2006;244(6):689-95.
7. Brusini P, Salvetat ML, Parisi L, et al. Discrimination between normal and early glaucomatous eyes with scanning laser polarimeter with fixed and variable corneal compensator settings. Eur J Ophthalmol. 2005;15(4): 468-76.
8. Tjon-Fo-Sang MJ, Lemij HG. The sensitivity and specificity of nerve fiber layer measurements in glaucoma as determined with scanning laser polarimetry. Am J Ophthalmol. 1997;123(1):62-9.
9. Ramakrishnan R, Krishnadas SR, Khrana M, et al. Diagnosis and Management of Glaucoma. New Delhi: Jaypee Brothers; 2013.
10. Wollstein G, Garway-Heath DF, Hitchings RA. Identification of early glaucoma cases with the scanning laser ophthalmoscope. Ophthalmology. 1998; 105(8):1557-63.
11. Zangwill LM, Weinreb RN, Berry CC, et al. The confocal scanning laser ophthalmoscopy ancillary study to the ocular hypertension treatment study: study design and baseline factors. Am J Ophthalmol. 2004;137(2): 219-27.
12. Zangwill LM, Weinreb RN, Berry CC, et al. Racial differences in optic disc topography: baseline results from the confocal scanning laser ophthalmoscopy ancillary study to the ocular hypertension treatment study. Arch Ophthalmol. 2004;122(1):22-8.

13. Mikelberg FS, Parfitt CM, Swindale NV, et al. Ability of the Heidelberg Retina Tomograph to detect early glaucomatous visual field loss. J Glaucoma. 1995;4(4):242-7.

14. Uchida H, Brigatti L, Caprioli J. Detection of structural damage from glaucoma with confocal laser image analysis. Invest Ophthalmol Vis Sci. 1996;37(12):2393-401.

15. Caprioli J, Park HJ, Ugurlu S, et al. Slope of the peripapillary nerve fiber layer surface in glaucoma. Invest Ophthalmol Vis Sci. 1998;39(12):2321-8.

16. Bathija R, Zangwill L, Berry CC, et al. Detection of early glaucomatous structural damage with confocal scanning laser tomography. J Glaucoma. 1998;7(2):121-7.

17. Bowd C, Weinreb RN, Lee B, et al. Optic disk topography after medical treatment to reduce intraocular pressure. Ophthalmol Vis Sci. 2000;41(3);775-82.

18. Swindale NV, Stjepanovic G, Chin A, et al. Automated analysis of normal and glaucomatous optic nerve head topography images. Invest Ophthalmol Vis Sci. 2000;41(7):1730-42.

19. Taibbi G, Fogagnolo P, Orzalesi N, et al. Reproducibility of the Heidelberg Retina Tomograph III Glaucoma Probability Score. J Glaucoma. 2009;18(3):247-52.

20. Moreno-Montañés J, Antón A, García N, et al. Glaucoma probability score vs Moorfields classification in normal, ocular hypertensive, and glaucomatous eyes. Am J Ophthalmol. 2008;145(2):360-8.

21. Fujimoto JG, Pitris C, Boppart SA et al. Optical coherence tomography: an emerging technology for biomedical imaging and optical biopsy. Neoplasia. 2000;2(1-2):9-25.

22. Nassif N, Cense B, Park BH, et al. In vivo human retinal imaging by ultra-high-speed spectral domain optical coherence tomography. Opt Lett. 2004;29(5):480-2.

23. Wojtkowski M, Srinivasan V, Ko T, et al. Ultra-high resolution, high speed, Fourier domain optical coherence tomography and methods of dispersion compensation. Opt Exp. 2004;12(11):2404-22.

24. Huang D, Swanson EA, Lin CP, et al. Optical coherence tomography. Science. 1991;254(5053):1178-181.

25. Mansoori T, Viswanath K, Balakrishna N, et al. Quantification of retinal nerve fiber layer thickness using spectral domain optical coherence tomography in normal Indian population. Indian J Ophthalmol. 2012;60(6):555-8.

26. Sowmya V, Venkataramanan VR, Vishnu Prasad KP. Analysis of retinal nerve fiber layer thickness using optical coherence tomography in normal South Indian population. Muller J Med Sci Res. 2014;5:5-10.

27. Appukuttan B, Giridhar A, Gopalakrishnan M. et al. Normative spectral domain optical coherence tomography data on macular and retinal nerve fiber layer thickness in Indians. Indian J Ophthalmol. 2014;62:316-21.

28. Pawar N, Maheshwari D, Ravindran M, et al. Retinal nerve fiber layer thickness in normal Indian pediatric population measured with optical coherence tomography. Indian J Ophthalmol. 2014;62:412-8.

29. Strouthidis NG, Yang H, Reynaud J, et al. Comparison of clinical and spectral domain optical coherence tomography optic disc margin anatomy. Invest Ophthalmol Vis Sci. 2009;50(10):4709-18.
30. Curcio CA, Allen KA. Topography of ganglion cells in human retina. J Comp Neurol. 1990;300(1):5-25.
31. Mwanza JC, Durbin MK, Budenz DI, et al. Glaucoma diagnostic accuracy of ganglion cell–inner plexiform layer thickness: Comparison with nerve fiber layer and optic nerve head. Ophthalmology. 2012;119(6):1151-8.
32. Wu Z, Vazeen M, Varma R, et al. Factors associated with variability in retinal nerve fiber layer thickness measurements obtained by optical coherence tomography. Ophthalmology. 2007;114(8):1505-12.
33. Wu Z, Huang J, Dustin L, et al. Signal strength is an important determinant of accuracy of nerve fiber layer thickness measurement by optical coherence tomography. J Glaucoma. 2009;18(3):213-6.
34. Lee JY, Hwang YH, Lee SM, et al. Age and retinal nerve fiber layer thickness measured by spectral domain optical coherence tomography. Korean J Ophthalmol. 2012;26(3):163-8.
35. Kim YW, Jeoung JW, Yu HG. Vitreopapillary traction in eyes with idiopathic epiretinal membrane: a spectral-domain optical coherence tomography study. Ophthalmology. 2014;121(10):1976-82.
36. Hood DC, Kardon RH. A framework for comparing structural and functional measures of glaucomatous damage. Progress in retinal and eye research. 2007;26(6):688-710.
37. Medeiros FA, Zangwill LM, Alencar LM, et al. Detection of glaucoma progression using stratus OCT retinal nerve fiber layer, optic nerve head and macular thickness measurements. Invest Ophthalmol Vis Sci. 2009;50(12):5741-8.
38. Strouthidis NG, Scott A, Peter NM, et al. Optic disc and visual field progression in ocular hypertensive subjects: detection rates, specificity, and agreement. Invest Ophthalmol Vis Sci. 2006;47(7):2904-10.
39. Bowd C, Balasubramanian M, Weinreb RN, et al. Performance of confocal scanning laser tomograph topographic change analysis (TCA) for assessing glaucomatous progression. Invest Ophthalmol Vis Sci. 2009;50(2):691-701.
40. Garas A, Vargha P, Hollo G. Reproducibility of retinal nerve fiber layer and macular thickness measurement with the RTVue-100 optical coherence tomograph. Ophthalmology. 2010;117(4):738-46.
41. Gonzalez-Garcia AO, Vizzeri G, Bowd C, et al. Reproducibility of RTVue retinal nerve fiber layer thickness and optic disc measurements and agreement with Stratus optical coherence tomography measurements. Am J Ophthalmol. 2009;147(6):1067-74.
42. Lee SH, Kim SH, Kim TW, et al. Reproducibility of retinal nerve fiber thickness measurements using the test-retest function of spectral OCT/SLO in normal and glaucomatous eyes. J Glaucoma. 2010;19(9):637-42.
43. Li JP, Wang XZ, Fu J, et al. Reproducibility of RTVue retinal nerve fiber layer thickness and optic nerve head measurements in normal and glaucoma eyes. Chin Med J (Engl). 2010;123:1898-1903.
44. Mwanza JC, Chang RT, Budenz DL, et al. Reproducibility of peripapillary retinal nerve fiber layer thickness and optic nerve head parameters measured

with CirrusTM HD-OCT in glaucomatous eyes. Invest Ophthalmol Vis Sci. 2010;51(11):5724-30.

45. Menke MN, Knecht P, Sturm V, et al. Reproducibility of nerve fiber layer thickness measurements using 3D fourier-domain OCT. Invest Ophthalmol Vis Sci. 2008;49:5386-91.

46. Schuman JS. Spectral domain optical coherence tomography for glaucoma (an AOS thesis). Trans Am Ophthalmol Soc. 2008;106:426-58.

47. Leung CK, Chiu V, Weinreb RN, et al. Evaluation of retinal nerve fiber layer progression in glaucoma: a comparison between spectral-domain and time-domain optical coherence tomography. Ophthalmology 2011;118(8):1558-62.

48. Leung CK, Cheung CY, Weinreb RN, et al. Retinal nerve fiber layer imaging with spectral-domain optical coherence tomography: a variability and diagnostic performance study. Ophthalmology. 2009;116(7):1257-63.

49. Kim JS, Ishikawa H, Sung KR, et al. Retinal nerve fibre layer thickness measurement reproducibility improved with spectral domain optical coherence tomography. Br J Ophthalmol. 2009;93(8):1057-63.

50. Bellezza AJ, Rintalan CJ, Thompson HW, et al. Deformation of the lamina cribrosa and anterior scleral canal wall in early experimental glaucoma. Invest Ophthalmol Vis Sci. 2003;44(2):623-37.

51. Takayama K, Hangai M, Kimura Y, et al. Three-dimensional imaging of lamina cribrosa defects in glaucoma using swept-source optical coherence tomography. Invest Optom Vis Sci. 2013;54(7):4799.

52. Wolbarsht ML, Walsh AW, George G. Melanin, a unique biological absorber. Appl Opt. 1981;20:2184-6.

53. Povazay B, Hermann B, Unterhuber A, et al. Three-dimensional optical coherence tomography at 1050 nm versus 800 nm in retinal pathologies: enhanced performance and choroidal penetration in cataract patients. J Biomed Opt. 2007;12:041211.

54. Esmaeelpour M, Povazay B, Hermann B, et al. Three-dimensional 1060-nm OCT: choroidal thickness maps in normal subjects and improved posterior segment visualization in cataract patients. Invest Ophthalmol Vis Sci. 2010;51:5260-6.

55. Povazay B, Hofer B, Torti C, et al. Impact of enhanced resolution, speed and penetration on three-dimensional retinal optical coherence tomography. Opt Express. 2009;17:4134-50.

56. Miller DT, Kocaoglu OP, Wang Q, et al. Adaptive optics and the eye (super resolution OCT). Eye. 2011;25(3):321-30.

57. Pircher M, Götzinger E, Leitgeb R, et al. Imaging of polarization properties of human retina in vivo with phase resolved transversal PS-OCT. Opt Express. 2004;12(24):5940-51.

58. Jia Y, Morrison JC, Tokayer J, Tran O, et al. Quantitative OCT angiography of optic nerve head blood flow. Biomed Opt Express. 2012;3(12):3127-37.

59. Jia Y, Wei E, Wang X, et al. Optical coherence tomography angiography of optic disc perfusion in glaucoma. Ophthalmology. 2014;7(121):1322-32.

16

Advances in the Management of Developmental Glaucoma

Mandal AK, Netland PA, Gothwal VK

INTRODUCTION

The primary objective in the management of the developmental glaucomas is to normalize and permanently control the intraocular pressure (IOP) to prevent loss of visual acuity, to preserve visual field and ocular integrity and to stimulate the development of binocular stereoscopic vision.

In 1939, Ringland Anderson stated 'the future of children with hydrophthalmia (primary infantile glaucoma) is bleak ... little hope of preserving sufficient sight to permit the earning of a livelihood.' The poor prognosis of the developmental glaucomas has changed dramatically with the introduction of the microsurgical techniques. Today a much more optimistic outlook has been reached. Pivotal to the new philosophy about the developmental glaucomas is accurate and early diagnosis, and prompt treatment.

Glaucoma in an infant is an uncommon disease but the impact on the visual development is extreme. Any vision during the child's formative years is worth even if it is ultimately lost in severe cases. As appropriate and early therapy of this relatively uncommon condition may improve the child's visual future.

The only effective and definitive form of treatment of most of the developmental glaucomas is surgical. Medical therapy has accorded a supportive role in reducing the IOP temporarily, to clear the cornea and to facilitate surgical intervention. Most patients who require long-term medical therapy have severe disease that had not responded to surgical therapy.

The aim of this chapter is to highlight the factors influencing therapeutic decisions, advances in medical therapy, surgical therapy with special emphasis on the recent microsurgical techniques and prognosis of the patients with the developmental glaucoma.

FACTORS INFLUENCING THERAPEUTIC DECISIONS

The choice of surgical therapy in developmental glaucomas (Fig. 16.1) is dependent on a variety of factors.[1] Most important of these is the structural defect[2,3] associated with the elevated IOP. In addition, age, corneal clarity and associated systemic syndromes can influence the choice of therapy.

Structural Defects

An isolated trabeculodysgenesis is the hallmark of primary developmental glaucoma (Fig. 16.2). In most instances, abnormal development of the trabecular meshwork increases the resistance to aqueous outflow, which causes elevated IOP. This condition is highly responsive to both goniotomy and trabeculotomy *ab externo*. The classic operation for the treatment of primary infantile glaucoma is Barkan's goniotomy,[4] a procedure that has changed little since its original description. In recent years, however, there has been a trend toward trabeculotomy *ab externo*.[5-7]

In iridotrabeculodysgenesis, the success rate for goniotomy and trabeculotomy decreases. When the only iris defect is hypoplasia of the anterior stroma, good response to goniotomy or trabeculotomy has been noted. However, when the iris defect includes abnormal vessels that appear to wander somewhat irregularly across the surface of the iris, then the prognosis is poor. In such cases, multiple surgeries are usually needed. If the angle can be easily

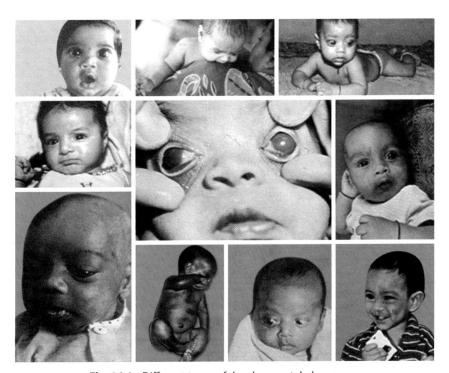

Fig. 16.1: Different types of developmental glaucomas.

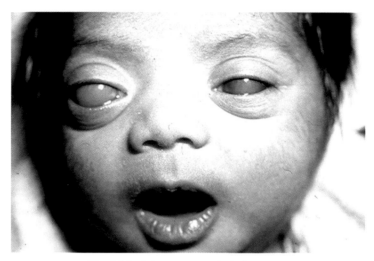

Fig. 16.2: Primary congenital glaucoma.

visualized, goniotomy may be attempted, but trabeculotomy is probably the better initial procedure of choice.

When there are extensive iris structural defects, careful evaluation of the angle is necessary. In aniridia, Grant and Walton[8] noted gradual folding up of the peripheral stump of the iris over the trabecular meshwork forming the peripheral anterior synechia that blocks aqueous outflow. They believe this is a common cause of glaucoma in aniridia and recommend prophylactic goniotomies to prevent the adhesion. Hoskins and associates frequently noted an anterior insertion of iris stroma in patients with aniridia, which is not an acquired process but present at birth. The stroma of the stump of the iris seems to sweep up across the angle. In the presence of this development anomaly, the authors prefer trabeculotomy *ab externo* for the initial operation when medical therapy fails.

In iridocorneotrabeculodysgenesis, the prognosis for surgical treatment is poor. Often medical therapy is unsuccessful, and surgical intervention becomes necessary. *Ab externo* combined trabeculotomy and trabeculectomy may be useful as the initial operation in these patients to control the IOP.

Angle-closure glaucoma is uncommon in childhood, but is important to recognize when it occurs. The surgical treatments are not effective for angle-closure glaucoma. Closure of the angle may be secondary to an underlying problem, which should be corrected.

Age

The age of the child at the onset of glaucoma is also a factor in choosing the appropriate therapy. In general, children under the age of 3 years are best treated surgically. Those with isolated trabeculodysgenesis respond well to both goniotomy and trabeculotomy *ab externo*. It has been observed that goniotomy is less successful after the age of 3 years, whereas trabeculotomy may be successful until later in life.

Children over 3 years of age deserve a trial of medical therapy unless a specific defect of trabeculodysgenesis is seen (including an anterior insertion of the iris, a thickened trabeculum, or a wrap round type of anterior iris stromal insertion). Such patients may be treated with trabeculotomy *ab externo*.

Systemic Syndromes

A number of systemic syndromes are associated with developmental glaucoma.

In Sturge-Weber Syndrome

In Sturge-Weber syndrome, glaucoma may be present at birth or appear at any time from infancy to adulthood (Fig. 16.3). The mechanism of glaucoma remains controversial.[9-12] Patients show varying response to surgical therapy depending on their age. When glaucoma is present in infancy, the developmental anomaly that obstructs aqueous outflow may predominate, which resembles primary congenital glaucoma.[9] Many surgeons prefer goniotomy or trabeculotomy as the operation of choice but report that the rate of success is consistently lower than that with primary congenital glaucoma.[10,11]

When glaucoma in Sturge-Weber syndrome has its onset in later life, it is thought to be primarily due to elevated episcleral venous pressure.[9] The angle defect is less severe and is sometimes minimal. In such patients, medical therapy should be tried first. If medical therapy fails, some surgeons

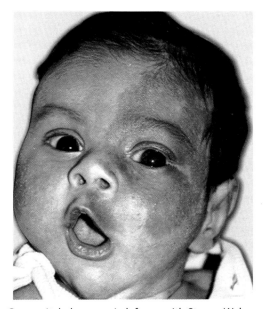

Fig.16.3: Congenital glaucoma in left eye with Sturge-Weber syndrome.

feel that filtering procedure, such as trabeculectomy, should be performed on these eyes.[12-14] We often use a technique combining *ab externo* trabeculotomy and trabeculectomy in such cases. Trabeculotomy is performed to remove the possible obstruction to aqueous outflow by a congenital angle deformity, while trabeculectomy is included to bypass the episcleral venous system. In other words, the combined procedure may address both possible mechanisms of glaucoma associated with this syndrome.[15]

There may be a rapid accumulation of a massive amount of supra-choroidal fluid during the operative procedure.[11,14] This will produce flattening of the anterior chamber, hardening of the globe and difficulty in repositing a prolapsed iris when the sclerotomy is made. After the iridectomy is done, it may be difficult to reposit ciliary processes that rotate anteriorly into the sclerotomy, and vitreous may be lost. These complications can be avoided or minimized if, before entering the anterior chamber, two posterior radial sclerotomies or a triangular sclerotomy is made in the inferior quadrants of the globe. This enables the supra-choroidal effusion to drain out of the eye.

To help avoid the complications of conventional glaucoma surgery in eyes with increased episcleral venous pressure, filtration techniques that do not require entry into the anterior chamber have been recommended by some surgeons. These include sinustomy[16] and nonpenetrating trabeculectomy with or without neodymium:yttrium-aluminum-garnet (Nd:YAG) laser trabeculotomy.[16,17]

Oculocerebrorenal Syndrome of Lowe

Oculocerebrorenal syndrome of Lowe is a rare syndrome, which may be associated with glaucoma and trabeculodysgenesis.[18] Hemorrhage may accompany surgery and, therefore, medical therapy should be tried initially. The success rate of surgery is lesser compared with the success for primary developmental glaucoma.

Homocysteinuria

In homoeysteinuria secondary glaucoma associated with angle closure may occur due to subluxation of the lens. Laser or surgical iridotomy or lens removal are surgical options in this situation. Intravascular thrombosis has been reported with general anesthesia in patients with homo-cysteinuria.[19]

Trisomy

In trisomy,[13] congenital glaucoma resulting from poor differentiation of the angle structures, has been reported.[20] However, most of these patients die within the first few weeks of life, and only 18% of patients survive upto first year. Thus, in this syndrome surgical intervention is warranted only in eyes that have a good prognosis and patients in whom longevity is likely to be good. Consultation with a pediatrician is useful in deciding management strategies.

Corneal Clarity

In situations where corneal clouding prevents adequate visualization of the trabecular meshwork by gonioscopy, trabeculotomy *ab externo* has to be performed in children with developmental glaucoma as the initial surgical procedure.[21,22]

Severity of Glaucoma

In advanced cases of developmental glaucomas (Figs. 16.4 and 16.5), initial goniotomy or trabeculotomy may be tried, but has a high failure rate. Combined trabeculotomy and trabeculectomy may offer a higher success rate than goniotomy or trabeculotomy. If the initial surgical procedure fails, it

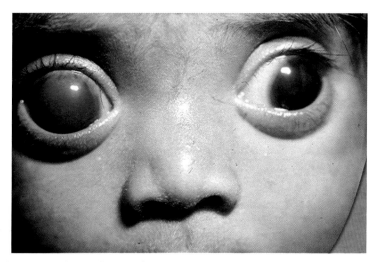

Fig. 16.4: Advanced stage of primary congenital glaucoma (before surgery).

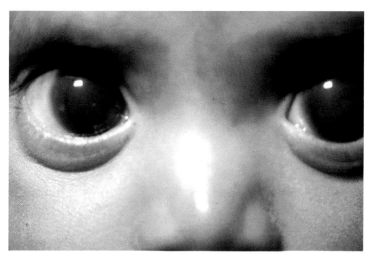

Fig. 16.5: Corneal edema cleared totally (after surgery).

may be necessary to perform trabeculectomy with adjunctive antifibrotic drug or glaucoma drainage implant.

Patients who present with bilateral cloudy corneas and severe glaucoma at birth often had surgery delayed until they were a week or so of age to reduce anesthetic risk. With current anesthetic techniques, surgery can be safely performed on the second or third day of life. We feel that early surgery salvage more eyes than delayed.

Corneal Diameter

Some authors have had an impression that corneal enlargement was a poor prognostic factor in trabeculotomy.[23] However, this had not been the experience of Luntz and Livingston in a prospective study of 86 treated eyes.[21,24] Quigley[25] reported a success rate of 67% in eyes with corneal diameter greater than 14 mm compared to 100% success in eyes less than 14 mm. McPherson and McFarland[26] noted that corneal diameter had little effect on the final outcome of the external trabeculotomy.

The success of goniotomy is decreased in eyes with significant buphthalmos. Barkan[27] felt that eyes with corneal diameters greater than 15 mm were not suitable for goniotomy. Similarly, Robertson[28] reported 13 of 15 successes in non-buphthalmic eyes compared with only 3 of 10 successes in buphthalmic eyes. In patients with a significant increase in corneal diameter, goniotomy is technically difficult to perform and the initial procedure of choice should be trabeculotomy *ab externo* or combined trabeculotomy and trabeculectomy.

Our impression has been that complications may occur with increased frequency in eyes with severe corneal enlargement and buphthalmos. Additional precautions to avoid complications improve safety during the postoperative period. These precautions include tightly sutured trabeculectomy flap and two-stage glaucoma drainage device implantation in order to minimize postoperative hypotony.

Surgical therapy is the most effective and definitive form of treatment for developmental glaucomas. The choice of surgical therapy is influenced by a variety of factors, including the structural defect, age of the patient, corneal clarity and associated systemic syndromes. Consideration of these factors may guide the ophthalmologist toward more effective treatment strategies.

MEDICAL TREATMENT

Primary congenital glaucoma responds poorly to medical therapy. When contemplating medical therapy in children, clinicians should evaluate the risks and benefits of the individual medication, use the minimum dosage required to achieve a therapeutic benefit and monitor ocular and systemic side effects.[29,30]

The commonly used medications are described briefly.

Beta Blockers

There is variable response to adjunctive treatment with timolol maleate in patients with a variety of pediatric glaucomas. It is reported that only one-third of the patients responded to treatment with good control of IOP.[31-34]

Plasma timolol levels in children after treatment with 0.25% timolol greatly exceed those in adults after instillation of 0.50% timolol.[35] Higher plasma levels of the drug would be expected to be associated with an increased risk of systemic side effects in children. In children over 5 years of age, reduction in resting pulse rate has been identified and is comparable to that in adults.[31] Side effects have been reported in 4–13% of children,[32,33] and timolol therapy had to be discontinued in 3–7% of patients.[29,30] Serious adverse events such as apnea have been reported in younger children with smaller body mass and blood volume.[36-38] Provocation of asthma may occur with topical timolol treatment. It is not known whether betaxolol, a selective beta-blocker, reduces the risk of pulmonary side effects in children. The effects of long-term use of topical beta blockers in children are not known.

Timolol in 0.25% and 0.50% solutions may be used with caution in young glaucoma patients, particularly in neonates, due to the possibility of apnea and other systemic side effects. A detailed pediatric examination should precede use of this drug, to determine the presence of systemic abnormalities such as bronchial asthma and cardiac disease. In these cases, beta blockers are contraindicated. Use of 0.25% timolol rather than 0.50% timolol is strongly recommended in order to minimize the risk of side effects. Once daily dosing with timolol 0.25% in gel-forming solution may help simplify medical regimen.

Carbonic Anhydrase Inhibitors

Systemic carbonic anhydrase inhibitors would be expected to have side effects in children similar to adults. In addition, growth suppression in children has been associated with oral acetazolamide therapy,[39] and infants may experience a severe metabolic acidosis.[40] Side effects due to systemic carbonic anhydrase inhibitors in infants and young children are not commonly reported as these patients may not verbalize these side effects. Oral administration of acetazolamide suspension in a dosage of 10 mg/kg/day (range 5–15 mg) given in divided doses (three times daily) is safe and well tolerated by children, lowers IOP and may reduce corneal edema prior to surgery.[41,42]

Topical versus oral carbonic anhydrase inhibitor therapy has been evaluated for pediatric glaucoma in a crossover design study.[43] The mean IOP reduction was 36% and 27% from the baseline after treatment with oral acetazolamide and topical dorzolamide, respectively. All eyes showed an increase in IOP when switched from acetazolamide to dorzolamide; the mean increase was 3.7 mm Hg. Although not as effective as acetazolamide in this group of patients, topical dorzolamide caused a significant reduction of IOP and was well tolerated.

At present, topical carbonic anhydrase inhibitors are more commonly prescribed than the systemic carbonic anhydrase inhibitors. Many clinicians recommend twice daily dosing, in order to minimize the discomfort associated with three times daily dosing. For older children, the fixed combination of dorzolamide with timolol may simplify medical regimens, reducing the number of drops instilled per day.

Prostaglandin-related Drugs

Prostaglandin-related drugs, specifically latanoprost, has been evaluated in a variety of glaucoma including glaucoma associated with Sturge-Weber syndrome.[44-48] Although the majority of children do not respond well to latanoprost, some children may have a significant ocular hypotensive effect with latanoprost treatment.[46] Side effects are infrequent and mild, and the dosage schedule is convenient. Parents and patients should be informed of the possible local side effects, including iris pigmentation, eyelash growth and hyperemia. When medical therapy prior to surgery or other short-term medical therapy is planned, these local side effects are generally not a problem.

Alpha-2 Agonists

Several noncomparative case series have described the use of brimonidine in pediatric glaucoma patients, but the use of apraclonidine is not described. In 30 patients with a mean age of 10 years, brimonidine treatment was associated with a mean reduction of IOP by 7%.[49] Two young children (ages 2 and 4 years) were transiently unarousable after administration of brimonidine, and five other children experienced extreme fatigue.[49] In 23 patients with a mean age of 8 years, 18% had systemic adverse effects sufficient to necessitate stopping the drug.[50] Four pediatric patients are reported to develop somnolence after treatment with brimonidine.[51] A 1-month-old infant developed recurrent episodes of 'coma' (unresponsiveness, hypotension, hypotonia, hypothermia and bradycardia) following treatment with brimonidine.[52]

Alpha-2-agonists are less commonly used in pediatric patients compared to adults. The potential for central nervous system-mediated side effects is greater with lipophilic drugs (e.g., brimonidine) compared with more hydrophilic drugs that are less likely to cross the blood–brain barrier (e.g., apraclonidine). Apraclonidine may help to minimize intraoperative hyphema in the setting of goniotomy.[53]

Other Adrenergic Agonists

Although uncommonly prescribed at present, epinephrine (1%) has been used in children.[54] Lack of efficacy and the potential for systemic toxicity (tachyarrythmia, hypertension) limit the use of this drug. A reactive conjunctival hyperemia may occur following the initial vasoconstriction. After prolonged use, melanin-like adrenochrome deposits may be noted in the conjunctiva and occasionally in the cornea. Dipivefrin hydrochloride 0.1%, a prodrug of epinephrine, may be used in children. Side effects may be attenuated compared to epinephrine, except for a high frequency of local allergic reactions. The drops are administered every 12–24 h. In aphakic or pseudophakic pediatric patients, these drugs should be avoided due to the risk of cystoid macular edema.

Cholinergic Drugs

Although miotic drugs increase the facility of aqueous outflow in normal persons as well as in glaucoma patients and thus lower the IOP, these drugs are probably not as effective in developmental glaucoma because of the abnormal insertion of ciliary muscle into the trabecular meshwork. In pediatric patients, the use of pilocarpine (2% concentration, topically applied every 6–8 h) is limited.[41] But, cholinergic drugs may be helpful in aphakic or pseudophakic children with elevated IOP. Also, these drugs may be useful in achieving miosis before and after goniotomy.[53]

The induced myopia caused by the miotics can produce disabling visual difficulties. A slow-release pilocarpine membrane delivery system (Ocusert), currently not available, was helpful in some young patients,[55] although sudden release of pilocarpine (burst effect) rarely induced myopic spasms. Ciliary spasm and angle-closure glaucoma have been precipitated by the use of phospholine iodide for esotropia in a child.[56]

The long-acting anticholinesterase drugs are not readily available, are associated with serious adverse effects and offer no advantages over pilocarpine for use in children. Echothiophate iodide (phospholine iodide), which is instilled every 12–24 h, is a potent and relatively irreversible inhibitor of cholinesterase. The systemic absorption of anticholinesterase agents can significantly reduce the serum cholinesterase and pseudo-cholinesterase levels. Affected children may show signs of weakness, diarrhoea, nausea, vomiting, salivation, decreased heart rate and other evidence of parasympathetic nervous system stimulation. This becomes particularly dangerous when surgery is contemplated, since succinyl-choline is commonly employed as a muscle relaxant during general anesthesia. This drug is normally promptly hydrolyzed by cholinesterase at the nerve endings. However, when the cholinesterase level is low, prolonged apnea can result.

Osmotic Drugs

Glycerol or glycerine is administered in a dose of 0.75–1.5 g/kg body weight, orally, in a 50% solution.[57] The very sweet taste may be partially masked by chilling the solution and by using fruit juice (lemon or orange) or flavored water to dilute it. This drug is rarely used in the treatment of developmental glaucomas. Mannitol (20% solution) is administered intravenously in a dose of 0.50–1.5 g/kg body weight, at approximately 60 drops per min. A rapid fall in pressure occurs in 20–30 min and lasts for 4–10 h. Mannitol may be administered to reduce the IOP before surgery in patients with developmental glaucomas when it remains very high even with standard medical therapy.

Medical therapy for pediatric glaucoma patients is often administered to reduce the IOP temporarily, to clear the cornea, and to facilitate surgical intervention. Most patients who require long-term medical therapy do usually have severe disease that has not responded to surgical therapy. Some patients with elevated IOP, however, may respond to therapy with various medications. Prior to initiating medical therapy, clinicians should carefully consider the potential for side effects. When using topical glaucoma medications, children may be at increased risk of systemic side effects compared with adults due to reduced body mass and blood volume for drug distribution.

INITIAL SURGICAL THERAPY

Early surgical intervention is of prime importance in the management of patients with developmental glaucoma. In some parts of the world, such as the United States, patients may have only mild or moderate corneal edema at referral for treatment. These patients may be candidates for goniotomy, which has a high success rate in Western populations. In other parts of the world, such as India or the Middle East, nearly all patients present with corneal clouding, and goniotomy is technically impossible. In these cases, external trabeculotomy is the initial procedure of choice. When initial trabeculotomy has a poor success rate, trabeculotomy may be combined with trabeculectomy. Another important consideration is that, although most patients have symptoms suggestive of congenital glaucoma at birth or within 6 months of birth, patients often present late due to various nonmedical factors. In such advanced cases, we prefer to perform *ab externo* combined trabeculotomy and trabeculectomy. which offers the best hope of success.

Goniotomy

After the introduction of clinical gonioscopy, Otto Barkan (1936) modified de Vincentis' operation (1892) by using a specially designed glass contact lens to visualize the angle structures while using a knife to create an internal cleft in trabecular tissue. He called the operation 'goniotomy.'[4,27,58-63] The objective of goniotomy is to remove obstructing tissue that causes resistance to aqueous flow, thereby restoring the access of aqueous to Schlemm's canal and maintaining the physiologic direction of outflow. Clinical and experimental evidence supports the belief that an improved facility of outflow after goniotomy is responsible for the lowering of IOP.[64]

In order to perform this surgery, special equipment is required, including a lens for gonioscopic surgery and a goniotomy knife. A variety of gonioscopy lenses are available for goniotomy, but the most popular and widely used one is the Swan-Jacob lens. It has a metal handle attached to the gonioscopy lens with a convex anterior surface, allowing observation of the angle with the microscope or with loupes. It does not require a viscous fluid space between the lens and the cornea because its corneal contact curvature is flatter than that of the cornea. The lens is small and permits insertion of goniotomy knife at the limbus without obstruction by the lens.

An ideal goniotomy knife should be sharp on both sides to allow it to cut in either direction, and it should have a sharp point for entering the trabecular meshwork. The average blade width should be 1–1.5 mm, and the paracentesis incision ideally should not leak after the withdrawal of knife. The blade is joined to a handle by a tapered shaft, to fill the paracentesis opening and prevent loss of aqueous with subsequent collapse of the anterior chamber when the shaft is fully inserted into the eye. The shaft and blade also should be slightly longer than the diameter of the anterior chamber. Some goniotomy knives have a fine metal cannula attached to the handle and to a tube running to a reservoir filled with balanced salt solution (BSS), which is infused during the operation to maintain a deep anterior chamber. Both the Barraquer knife and Worst knife fulfill all the above criteria and both are equally popular. A Swan spade or a long needle also may be used to perform goniotomy (Figs. 16.6 and 16.7).

Visualization of the anterior chamber angle can be achieved with various illumination and magnification techniques. The procedure can be performed with a headlamp and surgical loupes. The headlamp may be a conventional surgical headlamp or, alternatively, the surgeon may use the light source on an indirect ophthalmoscope. It is possible to use the conventional ophthalmic operating microscope by positioning the patient with a view of the anterior chamber angle. The system most commonly used by the authors is a neurosurgical microscope, which allows confocal viewing of the anterior chamber angle and can be adjusted to any viewing position without moving the patient.

After induction of general anesthesia, the eye is prepped and draped in the unusual manner for the surgical procedure. The Swan-Jacob goniotomy

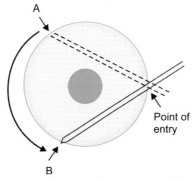

Fig. 16.6: Entry of goniotomy knife.

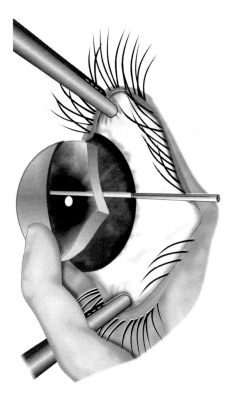

Fig. 16.7: Goniotomy in progress.

lens is placed on the cornea. For nasal goniotomy, the lens is placed on the cornea with approximately 2 mm of temporal corneal remaining exposed. The locking fixation forceps are placed by the assistant on the vertical recti for a goniotomy performed nasally or temporally.

Alternatively, the locking forceps are placed on the horizontal recti for a procedure done inferiorly or superiorly. A paracentesis is performed with a sharp blade or the goniotomy knife is used itself to enter the anterior chamber. The knife enters the anterior chamber through peripheral clear cornea, approximately 1 mm inside the corneo-limbal junction, at the previously selected site. Once in the anterior chamber, the knife is guided parallel to the iris, away from the pupil, toward the trabecular meshwork. The tip of the knife is engaged slightly anterior to the middle of the trabecular meshwork. With the operating microscope, the tip of the knife can be seen to indent the trabecular meshwork before it is cut by circumferential movement of the knife until comfortable visualization of the tissue is no longer possible.

During goniotomy, the tip of the knife should remain in a somewhat superficial position, cutting at the same depth along the incision. When the knife is at optimum depth, there is little or no perceptible tactile sensation of cutting trabecular tissue. If a coarse, grating sensation is felt, the knife is probably positioned too deep. As the incision proceeds, a white line develops behind the blade, the iris falls posteriorly and the angle deepens. Great care should be taken to avoid touching the iris on the knife edge or damaging the lens. The incision can encompass at least 110° with a maximum sweep. By rotation of the globe by the assistant surgeon, approximately 4–6 clock hours of meshwork can be incised.

Once the incision has been completed, the blade is withdrawn fairly rapidly taking care not to strike the corneal endothelium, iris, or lens. If the wound leaks, a single 10-0 nylon suture can be used to close the incision site. A moderate amount of bleeding following the surgery is typical and perhaps even a favorable sign indicating that communication has been created to the canal of Schlemm.[61,65-71] This bleeding is innocuous and usually rapidly clears following surgery. The whole procedure from the first grasping of the muscles by the assistant to the completion of suturing takes approximately 8–10 min. A drop of an antibiotic-corticosteroid preparation is instilled into the conjunctival sac and a patch and shield are applied to the eye. The following day the patch can be removed. Topical antibiotic-steroids drops are continued until the anterior chamber reaction resolves. The 10-0 nylon suture may be removed approximately 4–6 weeks after surgery.

The reported results of goniotomy surgery show a success rate of 80% in infantile glaucoma.[61,66-68,71-80] Goniotomy appears to be as effective as external trabeculotomy in this condition. It appears that goniotomy is most successful in patients whose glaucoma is recognized early and treated between one month and one year of age. Early diagnosis and prompt treatment of this disease are important if good results are to be obtained, although good success rates are achieved in patients up to 2 years of age. The severity of the filtration angle defect also determines the success rate of goniotomy.

To evaluate whether a more extensive incision of the tissue adjacent to the anterior trabecular meshwork can result in more effective control of IOP, Catalano et al.[81] performed one versus two simultaneous goniotomies as the initial surgical procedure for primary infantile glaucoma. Success of the two groups were not significantly different at 1 month or at 1 year postoperatively and the use of healon did not adversely affect IOP control. For the maintenance of a deep and stable anterior chamber during goniotomy, other surgeons also did prefer viscoelastic substances.[82-84]

Endoscopically controlled intraocular surgery has been evolving rapidly since the introduction of thinner endoprobes with increasing resolving power and higher image quality. The use of an endoscope for goniotomy surgery is a relatively new concept and only few animal studies and case reports were published in the literature.[85-89] Medow and Sauer[85] were the first to show that endoscopic goniotomy can be effective in treating primary congenital glaucoma. They performed endoscopic goniotomy in a 1500 g newborn with an IOP of 28 mm Hg and significant corneal clouding. The patient was followed for 2 years and IOP was controlled without medication, with pressure in the low teens. Recently, Bayaraktar and Koseoglu[86] reported 12 eyes of 7 patients treated with endoscopic goniotomy with anterior chamber maintainer and concluded that the procedure should be an effective treatment modality for congenital glaucoma even with totally opaque corneas. However, microendoscopy of the anterior segment of the eye creates a new surgical situation, so that great caution has to be exercised during the procedure. It demands technical adaptation, and the learning curve is steep.

Trabeculotomy Ab Externo

Trabeculotomy *ab externo* or external trabeculotomy as practiced today is an alternative to goniotomy for the surgical treatment of congenital and childhood glaucomas and can be used when corneal opacity prevents an adequate gonioscopic view. Simultaneously and independently described by Burian[5,7] and Smith[6] in 1960, trabeculotomy *ab externo* has given results better than those with goniotomy. On March 25, 1960, without the aid of an operating microscope, the first external trabeculotomy was performed by Burian on a young girl with Marfan's syndrome and glaucoma.[5] At about the same time in London, Redmond Smith developed an operation that he called 'nylon filament trabeculotomy.'[6] This involved cannulating Schlemm's canal with a nylon suture at one site and threading the suture circumferentially and then withdrawing it at another site and pulling it tight like a bowstring. The surgical technique of trabeculotomy *ab externo* is basically a combination of the procedures originally developed by Burian and Smith, and later modified by Harms,[90,91] Dannheim,[92,93] and McPherson.[26,78,94]

Trabeculotomy *ab externo* has a number of major advantages over goniotomy.[95] First, a trabeculotomy can be performed when the cornea is edematous or scarred and when there is poor visibility of the anterior chamber. Second, the procedure is anatomically precise in rupturing the inner wall of Schlemm's canal and the trabecular meshwork, creating continuity between the anterior chamber and Schlemm's canal. Third, trabeculotomy does not require the introduction of sharp instruments across the anterior chamber, which increases the risk of damage to other ocular tissues, especially for the inexperienced surgeon. Fourth, there is no need for the surgeon to adapt to the operating gonioprism, because the procedure is performed using a standard operating microscope and conventional anterior segment microsurgical technique.

Advocates of trabeculotomy argue that the success of trabeculotomy depends only on the type of angle anomaly and is not dependent on the severity of the glaucoma, the size of the cornea or the presence of corneal edema, which have been reported to influence the success of goniotomy.[96,97] A lower incidence of postoperative cataract and few postoperative complications have been reported after trabeculotomy compared with goniotomy. Furthermore, goniotomy controls the IOP in about 64[96] to 77%[97] of eyes having congenital glaucoma of all degrees of severity. If the eyes with corneal cloudiness are excluded, and in eyes where multiple goniotomies are performed, 85% of those operated can achieve control of IOP.[97] Trabeculotomy, on the other hand, will control IOP in over 90% of eyes with glaucoma of all

grades of severity, although some of these eyes may require two or three procedures. It seems that trabeculotomy achieves higher success rate compared
with goniotomy in eyes with all grades of severity. However, there are no prospective, controlled trials of trabeculotomy and goniotomy to confirm this
interpretation. Nonetheless, the popularity of trabeculotomy *ab externo* as an
initial procedure in the surgical management of primary infantile glaucoma
has been championed by a number of authorities.[7,21-24,26,66,78,90-94,98,99]

To perform trabeculotomy, a limbus-based conjunctival flap is prepared,
with the conjunctival incision approximately 7 mm from the limbus. Many
surgeons prefer a fornix-based conjunctival flap, with the incision at the limbus, and this approach is necessary when exposure is not adequate to allow
for a limbus-based conjunctival flap. Hemostasis is maintained throughout
the dissection of the conjunctival flap, although cautery should be minimized
to avoid excessive shrinkage of sclera. A partial thickness scleral flap is prepared, with its base at the limbus. The flap is usually an equilateral triangle,
measuring approximately three to four on each side, some surgeons prefer
a rectangular-shaped flap. The authors prefer a triangular flap as it allows
adequate exposure of the Schlemm's canal and involves less scleral dissection than a rectangular flap. The depth of the flap is approximately one-half
scleral thickness, bearing in mind that the sclera in buphthalmic eyes is usually much thinner than the adult eye.

The surgical landmarks and anatomy of the limbal region should be carefully identified during trabeculotomy. Closest to the limbus is a transparent
band of deep corneal lamellae. Behind that is a narrow grayish-blue band,
which represents the trabecular meshwork. Posterior to this area is white,
opaque sclera. The junction of the posterior border of the trabecular band
and the sclera is the external landmark of the scleral spur and the landmark
for finding the canal of Schlemm. In most eyes this is situated between 2 and
2.5 mm behind the surgical limbus. A radial incision is then made across the
scleral spur. The objective of this radial incision is to cut the external wall of
Schlemm's canal and to avoid entering the anterior chamber. It is important
to bear in mind that Schlemm's canal is separated from the anterior chamber
only by the trabecular meshwork. This is the most delicate step in the operation and demands the most microsurgical skill. Under high magnification,
the radial incision is gradually deepened with a sharp blade until it is carried
through the external wall of Schlemm's canal, at which point there is ooze of
aqueous, occasionally mixed with blood. The dissection is carefully continued through the external wall until the inner wall of the canal becomes visible. The inner wall is characteristically slightly pigmented and is composed
of crisscrossing fibers. Vannas scissors are used to enlarge the lumen of the
canal. Some surgeons confirm passage into the canal by passing a 6-0 nylon
suture into the canal, as described by Smith.[6]

The internal (lower or distal) arm of the trabeculotome is introduced into
the canal using the external (upper or proximal) parallel arm as a guide. Once
90% of the trabeculotome is within the canal, it is rotated into the anterior

chamber and rotation is continued until 75% of the probe arm length has entered the chamber, then the rotation is reversed and the instrument is withdrawn. About 2 to 2½ clock hours of the internal wall of Schlemm's canal and trabecular meshwork are disrupted by the rotation of the trabeculotome into the anterior chamber. The trabeculotome is then passed into the Schlemm's canal on the other side of the radial incision and rotated into the anterior chamber. In total, about 1000° to 1200° of trabecular meshwork is ruptured by this technique. It is important that no force be used when introducing the probe into the canal, as this will create a false passage. If the probe does not slip easily down the canal, it should be withdrawn and dissection of the outer wall continued until the surgeon is satisfied that all fibers of the outer wall are removed. The probe is then reintroduced into the canal.

As the probe passes into the anterior chamber, disrupting the inner wall of the canal, there should be some slight resistance and there may be a little intracameral bleeding from the inner wall.[26,78,94] This is a transient sign, usually resolving within a few days after the surgery. As the probe is swung from the canal into the anterior chamber, movement of the iris may indicate that the probe is too posterior. The probe should be repositioned to avoid iridodialysis. The cornea should also be carefully monitored to ensure that the probe is not passing anteriorly into the cornea, requiring repositioning of the probe. This is easy to detect because small air bubbles appear in the cornea as the probe ruptures corneal lamellae. In highly buphthalmic eyes, Schlemm's canal may not be located with certainty. In such cases it is possible to convert the procedure to a trabeculectomy by removing a block of deep limbal tissue beneath the scleral flap.

The alternative surgical technique of trabeculotomy *ab externo* is possible even in the presence of severe corneal edema. There are several successful reports of primary trabeculotomy for developmental glaucoma.[25,26,78,90-95,100]

While goniotomy is reported to be safe and successful when performed by experienced surgeons, trabeculotomy *ab externo* offers the advantage of being more predictable and technically easier. Anderson[77,101] and Shaffer[22] reported that the two procedures were equally effective. Shields and Krieglstein[102] recommended that the surgeon should focus on only one of the two procedures to gain experience in managing this rare disease. Filous and Brunova[103] reported the results of modified trabeculotomy in the treatment of primary congenital glaucoma employing trabeculotomy probes more closely corresponding to the variable course of Schlemm's canal. They reported a success rate of 87% over a mean follow-up of 38.4 ± 22.5 months and concluded that probing with the innovative instrument was easier and safer compared to standard trabeculotomy probes.

A newer trabeculotomy technique with a prolene suture was recently developed by Beck and Lynch.[104] They refined a technique for performing 360° trabeculotomy in a single procedure using a 6-0 polypropelene (Prolene) suture fragment and have used it in 15 patients (26 eyes) with primary congenital glaucoma. The refined technique can be performed via a single nasal surgical site. This procedure avoids many of the difficulties encountered with metal trabeculotomes and preserves conjunctiva should further glaucoma surgery be necessary. Recently, Mendicino et al.[105] compared the long-term surgical results of 360° trabeculotomy and goniotomy and reported significantly better IOP control with the former technique as they believed that it is more standardized than the latter technique. Perhaps more controlled and randomized studies comparing the two techniques will reveal which one is more efficient and safer in the management of congenital glaucoma.

Primary Trabeculectomy

Trabeculectomy is a procedure that most ophthalmologists are familiar with and it is technically easier than goniotomy or trabeculotomy. However, primary trabeculectomy is not a first-line procedure in congenital glaucoma in view of a higher incidence of complications and lower success rate in normalizing the IOP.[106-108] In contrast several published reports documented successful results following primary trabeculectomy for congenital glaucoma that are comparable to or are higher than some of the reported series on goniotomy or trabeculotomy.[109-114]

Ab externo Combined Trabeculotomy-Trabeculectomy

Combined trabeculotomy and trabeculectomy may be performed as a primary or secondary procedure. The procedure is used as a primary procedure in patients that have a poor prognosis for success of initial goniotomy or trabeculotomy, such as patients in the Middle East or India, or patients over 2 years of age.

After performing trabeculotomy as described above, trabeculectomy may be performed by making an incision at the surgical limbus with a sharp blade and using the Descemet's punch. Alternatively, a block of sclera may be removed using a sharp blade and Vannas scissors. After performing a surgical iridectomy, the partial thickness flap is closed with interrupted sutures, usually one at the apex and one on each lateral side of the triangular flap. These may be 10-0 nylon sutures, or, alternatively, absorbable sutures, such as 9-0 vicryl (polyglactin) sutures may be used to encourage aqueous flow during the postoperative period. Conjunctiva and Tenon's capsule are then closed with a running suture using 8-0 or 9-0 vicryl (Figs. 16.8 to 16.19).

Most surgeons perform a paracentesis opening with a beveled corneal incision at the beginning of the surgery. Through the paracentesis, the anterior chamber can be reformed with BSS and patency of trabeculectomy can be tested at the conclusion of the surgery. Also, identification of Schlemm's canal may be facilitated when the IOP is lowered after the paracentesis. Subconjunctival injection of an antibiotic-steroid preparation is performed, topical antibiotic-steroid medications are placed into the conjunctival sac, and a patch and shield are applied to the eye.

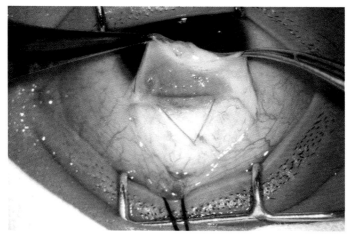

Fig. 16.8: Partial thickness triangular scleral flap delineated.

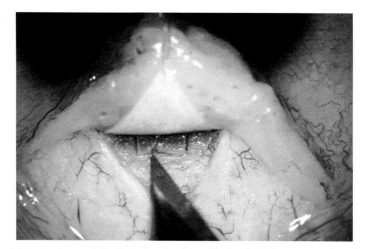

Fig. 16.9: Anatomy of the limbal region identified and Schlemm's canal explored.

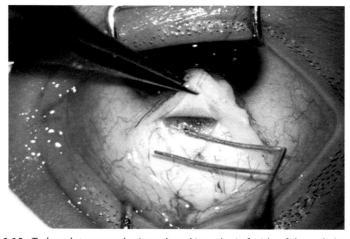

Fig. 16.10: Trabeculotomy probe introduced into the Left side of the radial incision.

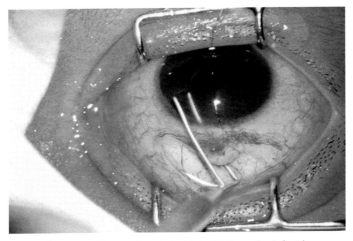

Fig. 16.11: The probe rotated into AC from the left side.

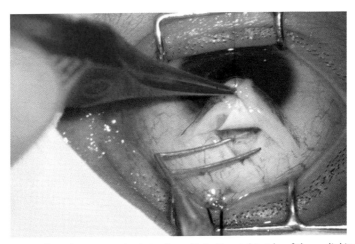

Fig. 16.12: Trabeculotomy probe introduced into the right side of the radial incision.

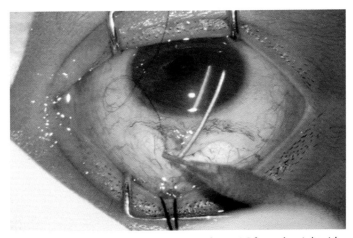

Fig. 16.13: Trabeculotomy probe rotated into AC from the right side.

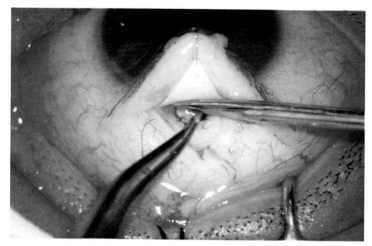

Fig. 16.14: The deeper trabecular block removed.

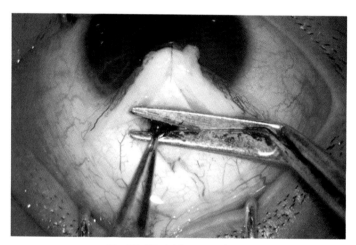

Fig. 16.15: Iridectomy done.

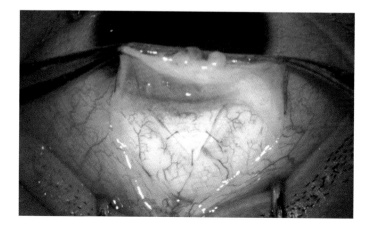

Fig. 16.16: Closure of the triangular scleral flap with 10-0 nylon.

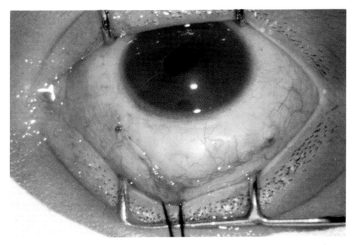

Fig. 16.17: Closure of the conjunctival incision with 8-0 vicryl.

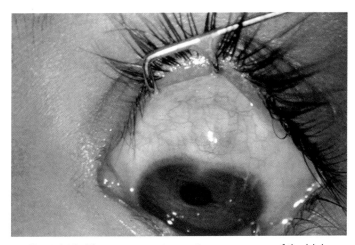

Fig. 16.18: Three years postoperative appearance of the bleb.

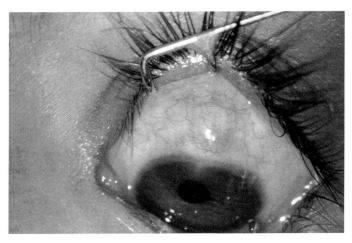

Fig. 16.19: Three years postoperative appearance of Anterior segment showing clear cornea with Haab's striae.

The dressing is removed on the first postoperative day. A steroid-antibiotic combination is prescribed four times a day. A cycloplegic is used only if the eye has a shallow anterior chamber and is frequently monitored. Examination of the patient under anesthesia is performed approximately 3–4 weeks after surgery. If all is stable, the patient is scheduled for another evaluation under anesthesia in approximately 3 months. The evaluations are repeated at quarterly intervals for the first year after surgery. After the first year, the examinations are bi-annual until the child is old enough to cooperate fully with an office examination. Office visits may be scheduled between examinations under anesthesia as needed. These patients should be followed up for an indefinite period to determine whether or not adequate control of IOP has been achieved. The success rate is high for children with infantile glaucoma and surgery within the first year of life, whereas patients with Sturge-Weber syndrome have increased failure with longer follow-up.

Whether combined trabeculotomy-trabeculectomy is superior to trabeculotomy alone is debatable. Binder and Rothkoff[115] found no difference between trabeculotomy and combined trabeculotomy-trabeculectomy in a small series of 7 patients with congenital glaucoma. Dietlein et al.[116] investigated the outcome of trabeculotomy, trabeculectomy and a combined procedure as initial surgical treatment approaches in primary congenital glaucoma. Although the combined procedure seemed to have a favorable outcome, after 2 years the advantages of this procedure over trabeculotomy or trabeculectomy was not statistically significant according to the life table analysis. Elder[117] compared primary trabeculectomy with combined trabeculotomy-trabeculectomy and found the combined procedure to be superior. The superior results of the combined procedure may be because of the dual outflow pathway as explained by Elder. Mullaney et al.[118] and Al-Hazmi et al.[119] used mitomycin-C (MMC) in primary combined trabeculotomy-trabeculectomy and reported a higher success rate. The results reported by Mandal et al.[120-126] from India are comparable to that reported by Mullaney et al. and Al-Hazmi et al. from Saudi Arabia but Mandal et al. do not believe in using MMC in primary surgery. A higher incidence of successful IOP control has been reported from India (Figs. 16.20 to 16.22) and Saudi Arabia with a single operative procedure. O'Connor[127] commented that combined trabeculotomy-trabeculectomy is potentially a very successful surgical procedure in the management of congenital glaucoma and may represent the next step in the search for the best surgical treatment of congenital glaucoma. Further prospective randomized studies are required to explore the surgical results of trabeculotomy, primary combined trabeculotomy and trabeculectomy and 360° trabeculotomy. However, such a study is difficult to conduct because most glaucoma specialists are better trained in and more comfortable with one angle procedure than the other.

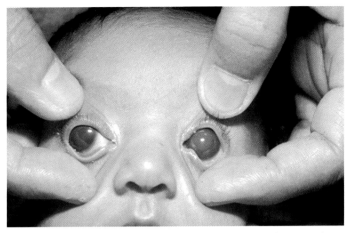

Fig. 16.20: Primary congenital glaucoma operated at the age of one week.

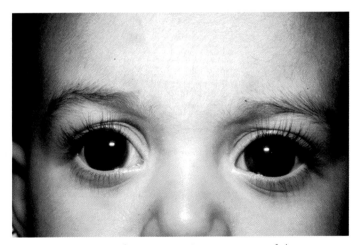

Fig. 16.21: Six months postoperative appearance of clear cornea.

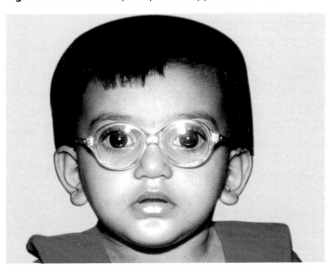

Fig. 16.22: Three years postoperative appearance of the same child with normal vision.

SIMULTANEOUS BILATERAL SURGERY FOR DEVELOPMENTAL GLAUCOMA

One hundred and nine consecutive patients who underwent planned simultaneous bilateral primary combined trabeculectomy and trabeculotomy were evaluated for intraoperative and postoperative ocular and anesthetic complications.[124] The reasons for performing simultaneous bilateral surgeries were bilateral presentation of the disease and the anesthetic risks involved in two surgeries versus one. Success (IOP < 16 mm Hg) probabilities were 91%, 88% and 69% at 1, 2 and 3 years, respectively. The success probability of 69% was maintained up to 6 years on follow-up (Figs. 16.23 and 16.24).

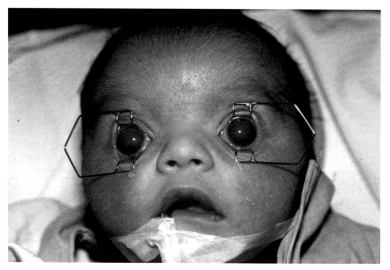

Fig. 16.23: Simultaneous bilateral primary trabeculotomy-trabeculectomy at the age of 3 days.

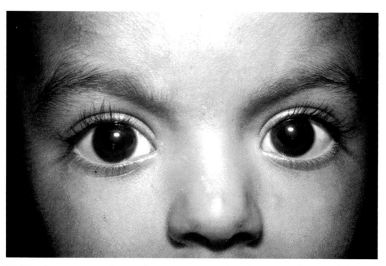

Fig. 16.24: Four years postoperative appearance showing normal corneal clarity.

There were no endophthalmitis or any other sight-threatening complications. Eight eyes developed a shallow anterior chamber, which required reformation in three of these eyes. During anesthesia apnea occurred in 16% of patients and all were resuscitated. Two children had delayed recovery. Cardiopulmonary arrest occurred 5 h postoperatively during feeding in one child who could not be resuscitated. In this series, simultaneous bilateral primary combined trabeculotomy and trabeculectomy was found to be safe and effective for treatment of the developmental glaucoma.[124]

Simultaneous bilateral surgeries for congenital glaucoma may be planned to avoid risks associated with repeat anesthesia[124,128] and an urge to visually rehabilitate the afflicted children as early as possible and to prevent deprivation amblyopia. Additionally, simultaneous surgery is cost effective because it reduces the hospital stay with greater satisfaction to the parents. The treating surgeon has to balance the risk of bilateral endophthalmitis against the reduced risk of one anesthesia versus two, reduced cost and the advantages of simultaneous early visual rehabilitation. A clear understanding of these factors is mandatory for the treating physician as well as the parents.

MANAGEMENT OF REFRACTORY PEDIATRIC GLAUCOMA

Surgical treatment is usually required for developmental glaucoma, using goniotomy or trabeculotomy as primary surgical therapy. Both of these procedures have a high success rate, are equally effective as initial surgical treatment, and have been assessed in a large number of patients over long periods of time.[79,101] However, at least 10–20% of patients fail to responds to the initial surgical procedure and some patients have a poor prognosis for the success of initial goniotomy or trabeculotomy. When the IOP is not controlled after primary surgery, the next step varies according to individual patient factors and surgeon preferences. The surgical options available to treat these children include filtering surgery, glaucoma drainage implants and cyclodestructive procedures.

Filtration Surgery with Antifibrotic Drugs

Children or young adults undergoing filtering surgery do not enjoy the same success rate compared with the older age group. The barriers to success of filtering surgery in children include a thick and active Tenon's capsule, rapid wound healing response, lower scleral rigidity and a large buphthalmic eye with thin sclera.[106] Additionally, conjunctival scarring from previous ocular surgery may limit the success of repeat surgery in children with congenital glaucoma. Trabeculectomy without antifibrotic drugs in young patients has been unsuccessful in most,[106,107,129,130] but not all,[112] reports.

Antifibrotic drugs have been widely used in adult glaucoma filtering surgery to improve the success rate and produce lower mean postoperative IOP. The initial experience with antifibrotic drugs as adjunctive treatment for trabeculectomy was with postoperative subconjunctival 5-fluorouracil (5-FU) injections. Adjunctive use of 5-FU has been described in young patients, with some success in achieving IOP levels in the low teens.[131,132] However, 5-FU has disadvantages, including the need for multiple subconjunctival injections (requiring multiple general anesthesias in children) and the possibility of ocular complications such as hypotony and recalcitrant corneal epithelial defects. A small, prospective, randomized trial showed that 5-FU was less effective compared with MMC in achieving successful control of IOP in pediatric filtration surgery.[133]

Mitomycin C has emerged as an effective antimetabolite for topical use during trabeculectomy. It is an antineoplastic antibiotic isolated from the fermentation filtrate of *Streptomyces caespitosus*, which has the ability to significantly suppress fibrosis and vascular ingrowth after intraoperative application at the site of filtration surgery. Mitomycin C is a more potent anti-fibrotic drug compared with 5-FU. In adults, eyes treated with MMC have lower mean IOP on fewer medications compared with eyes treated with 5-FU. Also, MMC is administered in a single intraoperative application, which is more convenient for the patient and surgeon compared with 5-FU.

Studies of trabeculectomy with adjunctive MMC in pediatric patients are summarized in Table 16.1.[118,119,134-141] The success rate reported in these

Table 16.1: Studies of trabeculectomy with adjunctive mitomycin C in children.

Reference	No. of eyes	MMC procedure	Success criteria	Success
Susanna et al. (1995)[134]	79	0.2 mg/mL, 5 min	IOP # 21 mm Hg	67%
Mandal et al. (1997)[135]	19	0.4 mg/mL, 3 min	IOP <21 mm Hg	95%
Agarwal et al. (1997)[136]	30	0.2 mg/mL, 4 min 0.4 mg/mL, 4 min	IOP <21 mm Hg without meds	60% 87%
Beck et al. (1995)[137]	60	0.25 or 0.5 mg/mL, 5 min	IOP # 22 mm Hg without meds	67%
Al-Hazmi et al. (1998)[119]	254	0.2 to 0.4 mg/mL, 2 to 5 min	IOP # 21 mm Hg without meds	48- 85%
Mullaney et al. (1999)[118]	100	0.2 to 0.4 mg/mL, 2 to 5 min	IOP <21 mm Hg	67%
Azuara-Blanco et al. (1999)[138]	21	0.4 mg/mL, 1-5 min	IOP <21 mm Hg without meds	76%
Mandal et al. (1999)[139]	38	0.4 mg/mL, 3 min	IOP <21 mm Hg	65%
Freedman et al. (1999)[140]	21	0.4 mg/mL, 3-5 min	IOP = 4-16 mm Hg	52%
Sidoti et al. (2000)[141]	29	0.5 mg/mL, 1.5-5 min	IOP <21 mm Hg without meds	82-59%

MMC: Mitomycin C; IOP: Intraocular pressure; meds: Glaucoma medications.

studies ranged from 48 to 95%, depending on the patient age, the definition of success, length of follow-up and other factors. It is clear that trabeculectomy with MMC has a higher success rate than trabeculectomy alone in pediatric patients (Figs. 16.25 and 16.26). However, complications were reported in these studies, including hypotony with shallow anterior chamber, choroidal detachment, retinal detachment, cataract, bleb leak and bleb-related infection (blebitis and endophthalmitis). Sidoti and coworkers[141] showed a high (17%) long-term incidence of bleb-related infection in children after trabeculectomy with MMC.

Late bleb-related ocular infection and vision loss may occur in children after trabeculectomy with MMC.[142,143] These infections are characterized by abrupt

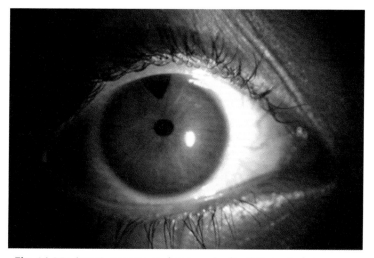

Fig. 16.25: Anterior segment photograph after failed primary surgery.

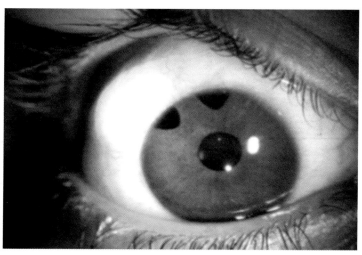

Fig. 16.26: Anterior segment photograph showing bleb appearance after MMC augmented trabeculectomy.

onset, bleb infiltration and rapid progression. In one report, staphylococcus grew in all the three eyes that developed bleb-related ocular infection.[142] In another report, surgical technique in young patients using limbus-based conjunctival flap was more likely to result in cystic bleb appearance and bleb-related ocular infection compared with fornix-based conjunctival flap.[143] After trabeculectomy with MMC, patients develop thin-walled, avascular blebs, which may predispose patients to an increased incidence of late complications. A life-long periodic follow-up of these eyes is required. The parents of children treated with MMC augmented trabeculectomy should be instructed to report to the ophthalmologist on an emergency basis, if the operated eye develops redness, discharge, decreased vision, or any other symptoms.

The optimal dosing and administration of MMC in children is yet unknown. Since children are known to have more fibroblastic activity compared to young adults and elderly patients, most clinicians use a standard dose of MMC, similar to the concentration and exposure time used in elderly patients or young adults. The usual range of concentration used is from 0.2 to 0.4 mg/mL, with an exposure time of 2–4 min. In adults, no definite differences in efficacy or success rate have been identified in this dose range.[144,145] Further studies are needed for the dosing and administration of MMC in pediatric patients.

Despite achieving good results with the use of MMC with trabeculectomy, we do not recommend its use during primary surgery in children afflicted with congenital glaucomas. Adjunctive use of MMC is associated with potentially serious ocular complications and its long-term effects are not yet known. Additionally, conventional primary surgery such as goniotomy, trabeculotomy or combined trabeculotomy-trabeculectomy has been very effective. However, intraoperative application of MMC is a useful option in children with refractory congenital glaucoma with previously failed primary surgery. After trabeculectomy with MMC, children require periodic examination and the parents should be educated about the possible late complications.

Glaucoma Drainage Implants

Glaucoma drainage implants are useful when other surgical treatments have a poor prognosis for success, prior conventional surgery fails or when significant conjunctival scarring precludes filtration surgery. Smaller sized drainage implants have been marketed for use in pediatric patients, but adult-sized devices are commonly implanted. Available types of drainage implants are either an open tube (nonrestrictive) device or a valved (flow-restrictive) device. Examples of open tube implants include the Molteno and Baerveldt implants, whereas the Krupin implant and the Ahmed glaucoma valve are flow-restrictive devices. The flow-restrictive devices are intended to reduce the incidence of complications associated with hypotony during the immediate postoperative period. Glaucoma drainage implants are most usually placed in the supero-temporal quadrant, but may be surgically positioned in any quadrant.

Studies of glaucoma drainage implants in pediatric patients are summarized in Table 16.2.[146-162] The success rate reported in these studies ranged from 56–95%, depending on the patient age, the definition of success, length of follow-up and other factors. Glaucoma drainage implants may be effective in controlling the IOP, even in patients who have failed previous glaucoma surgery. However, complications have been associated with glaucoma drainage implants in pediatric patients. Reported complications include hypotony with shallow anterior chamber and choroidal detachments, tube-cornea touch and corneal edema, obstructed tube, exposed tube or plate, endophthalmitis and retinal detachment. Most of these complications did not affect the outcomes, but a few of them were associated with vision loss.

Postoperatively, patients often require adjunctive glaucoma medications and close monitoring for complications. Iris creep around the tube insertion

Table 16.2: Studies of glaucoma drainage implants in pediatric patients.

Author (year)	No. of eyes	Implant type	Success criteria	Success
Molteno et al. (1984)[146]	83	Molteno	IOP < 20 mm Hg no meds	73%
			IOP < 20 mm Hg with meds	95%
Billson et al. (1989)[147]	23	Molteno	IOP < 21 mm Hg with meds	78%
Hill et al. (1991)[148]	65	Molteno	5 mm Hg < IOP < 22 mm Hg	62%
Munoz et al. (1991)[149]	53	Molteno	IOP < 22 mm Hg	68%
Lloyd et al. (1992)[150]	16	Molteno	5 mm Hg < IOP < 22 mm Hg	56%
Nesher et al. (1992)[151]	27	Molteno	IOP < 21 mm Hg "meds	57%
Netland and Walton (1993)[152]	20	Molteno, Baerveldt	IOP < 21 mm Hg	80%
Fellenbaum et al. (1995)[153]	30	Baerveldt	5 mm Hg < IOP < 22 mm Hg	86%
Siegner et al. (1995)[154]	15	Baerveldt	5 mm Hg < IOP < 22 mm Hg	80%
Coleman et al. (1997)[155]	24	Ahmed	IOP < 22 mm Hg 1 year:	78%
			1 year:	61%
Eid et al. (1997)[156]	18	Molteno Schocket, Baerveldt	6 mm Hg < IOP < 21 mm Hg	72%
Donahue et al. (1997)[157]	23	Baerveldt	IOP < 21 mm Hg with meds	61%
Huang et al. (1999)[158]	11	Ahmed	5 mm Hg < IOP < 22 mm Hg	91%
Englert et al, 1999[159]	27	Ahmed	IOP < 22 mm Hg	85%
Djodeyre et al. (2001)[160]	35	Ahmed	IOP < 22 mm Hg 1 year:	70%
			2 year:	64%
Pereira et al. (2002)[161]	10	NS	NS	80%
Morad et al. (2003)[162]	60	Ahmed	IOP < 21 mm Hg 1 year:	93%
			2 year:	86%

IOP: Intraocular pressure: meds: Glaucoma medications, NS: Not specified.

site may cause correctopia.[163] Extraocular muscle imbalance was reported after Baerveldt implant,[164] but it may occur after any type of drainage implant. Conjunctival and transcorneal[165] tube erosion was reported, which may lead to delayed endophthalmiti.[166,167] Episodes of postoperative hypotony are common with open-tube implants, whereas the flow-resistive implants have reduced rate of hypotony in the immediate postoperative period.

Two-stage implantation of glaucoma drainage device should be considered in eyes at high risk for complications due to hypotony.[146,147] In the first stage, the plate is implanted and the tube is left under the conjunctiva near the limbus. A period of 4–6 weeks prior to the second stage allows a pseudocapsule to form, which offers some resistance to aqueous flow in the immediate postoperative period after tube insertion. In the second stage, the tube is inserted into the anterior chamber. This approach is most commonly used for open tube implants, such as the Molteno[146,147] and Baerveldt[168] implants, but may also be used for flow-resistive valves.

Goniotomy and trabeculotomy often fail in patients of Sturge-Weber syndrome with glaucoma but these procedures are preferred as primary surgery, because of a lower complication rate compared with trabeculectomy.[169] Glaucoma drainage implants have been helpful in patients with Sturge-Weber syndrome requiring additional surgical treatment. Satisfactory results have been reported using a two-stage Baerveldt implant[168] or a single-stage Ahmed glaucoma valve.[170]

If the IOP increases after glaucoma drainage implant, most clinicians recommend adjunctive medical therapy. If adjunctive medical therapy fails to control the IOP, supplemental laser cyclophotocoagulation may be useful.[171] Another alternative is revision of the drainage implant, excising a portion of the pseudocapsule around the implant plate.[172] This approach is similar in concept to needling of encapsulated blebs and has a similar success rate. Additional glaucoma drainage devices may be implanted in an unused quadrant, which may control the IOP.[173,174]

The initial surgery for developmental glaucoma fails in 10–20% of patients, the clinician often chooses trabeculectomy with MMC or a drainage implant as a subsequent surgical treatment. In one study comparing outcomes of trabeculectomy with MMC and glaucoma drainage implant, the success rate was higher after drainage implant,[175] whereas another study found similar success rates after these two procedures.[176] Both procedures are useful in patients with developmental glaucoma refractory to initial surgical treatment. We recommend trabeculectomy with MMC in such cases and, if this procedure fails too, a drainage implant is placed.

Cyclodestructive Procedures

If initial and secondary surgical procedures fail to control the IOP, a cyclodestructive procedure should be considered. In some instances, these procedures may be performed as adjunctive therapy or as primary therapy.

Cyclodestructive procedures cause damage to the ciliary epithelium, reduce aqueous production and thereby lower the IOP. The most commonly performed procedures are cyclocryotherapy and cyclophotocoagulation. When available, cyclophotocoagulation is usually the preferred procedure because it is associated with less postoperative inflammation and less discomfort to the patient compared with cyclocryotherapy.

In cyclodestructive procedures, the amount of treatment required to achieve the desired degree of IOP reduction may be difficult to titrate.[177] Retreatments are often necessary after cyclo-destructive procedures and these procedures may be associated with vision-threatening complications. The risk of hypotony, vision loss and even phthisis is substantial. Parents should be informed about these possibilities and IOP should be monitored.

In cyclocryotherapy, a probe is applied just posterior to the limbus to freeze the ciliary body and ciliary epithelium. Al-Faran and coworkers178 reported a 30% success rate, with no difference between the success rates in eyes that had been treated with other glaucoma procedures prior to cyclocryotherapy and with no previous glaucoma surgery. Wagle and coworkers179 reported 44% success after cyclocryotherapy in refractory pediatric glaucoma, requiring an average of 4.1 treatments. Devastating complications occurred even more frequently among eyes with aniridia (50%) compared with other eyes (11%). Vision-threatening complications include retinal detachment, hypotony, and phthisis.

Cyclophotocoagulation can be performed with a variety of lasers, including the Nd:YAG, 810 nm diode, and krypton laser. Although noncontact procedures have been described, the procedure is usually performed with a specially designed contact probe, which is applied near the limbus over the ciliary body. The procedure is usually performed under general anesthesia in the supine position.

Table 16.3 summarizes the results of studies of cyclophotocoagulation in pediatric patients.[180-186] In general, success rate with a single treatment is low, retreatment is often required and complications are perhaps less frequent but are similar to those found after cyclocryotherapy.

Cyclophotocoagulation may be performed with an endolaser and an endoscope, although this approach is not widely available. The procedure requires intraocular surgery, but the laser energy is delivered more precisely to the target tissue.[187-190] In a study on 36 eyes, Neely and Plager[188] reported a success rate of 34% in the initial procedure (IOP 21 mm Hg, with or without adjunctive glaucoma medications), which increased to 43% after retreatments. There is no clear benefit of this procedure compared with contact transscleral cyclophotocoagulation.

Cyclodestructive procedures are usually reserved for children who do not respond to other surgical treatments for intractable elevation of IOP. These procedures have limited success rates often require retreatment, and may be associated with vision-threatening complications. Some clinicians advocate cyclodestructive procedures early in the surgical treatment

Table 16.3: Studies of contact transscleral cyclophotocoagulation in pediatric patients.

Author, year	No. of eyes	Laser	Success criteria	Success
Phelan and Higginbotham (1995)[180]	10	Nd:YAG	IOP <21 mm Hg	50%
Bock et al. (1997)[181]	26	Diode	IOP <21 mm Hg	38%, 50%*
Hamard et al. (2000)[182]	28	Diode	6 mm Hg <IOP <20 mm Hg	28%*
Izgi et al. (2001)[183]	41	Diode	NS	59%, 75%*
Raivio et al. (2001)[184]	27	Krypton	8 mm Hg <IOP <21 mm Hg	64%*
Kirwan et al. (2002)[185]	77	Diode	<22 mm Hg	37%, 72%*
Autrata and Rehurek (2003)[186]	69	Diode	IOP <21 mm Hg	41%, 79%*

*Success rate allowing retreatment.

Nd:YAG: Neodymium:yttrium-aluminum-garnet; IOP: Intraocular pressure,

NS: Not specified.

regimen, while most reserve cycloablation until after other primary and secondary treatments have failed. Supplemental sub-maximal or full treatment with cyclophotocoagulation may be useful if the IOP remains uncontrolled despite glaucoma drainage implants or other glaucoma surgical treatments.[171]

LONG-TERM FOLLOW-UP AND PROGNOSIS

Between 3 and 6 weeks after surgery, the postoperative control of the glaucoma must be judged. The degree of relief from photophobia, tearing and blepharospasm usually reflect the effectiveness of surgery and may reasonably predict whether or not additional surgery will be required. Children with the developmental glaucoma must be periodically examined for a long time to determine whether or not adequate control of intraocular pressure has been achieved. Most of the examination can be done in an office setting. Examination under anesthesia often allows more accurate gonioscopy and measurements. Each follow-up evaluation should include vision testing, external examination, refraction, ophthalmoscopy, corneal assessment, tonometry, gonioscopy, ultrasonographic biometry and disc photography.

Vision testing techniques vary greatly with the age of the patient. In infants, good fixation and flash light following as well as the absence of nystagmus are important indicators of good visual function. In children over 3 years of age, visual acuity and visual fields should also be determined. The external examination is important in order to detect evidence of associated abnormalities, inflammation and lacrimal duct obstruction. Subjective refraction is generally not possible, but retinoscopy of the eye can be compared to the previous refractive error. The optic disk should be examined by ophthalmoscopy to determine if the optic cup has remained the same, enlarged, or regressed.[25] The cornea is assessed, the degree of corneal haze or edema is noted, and the calipers are used to measure the corneal diameter. A problem with the calipers in measuring the corneal diameter is that it is difficult to distinguish the actual corneal diameter from a chord length. Accurate measurements of the corneal diameter is facilitated by the use of a plastic gauge with calibrated holes.[191]

Tonometry is best performed on a peaceful, awake infant. If an examination under anesthesia is required, tonometry is performed at an appropriate stage of anesthesia,[192] but the significance of the IOP reading must be balanced carefully against the other clinical signs. Many anesthetic drugs alter IOP of patients with developmental glaucomas. Postoperatively, gonioscopy provides important anatomic information about the status of the anterior chamber angle treated with goniotomy or trabeculotomy *ab externo*. Ultrasonographic biometry may be performed, utilizing the A-scan ultrasound to measure the axial length and to compare with presurgical readings. Sampaolesi[193] and other authors[194-196] have stressed the clinical importance of echography in the diagnosis and follow-up of the developmental glaucomas.

Disk photography may provide a record for future comparisons. A decrease in cupping can occur within hours or days after IOP control in a very young patient, especially marked in infants below 1 year of age. The prognosis of this disease is related to the time of its initial presentation, initial surgical intervention, degree of optic nerve damage, nature of corneal enlargement, astigmatism, progressive refractive error and anisometropic amblyopia.[197] The inability to easily quantitate visual acuity and extent of visual loss in neonates and children makes these variables less helpful in following patients than measurements of corneal diameter and IOP. However, these data should not be relied upon exclusively to determine the success of treatment in developmental glaucoma.

Because of difficulties in measuring the IOP and recording the visual fields in children, ophthalmoscopy often provides the most reliable information of elevated IOP as seen by cupping of the optic nerve. Continued enlargement of the globe, as seen by retinoscopy or ultrasonography, signifies inadequately controlled pressure; while stability (and sometimes slight reduction)[198] of ocular size suggests adequate control of IOP during the long-term follow-up.

In properly selected patients, namely those with isolated trabeculo-dysgenesis, surgical treatment (trabeculotomy *ab externo* or goniotomy) is often successful. It should be remembered that increased IOP can occur at any time in the life of the patient and, therefore, a lifelong follow-up is necessary. The most important variables in the follow-up examinations are cupping of the optic disk visualized by ophthalmoscopy, axial length value measured by ultrasonographic biometry, IOP measured by applanation tonometry and visual field evaluation (if possible).

There are only a few reports in the literature regarding the long-term surgical and visual outcomes in children with developmental glaucoma. Recently Mandal et al.[126] reported a long-term outcome of 299 eyes of 157 consecutive patients who underwent primary combined trabeculotomy-trabeculectomy for developmental glaucoma by a single surgeon over a 12-year period. Kaplan-Meier survival analysis demonstrated the success probabilities of 94.4%, 92.0%, 86.7%, 79.4%, 72.9% and 63% at the 1st, 2nd, 3rd, 4th, 5th and 6th year respectively (Figs. 16.27 to 16.30). The success rate

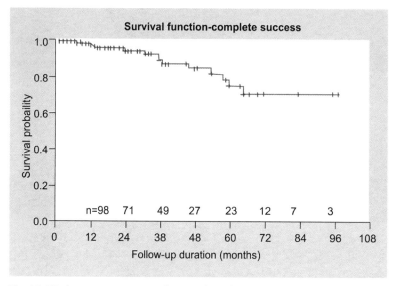

Fig. 16.27: Long-term success after combined trabeculotomy-trabeculectomy.

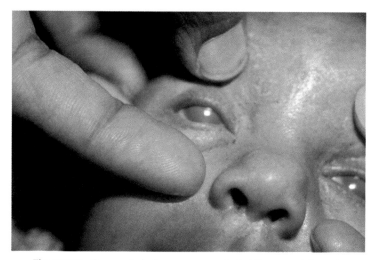

Fig. 16.28: Congenital glaucoma operated at the age of 1 week.

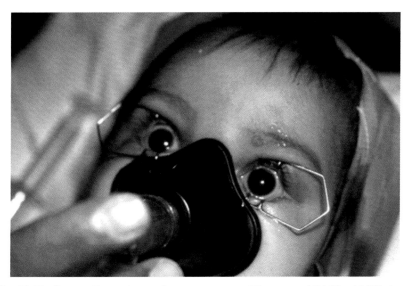

Fig. 16.29: Six months postoperative appearance of the same child (Fig. 19.20) showing clear cornea.

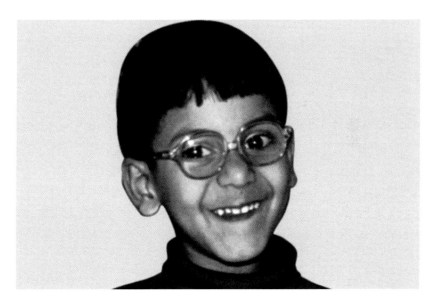

Fig. 16.30: Ten years postoperative appearance of the same child (Fig. 19.21) with normal vision.

of 63.1% was maintained till 8 years of follow-up. Data on visual acuity was available in 49 patients (3.2%). At the final follow-up visit, 20 patients (40.8%) had normal visual acuity (best-corrected visual acuity of better than or equal to 20/60 in the better eye). The visual outcome reported by them was better than the earlier reports (Table 16.4).[65,75,76,79,100,103,105,120,124,126,199,200-204]

Table 16.4: Studies of visual outcome for developmental glaucoma.

Author(s)	Year of publication	IType of developmental glaucoma	No. of subjects/eyes studied	Best-corrected visual acuity
Scheie[199]	1959	Infantile glaucoma	53 eyes	≥20/50 (60% eyes)
Richardson etal.[75]	1967	Infantile glaucoma	—	≥20/50 (39% eyes) ≥20/200 (40% eyes)
Hass [65]	1968	Infantile glaucoma	—	> 20/50 (39%)
Biglan and Hiles[200]	1979	Infantile glaucoma	25 eyes	≥20/50 (64% eyes)
Robin et al.[202]	1979	Infantile glaucoma	102 eyes	> 20/50 (41%; 30 eyes) < 20/200 (41%; 30 eyes) ≥20/40 (15 eyes)
Broughton and Parks [76]	1981	Congenital glaucoma	29 eyes	≥20/60 (20 eyes) ≥20/50 (58%; 7 eyes)
Morgan etal [201]	1981	Congenital glaucoma	12 eyes	20/100 (9 eyes)
Shaffer [79]	1982	Developmental glaucoma	287 eyes	20/20-20/40 (28eyes) 20/50-20/200(11 eyes) ≥20/200 (13 eyes)
Akimoto etal.[100]	1994	Developmental glaucoma	111 eyes	> 20/40 (68 eyes) 20/200 −20/40 (23 eyes) <20/200 (20 eyes)
Mandal et al.[120]	1998	Juvenile-onset developmental glaucoma	38 eyes	<20/200 (50%;19 eyes) 20/200 (26.3%; 10 eyes) 20/100 − 20/40 (7.8%; 3 eyes) >20/40 (15.7%; 6 eyes)
Mendicino etal.[105]	2000	Congenital glaucoma	24 eyes (trab) 40 eyes (gonio)	≥20/50 (79.2%; 19 eyes) ≥20/50 (52.5%; 21 eyes)
Meyer et al.[203]	2000	Congenital glaucoma	35 eyes	Within normal nomogram range in 12 eyes
Mandal et al.[124]	2002	Developmental glaucoma	28 eyes	<20/200 (28.6%; 8 eyes) 20/200-20/50 (28.6%; 8 eyes) >20/50 (42.9%; 12 eyes)
Filous and Brunova[103]	2002	Congenital glaucoma	78 eyes	20/20 −20/40 (64.1%) 0.35- 0.1 (29.5%) 0.08 − 0.04 (6.4%)
MacKinnon et al.[204]	2004	Infantile glaucoma	83 eyes	20/40 or better (61.8%)
Mandal et al.[126]	2004	Developmental glaucoma	49 patients	20/60 or better (40.8%)

CONCLUSION

The responsibility of the surgeon does not end with surgery, and it is important not to be lulled into a false sense of security by surgical control of IOP in patients with developmental glaucoma. Visual rehabilitation is as important in the management of the disease as is IOP control. Visual rehabilitation involves correction of refractive errors, correction of opacities in the media, including corneal scarring and cataract, and orthoptic treatment to stimulate the development of binocular stereoscopic vision. Anisometropia and amblyopia must be aggressively managed to give these children the best chance for good vision in both eyes.

An attempt should be made to familiarize the parents with the protracted nature of the illness, the prognosis, the frequent possible necessity for repeat surgery and a lifelong continued follow-up examination. The parents may be quite young and may be emotionally and economically ill-equipped to cope with the problems that have suddenly and dramatically occurred. Their guilt problems must be assuaged, particularly if a family history of congenital glaucoma exists. The parents should also be familiarized with the various agencies that will provide financial assistance when necessary. Time and effort well-spent will reward the ophthalmologist.[205]

Fortunately, with early diagnosis and microsurgical techniques, the large majority of these eyes can be controlled if not completely cured. However, in few patients who continue to show poor response to surgery such operations may delay loss of vision and allow the child to develop visual images that will be valuable to him or her in later life. Eventually, the social aspects of the glaucomatous child will require repeated counselling. Poor vision will need explanation to the parents and teachers, the child may require the help of visual aids, and cosmetic blemishes will need correction where possible. Continued clinical monitoring combined with adequate social support should allow the best possible outcome for the child.

REFERENCES

1. Mandal AK, Netland PA. The Pediatric Glaucomas. Edinburgh, UK: Elsevier; 2006.
2. Hoskins HD, Jr, Shaffer RN, Hetherington J. Anatomical classification of the developmental glaucomas. Arch Ophthalmol. 1984;102(9):133-6.
3. Hoskins, HD Jr, et al. Developmental glaucoma: Diagnosis and classification. In: The New Orleans Academy of Ophthalmology Symposium on Glaucoma. St Louis, MO: The CV Mosby Company; 1981.
4. Barkan O. Technique of goniotomy. Arch Ophthalmol. 1938;19:217-21.
5. Burian HM. A case of Marfan's syndrome with bilateral glaucoma with a description of a new type of operation for developmental glaucoma. Am J Ophthalmol. 1960;50:1187-92.
6. Smith R. A new technique for opening the canal of Schlemm. Br J Ophthalmol. 1960;44:370-3.

7. Burian HM, Allen L. Trabeculotomy *ab externo*; a new glaucoma operation: Technique and results of experimental surgery. Am J Ophthalmol. 1962;53: 19-26.

8. Grant WM, Walton DS. Progressive changes in the angle in congenital aniridia with development of glaucoma. Am J Ophthalmol. 1974;78(5):842.

9. Weiss DL. Dual origin of glaucoma in encephalotrigeminal hemangiomatosis. Trans Ophthalmol Soc UK. 1973;93(0):477-91.

10. Barkan O. Goniotomy for glaucoma associated with nevus flammeus. Am J Ophthalmol. 1957;43(Part 1):545-9.

11. Christensen GR, Records RE. Glaucoma and expulsive hemorrhage mechanism in the Sturge-Weber syndrome. Ophthalmology. 1979;86(7):1360-6.

12. Phelps CD. The pathogenesis of glaucoma in Sturge-Weber syndrome. Ophthalmology. 1978;85(3):276-86.

13. Keverline DO, Hills DA. Trabeculectomy for adolescent glaucoma in Sturge-Weber syndrome. J Pediatr Ophthalmol Strabismus. 1977;13(3):144-8.

14. Bellows AR, Chylark LT, Epstein DL, et al. Choroidal effusion during glaucoma surgery in patients with prominent episcleral vessels. Arch Ophthalmol. 1979;97(3):493-7.

15. Board RJ, Shields MB. Combined trabeculotomy-trabeculectomy for the management of glaucoma associated with Sturge-Weber syndrome. Ophthal Surg. 1981;12(11):813-7.

16. Krasnov MM. Microsurgery of the Glaucomas. St Louis, MO: The CV Mosby Company; 1979.

17. Zimmerman TJ, Kooner KS, Ford VJ, et al. Trabeculectomy vs nonpenetrating trabeculectomy: A retrospective study of two procedures in phakic patients with glaucoma. Ophthalmic Surg. 1984;15(9):734-40.

18. Curtin VT, Joyee EE, Ballin N. Ocular pathology in the oculocerebrorenal syndrome of Lowe. Am J Ophthalmol. 1967;64:533.

19. Komrower GM, Wilson VK. Homocysteinuria. Proc R Soc Med. 1963;56: 996-7.

20. Lichter PR, Schmeikel RD. Posterior vortex vein and congenital glaucoma in a patient with trisomy-13 syndrome. Am J Ophthalmol. 1975;80(5):939-42.

21. Luntz MH, Livingston DG. Trabeculotomy *ab externo* and trabeculectomy in congenital and adult-onset glaucoma. Am J Ophthalmol. 1977;83(2): 174-9.

22. Hoskins HD, Shaffer RN, Hetherington J. Goniotomy vs trabeculotomy. J Pediatr Ophthalmol Strabismus 1984;21(4):153-8.

23. Gregerson E, Kessing SVV. Congenital glaucoma before and after the introduction of microsurgery. Results of 'Macro-surgery' 1943-1963 and of microsurgery (Trabeculotomy/ectomy) 1970-1974. Acta Ophthalmol. 1977; 55(3): 422-30.

24. Luntz MH. Primary buphthalmos (infantile glaucoma) treated by trabeculotomy *ab externo*. S Afr Arch Ophthalmol. 1974;2:319-34.

25. Quigley HA. Childhood glaucoma: results with trabeculotomy and study of reversible cupping. Ophthalmology. 1982;89(3):219-25.

26. McPherson SD, McFarland D. External trabeculotomy for developmental glaucoma. Ophthalmology. 1980;87(4):302-5.
27. Barkan O. Goniotomy for the relief of congenital glaucoma. Br J Ophthalmol. 1948;32(9):701-28.
28. Robertson EN, Jr. Therapy of congenital glaucoma. AMA Arch Ophthalmol. 1955;54(1):55-8.
29. Wallace DK, Steinkuller PG. Ocular medications in children. Clin Pediatr. 1998;37(11):645-52.
30. Palmer EA. How safe are ocular drugs in pediatrics? Ophthalmology. 1986; 93(8):1038-40.
31. Boger WP III, Walton DS. Timolol in uncontrolled childhood glaucomas. Ophthalmology. 1981;88(3):253-58.
32. McMahon CD, Hetherington J Jr, Hoskins HD Jr, et al. Timolol and pediatric glaucomas. Ophthalmology. 1981;88(3):249-52.
33. Zimmerman TJ, Kooner KS, Morgan KS. Safety and efficacy of timolol in pediatric glaucoma. Surv Ophthalmol 1983;28 (Suppl 2):262-4.
34. Hoskins HD Jr, Hetherington J Jr, Magee SD, et al. Clinical experience with timolol in childhood glaucoma. Arch Ophthalmol. 1985;103(8):1163-5.
35. Passo MS, Palmer EA, Van Buskirk EM. Plasma timolol in glaucoma patients. Ophthalmology. 1984;91(11):1361-3.
36. Burnstine RA, Felton JL, Ginther WH. Cardiorespiratory reaction to timolol maleate in a pediatric patient: a case report. Ann Ophthalmol. 1982;14(10): 905-6.
37. Bailey PL. Timolol and postoperative apnea in neonates and young infants. Anesthesiology. 1984;61(5):622.
38. Olsen RJ, Bromberg BB, Zimmerman TJ. Apneic cells associated with timolol therapy in a neonate. Am J Ophthalmol. 1979;88(1):120-2.
39. Futagi Y, Otani K, Abe J. Growth suppression in children receiving acetazolamide with antiepileptic drugs. Pediatr Neurol. 1996;15(4):323-6.
40. Ritch R. Special therapeutic situations. In: Netland PA, Allen RC (Eds). Glaucoma Medical Therapy: Principles and Management. San Francisco, CA: American Academy of Ophthalmology; 1999. pp. 193-211.
41. Hass J. Principles and problems of therapy in congenital glaucoma. Invest Ophthalmol. 1968;7(2):140-6.
42. Shaffer RN. New concepts in infant glaucoma. Trans Ophthalmol Soc UK. 1967;87:581-90.
43. Portellos M, Buckley EG, Freedman SF. Topical versus oral carbonic anhydrase inhibitor therapy for pediatric glaucoma. J AAPOS. 1998;2(1):43-7.
44. Enyedi LB, Freedman SF, Buckley EG. The effectiveness of latanoprost for the treatment of pediatric glaucoma. J AAPOS. 1999;3(1):33-9.
45. Yang CB, Freedman SF, Myers JS, et al. Use of latanoprost in the treatment of glaucoma associated with Sturge-Weber syndrome. Am J Ophthalmol. 1998;126(4):600-2.
46. Altuna JC, Greenfield DS, Wand M, et al. Latanoprost in glaucoma associated with Sturge-Weber syndrome: benefits and side-effects. J Glaucoma. 1999;8(3):99-203.

47. Ong T, Chia A, Nischal KK. Latanoprost in port wine stain related paediatric glaucoma. Br J Ophthalmol. 2003;87(9):1091-3.
48. Enyedi LB, Freedman SF. Latanoprost for the treatment of pediatric glaucoma. Surv Ophthalmol. 2002;(Suppl 1): S129-32.
49. Enyedi LB, Freedman SF. Safety and efficacy of brimonidine in children with glaucoma. J AAPOS. 2001;5(5):281-4.
50. Bowman RJ, Cope J, Nischal KK. Ocular and systemic side effects of brimonidine 0.2% eye drops (Alphagan) in children. Eye. 2004;18(1):24-6.
51. Levy Y, Zadok D. Systemic side effects of ophthalmic drops. Clin Pediatr (Phila). 2004;43(1):99-101.
52. Berlin RJ, Lee UT, Samples JR, et al. Ophthalmic drops causing coma in an infant. J Pediatr. 2001;138(3):441-3.
53. Freedman SF. Medical and surgical treatments for childhood glaucomas. In: Epstein DL, Allingham RR, Schuman JS (Eds). Chandler and Grant's Glaucoma (4th edition). Baltimore, MD: Williams & Wilkins; 1997. p 636.
54. Raab EL. Congenital glaucoma. Persp Ophthalmol. 1978;2:35-41.
55. Pollack IP, Quigley HA, Harbin TS. The Ocusert pilocarpine system: advantages and disadvantages. South Med J. 1976;69(10):1296-8.
56. Jones DE, Watson DM. Angle-closure glaucoma precipitated by the use of phospholine iodide for esotropia in child. Br J Ophthalmol. 1967; 51(11):783-5.
57. Netland PA, Kolker AE. Osmotic drugs. In: Netland PA, Allen RC (Eds): Glaucoma Medical Therapy: Principles and Management. San Francisco, CA: American Academy of Ophthalmology, 1999. pp. 133-47.
58. Barkan O. A new operation for chronic glaucoma. Am J Ophthalmol. 1936; 19:951.
59. Barkan O. Operation for congenital glaucoma. Am J Ophthalmol. 1942; 25: 552-68.
60. Barkan O. Techniques of goniotomy for congenital glaucoma. Arch Ophthamol. 1949;41:65-8.
61. Barkan O. Surgery of congenital glaucoma. Review of 196 eyes operated by goniotomy. Am J Ophthalmol. 1953;36:1523-34.
62. Barkan O. Pathogenesis of congenital glaucoma. Gonioscopic and anatomic observation of the angle of the anterior chamber in the normal eye and in congenital glaucoma. Am J Ophthalmol. 1955;40:11.
63. Barkan O. Goniotomy. Trans Am Acad Ophthalmol. 1955;589:322-32.
64. Maumenee AE. Further observations on the pathogenesis of congenital glaucoma. Trans Am Ophthalmol Soc. 1962;60:140-6.
65. Hass J. Principles and problems of therapy in congenital glaucoma. Invest Ophthalmol. 1968;7(2):140-6.
66. Haas JS. End results of treatment. Trans Am Acad Ophthalmol Otolaryngol. 1955;59:333-40.
67. Scheie HG. Management of infantile glaucoma. Arch Ophthalmol. 1959; 62(1):35-54.
68. Shaffer RN. New concepts in infantile glaucoma. Can J Ophthalmol. 1967;2: 243-7.

69. Shaffer RN, Hetherington J. Glaucomatous disc in infants, a suggested hypothesis for disc cupping. Trans Am Acad Ophthalmol Otolaryngol. 1969; 73:929-35.
70. Shaffer RN, Weiss DI. The Congenital and Pediatric Glaucomas. St Louis, MO: CV Mosby; 1970.
71. Bietti GB. Contribution a la connaissance des resultats de la goniotomie dans le glaucoma congenitable. Ann Ocul (Paris). 1966;199:481-5.
72. Morgan KS, Black B, Ellis FD, et al. Treatment of congenital glaucoma. Am J Ophthalmol. 1981;92(6):799-803.
73. Moller PM. Goniotomy and congenital glaucoma. Acta Ophthalmol. 1977;55(3): 436-42.
74. Morin JD. Congenital glaucoma. Trans Am Ophthalmol Soc. 1980;78: 123-31.
75. Richardson KT, Ferguson WJ Jr. Shaffer RN. Long-term functional results in infantile glaucoma. Trans Am Acad Ophthalmol Otolaryngol. 1967;71(5): 833-7.
76. Broughton WL, Parks MM. Analysis of treatment of congenital glaucoma by goniotomy. Am J Ophthalmol. 1981;91(5):566-72.
77. Anderson DR. In discussion of Quigley HA: Childhood glaucoma. Ophthalmology. 1982;90:225-6.
78. McPherson SD Jr, Berry DP. Goniotomy vs external trabeculotomy for developmental glaucoma. Am J Ophthalmol. 1983;95(4):427-31.
79. Shaffer RN. Prognosis of goniotomy in primary infantile glaucoma (trabeculo-dysgenesis). Trans Am Ophthalmol Soc. 1982; 80:321-5.
80. Shaffer RN, Hoskins HD. Montgomery lecture. Goniotomy in the treatment of isolated trabeculodysgenesis (primary congenital [infantile] developmental glaucoma). Trans Ophthalmol Soc UK. 1983;103:581-5.
81. Catalano RA, King RA, Calhoun JH, et al. One versus two simultaneous goniotomies as the initial surgical procedure for primary infantile glaucoma. J Pediatr Ophthalmol Strabismus. 1989;26(1):9-13.
82. Arnoult J, Vila Coro A, Mazow M. Goniotomy with sodium hyaluronate. J Pediatr Ophthalmol Strabismus. 1988;25(1):18-22.
83. Winter R. Technical modification in goniotomy using high viscous hyaluronic acid. Dev Ophthalmol. 1985; 11: 136-8.
84. Hodapp E, Heuer DK. A simple technique for goniotomy. Am J Ophthalmol. 1986;102(4):537.
85. Medow NB, Sauer HL. Endoscopic goniotomy for congenital glaucoma. J Pediatr Ophthalmol Strabismus. 1997;34(4):258-9.
86. Bayraktar S, Koseoglu T. Endoscopic goniotomy with anterior chamber maintainer: Surgical technique and one year results. Ophthal Surg Lasers. 2001;32(6):496-502.
87. Joos KM, Alward WL, Folberg R. Experimental endoscopic goniotomy. A potential treatment for primary infantile glaucoma. Ophthalmology. 1993;100(7):1066-70.
88. Joos KM, Shen JH. An ocular endoscope enables a goiniotomy despite a cloudy cornea. Arch Ophthalmol. 2001;119(1):134-5.

89. Sun W, Shen JH, Shetlar DJ, et al. Endoscopic goniotomy with the free electron laser in congenital glaucoma rabbits. J Glaucoma. 2000;9(4):325-33.
90. Harms H. Dannheim R. Epicritical consideration of 300 cases of trabeculotomy *ab externo*. Trans Ophthalmol Soc UK. 1970;89:491-9.
91. Harms H, Dannheim R. Trabeculotomy—results and problems. Bibl Ophthalmol. 1970;81:121-31.
92. Dannheim R. Trabeculotomy. Techniques and results. Arch Chili Oftal. 1971;28:149-57.
93. Dannheim R. Trabeculotomy. Trans Am Acad Ophthalmol Otolarynogol. 1972;76:375-83.
94. McPherson SD Jr. Results of external trabeculotomy. Am J Ophthalmol. 1973;76(6):918-20.
95. Luntz MH. The advantages of trabeculotomy over goniotomy. J Pediatr Ophthalmol Strabismus. 1984;4:150-3.
96. Hetherington J Jr. Congenital glaucoma, in Duane TD (Ed): Clinical Ophthal-mology. New York: Harper and Row; 1982. Vol. 3 pp. 51,4.
97. Hass H. in Kwitko MC (Ed). Glaucoma in Infants and Children. New York: Appleton-Century-Crofts; 1973;12,591.
98. Kiffney GT, Meyers GW, McPherson SD Jr. The surgical management of congenital glaucoma. South Med J. 1960;53:989-95.
99. Luntz MH. Congenital, infantile, and juvenile glaucoma. Ophthalmology. 1979;86(5):793-802.
100. Akimoto M, Tanihara H, Negi A, et al. Surgical results of trabeculotomy *ab externo* for developmental glaucoma. Arch Ophthalmol. 1994;112(12):1540-4.
101. Anderson DR. Trabeculotomy compared to goniotomy of glaucoma in children. Ophthalmology. 1983;90(7):805-6.
102. Shields MB, Krieglstein GK. Glaukom: Grundlagen. Differentialdiagnose, Threapie. Berlin: Springer. 1993;50-78,211-25, 527-32.
103. Filous A, Brunova B. Results of the modified trabeculotomy in the treatment of primary congenital glaucoma. J AAPOS. 2002;6(3):182-6.
104. Beck AD, Lynch MG. 360° trabeculotomy for primary congenital glaucoma. Arch Ophthalmol. 1995;113(9):1200-2.
105. Mendicino ME, Lynch MG, Drack A, et al. Long-term surgical and visual outcomes in primary congenital glaucoma: 3600 trabeculotomy versus goniotomy. J AAPOS. 2000;4(4):205-10.
106. Beauchamp GR, Parks MM. Filtering surgery in children: barriers to success. Ophthalmology. 1979;86(1):170-80.
107. Cadera W, Pachtman MA, Cantor LB, et al. Filtering surgery in childhood glaucoma. Ophthal Surg. 1984;15(4):319-22.
108. Levene RZ. Glaucoma filtering surgery: factors that determine pressure control. Ophthal Surg. 1984;15(6):475-83.
109. Joseph A. Trabeculectomy in congenital glaucoma. Indian J Ophthalmol. 1981;29(2):81-2.
110. Debnath SC, Teichmann KD, Salamah K. Trabeculectomy versus trabeculectomy in congenital glaucoma. Br J Ophthalmol. 1989;73(8):608-11.

111. Rao KV, Sai CM, Babu BVN. Trabeculectomy in congenital glaucoma. Indian J Ophthalmol. 1984;32(5):439-40.
112. Burke JP, Bowell R. Primary trabeculectomy in congenital glaucoma. Br J Ophthalmol. 1989;73(3):186-90.
113. Miller MH, Rice NSC. Trabeculectomy combined with beta irradiation for congenital glaucoma. Br J Ophthalmol. 1991;75(10):584-90.
114. Fulcher T, Chan J, Lanigan B, et al. Long-term follow up of primary trabeculectomy for infantile glaucoma. Br J Ophthalmol. 1996;80(6):499-502.
115. Biedner BZ, Rothkoff L. Combined trabeculotomy-trabeculectomy compared with primary trabeculotomy for congenital glaucoma. J Pediatr Ophthalmol Strabismus. 1998;35(1):49-50.
116. Dietlein TS, Jacob PC, Krieglstein GK. Prognosis of primary *ab externo* surgery for Primary congenital glaucoma. Br J Ophthalmol. 1999;83(3): 317-22.
117. Elder MJ. Combined trabeculotomy-trabeculectomy compared with primary trabeculectomy for congenital glaucoma. Br J Ophthalmol. 1994; 78(10): 745-8.
118. Mullaney PB, Selleck, Al-Award A, et al. Combined trabeculotomy and trabeculectomy as initial procedure in uncomplicated congenital glaucoma. Arch Ophthalmol. 1999;117(4):457-60.
119. Al-Hazmi A, Zwaan J, Awad A, et al. Effectiveness and complications of mitomycin-C use during pediatric glaucoma surgery. Ophthalmology. 1998;105(10):1915-20.
120. Mandal AK, Naduvilath TJ, Jayagandhan A. Surgical results of combined trabeculotomy-trabeculectomy for developmental glaucoma. Ophthalmology. 1998;105(6):974-82.
121. Mandal AK. Current concepts in the diagnosis and management of developmental glaucomas. Indian J Ophthalmol. 1993;41(2):51-70.
122. Mandal AK. Microsurgical technique combines trabeculotomy and trabeculectomy to treat developmental glaucoma. Ocular Surg News. Int ed. 1994;8: 38-43.
123. Mandal AK. Primary combined trabeculotomy-trabeculectomy for early onset glaucoma in Sturge-Weber syndrome. Ophthalmology. 1999;106(8): 1621-7.
124. Mandal AK, Bhatia PG, Gothwal VK, et al. Safety and efficacy of simultaneous bilateral primary combined trabeculotomy-trabeculectomy for developmental glaucoma in India. Indian J Ophthalmol. 2002;50(1): 13-9.
125. Mandal AK, Gothwal VK, Bagga H, et al. Outcome of surgery on infants younger than 1 month with congenital glaucoma. Ophthalmology. 2003; 110(10): 1909-15.
126. Mandal AK, Bhatia PG, Bhaskar A, et al. Long-term surgical and visual outcomes in Indian children with developmental glaucoma operated on within 6 months of birth. Ophthalmology. 2004;111(2):283-90.

127. O' Connor G. Combined trabeculotomy-trabeculectomy for congenital glaucoma (Editorial). Br J Ophthalmol. 1994;78(10):735.

128. Mandal AK, Matalia JH, Nutheti R, et al. Combined trabeculotomy and trabeculectomy in advanced primary developmental glaucoma with corneal diameter of 14 mm or more. Eye 2006;20:135-43.

129. Gressel MG, Heuer DK, Parrish RK II. Trabeculectomy in young patients. Ophthalmology. 1984;91(10):1242-6.

130. Veldman E, Greve EL. Glaucoma filtering surgery, a retrospective study of 300 operations. Doc Ophthalmol. 1987;67(1-2):151-70.

131. Zalish M, Leiba H, Oliver M. Subconjunctival injection of 5-fluorouracil following trabeculectomy for congenital and infantile glaucoma. Ophthalmic Surg. 1992;23(3):203-5.

132. Michel JW, Liebmann JM, Ritch R. Initial 5-Fluorouracil trabeculectomy in young patients. Ophthalmology. 1992;99(1):7-13.

133. Snir M, Lusky M, Shalev B, et al. Mitomycin C and 5-fluorouracil antimetabolite therapy for pediatric glaucoma filtration surgery. Ophthal Surg Lasers. 2000;31(1):31-7.

134. Susanna R Jr, Oltrogge EW, Carani JCE, et al. Mitomycin as adjunct chemotherapy with trabeculectomy in congenital and developmental glaucomas. J Glaucoma. 1995;4(3):151-7.

135. Mandal AK, Walton DS, John T, et al. Mitomycin C-augmented trabeculectomy in refractory congenital glaucoma. Ophthalmology. 1997;104(6):996-1001.

136. Agarwal HC, Sood NN, Sihota R, et al. Mitomycin-C in congenital glaucoma. Ophthal Surg Lasers. 1997;28(12):979-85.

137. Beck AD, Wilson WR, Lynch MG, et al. Trabeculectomy with adjunctive mitomycin C in pediatric glaucoma. Am J Ophthalmol. 1998;126(5):648-57.

138. Azuara-Blanco A, Wilson RP, Spaeth GL, et al. Filtration procedures supplemented with mitomycin C in the management of childhood glaucomas. Br J Ophthalmol. 1999;83(2):151-6.

139. Mandal AK, Prasad K, Naduvilath TJ. Surgical results and complications of mitomycin C-augmented trabeculectoy in refractory developmental glaucoma. Ophthal Surg Lasers. 1999;30(6):473-80.

140. Freedman SF, McCormick K, Cox TA. Mitomycin C-augmented trabeculectomy with postoperative wound modulation in pediatric glaucoma. J AAPOS. 1999;3(2):117-24.

141. Sidoti PA, Belmonte SJ, Liebmann JM, Ritch R. Trabeculectomy with mitomycin-C in the treatment of pediatric glaucomas. Ophthalmology. 2000; 107(3):422-9.

142. Waheed S, Ritterband DC, Greenfield DS, et al. Bleb-related ocular infection in children after trabeculectomy with mitomycin C. Ophthalmology. 1997;104(12):2117-20.

143. Wells AP, Cordeiro MF, Bunce C, et al. Cystic bleb formation and related complications in limbus- versus fornix-based conjunctival flaps in pediatric and young adult trabeculectomy with mitomycin C. Ophthalmology. 2003;110(11):2192-7.

144. Megevand GS, Salmon JF, Scholtz RP, et al. The effect of reducing the exposure time of mitomycin-C in glaucoma filtering surgery. Ophthalmology. 1995;102(1):84-90.

145.Lee JJ, Park KH, Youn DH. The effect of low- and high-dose adjunctive mitomy-cin C in trabeculectomy. Korean J Ophthalmol. 1996;10(1):42-7.

146.Molteno AC, Ancker E, Van Biljon G. Surgical technique for advanced juvenile glaucoma. Arch Ophthalmol. 1984;102(1):51-7.

147.Billson F, Thomas R, Aylward W. The use of two-stage Molteno implants in developmental glaucoma. J Pediatr Ophthalmol Strabismus. 1989;26(1): 3-8.

148.Hill RA, Heuer DK, Baerveldt G, et al. Molteno implantation for glaucoma in young patients. Ophthalmology. 1991;98(7):1042-6.

149.Munoz M, Tomey KF, Traverso C, et al. Clinical experience with the Molteno implant in advanced infantile glaucoma. J Pediatr Ophthalmol Strabismus. 1991;28(2):68-72.

150.Lloyd MA, Sedlak T, Heuer DK, et al. Clinical experience with the single-plate Molteno implant in complicated glaucomas. Update of a pilot study. Ophthalmology. 1992;99(5):679-87.

151.Nesher R, Sherwood MB, Kass MA, et al. Molteno implants in children. J Glaucoma. 1992;1(4):228-32.

152.Netland PA, Walton DS. Glaucoma Drainage implants in pediatric patients. Ophthalmic Surg. 1993;24(11):723-9.

153.Fellenbaum PS, Sidoti PA, Heuer DK, et al. Experience with the Baerveldt implant in young patients with complicated glaucomas. J Glaucoma. 1995; 4(2):91-7.

154.Siegner SW, Netland PA, Urban RC Jr, et al. Clinical experience with the Baerveldt glaucoma drainage implant. Ophthalmology. 1995;102(9):1298-307.

155.Coleman AL, Smyth RJ, Wilson MR, et al. Initial clinical experience with the Ahmed Glaucoma Valve implant in pediatric patients. Arch Ophthalmol. 1997;115(2):186-91.

156.Eid TE, Katz LJ, Spaeth GL, et al. Long-term effects of tube-shunt procedures on management of refractory childhood glaucoma. Ophthalmology. 1997;104(6):1011-6.

157.Donahue SP, Keech RV, Munden P, et al. Baerveldt implant surgery in the treatment of advanced childhood glaucoma. J AAPOS. 1997;1(1):41-5.

158.Huang MC, Netland PA, Coleman AL, et al. Intermediate-term clinical experience with the Ahmed glaucoma valve implant. Am J Ophthalmol. 1999; 127(1):27-33.

159.Englert JA, Freedman SF, Cox TA. The Ahmed valve in refractory pediatric glaucoma. Am J Ophthalmol. 1999;127(1):34-42.

160.Djodeyre MR, Peralta Calvo J, Abelairas Gomez J. Clinical evaluation and risk factors of time to failure of Ahmed Glaucoma Valve implant in pediatric patients. Ophthalmology. 2001;108(3):614-20.

161.Pereira ML, Araujo SV, Wilson RP, et al. Aqueous shunts for intractable glaucoma in infants. Ophthalmic Surg Lasers. 2002;33(1):19-29.

162.Morad Y, Donaldson CE, Kim YM, et al. The Ahmed drainage implant in the treatment of pediatric glaucoma. Am J Ophthalmol. 2003;135(6): 821-9.

163.Fuller JR, Molteno AC, Bevin TH. Iris creep producing correctopia in response to Molteno implants. Arch Ophthalmol. 2001;119(2):304.

164. Smith SL, Starita RJ, Fellman RL, et al. Early clinical experience with the Baerveldt 350-mm2 glaucoma implant and associated extraocular muscle imbalance. Ophthalmology. 1993;100:914-8.

165. Al-Torbak A, Edward DP. Transcorneal tube erosion of an Ahmed valve implant in a child. Arch Ophthalmol. 2001;119(10):1558-9.

166. Al-Torbaq AA, Edward DP. Delayed endophthalmitis in a child following an Ahmed glaucoma valve implant. J AAPOS. 2002;6(2):123-5.

167. Gedde SJ, Scott IU, Tabandeh H, et al. Late endophthalmitis associated with glaucoma drainage implants. Ophthalmology. 2001;108(7):1323-7.

168. Budenz DL, Sakamoto D, Eliezer R, et al. Two-staged Baerveldt glaucoma implant for childhood glaucoma associated with Sturge-Weber syndrome. Ophthalmology. 2000;107(11):2105-10.

169. Iwach AG, Hoskins HD Jr, Hetherington J Jr, et al. Analysis of surgical and medical management of glaucoma in Sturge-Weber syndrome. Ophthalmology. 1990;97(7):904-9.

170. Hamush NG, Coleman AL, Wilson MR. Ahmed glaucoma valve implant for management of glaucoma in Sturge-Weber syndrome. Am J Ophthalmol. 1999;128(6):758-60.

171. Semchyshyn TM, Tsay JC, Joos KM. Supplemental transscleral diode laser cyclophotocoagulation after aqueous shunt placement in refractory glaucoma. Ophthalmology. 2002;109(6):1078-84.

172. Tsai JC, Grajewski AL, Parrish RK II. Surgical revision of glaucoma shunt implants. Ophthalmic Surg Lasers. 1999;30(1):41-6.

173. Shah AA, WuDunn D, Cantor LB. Shunt revision versus additional tube shunt implantation after failed tube shunt surgery in refractory glaucoma. Am J Ophthalmol. 2000;129(4):455-60.

174. Burgoyne JK, WuDunn D, Lakhani V, Cantor LB. Outcomes of sequential tube shunts in complicated glaucoma. Ophthalmology. 2000;107(2):309-14.

175. Beck AD, Freedman S, Kammer J, et al. Aqueous shunt devices compared with trabeculectomy with mitomycin-C for children in the first two years of life. Am J Ophthalmol. 2003;136(6):994-1000.

176. Hill R, Ohanesian R, Voskanyan L, et al. The Armenian Eye Care Project: surgical outcomes of complicated paediatric glaucoma. Br J Ophthalmol. 2003;87(6):673-6.

177. Terraciano AJ, Sidoti PA. Management of refractory glaucoma in childhood. Curr Opin Ophthalmol. 2002;13(2):97-102.

178. Al Faran MF, Tomey KF, Al Mutlaq FA. Cyclocryotherapy in selected cases of congenital glaucoma. Ophthalmic Surg. 1990;21(11):794-8.

179. Wagle NS, Freedman SF, Buckley EG, et al. Long-term outcome of cyclocryotherapy for refractory pediatric glaucoma. Ophthalmology. 1998; 105(10):1921-6.

180. Phelan MJ, Higginbotham EJ. Contact transscleral Nd:YAG laser cyclophoto-coagulation for the treatment of refractory pediatric glaucoma. Ophthalmic Surg Lasers. 1995;26(5):401-3.

181. Bock CJ, Freedman SF, Buckley EG, et al. Transscleral diode laser cyclopho-tocoagulation for refractory pediatric glaucomas. J Pediatr Ophthalmol Strabismus. 1997;34:235-9.

182. Hamard P, May F, Quesnot S, et al. [Transscleral diode laser cyclophoto-coagulation for the treatment of refractory pediatric glaucoma]. J Fr Ophtalmol. 2000;23(8):773-80.

183. Izgi B, Demirci H, Demirci FY, et al. Diode laser cyclophotocoagulation in refractory glaucoma: comparison between pediatric and adult glaucomas. Ophthalmic Surg Lasers. 2001;32(2):100-7.

184. Raivio VE, Immonen IJ, Puska PM. Transscleral contact krypton laser cyclophotocoagulation for treatment of glaucoma in children and young adults. Ophthalmology. 2001;108(10):1801-7.

185. Kirwin JF, Shah P, Khaw PT. Diode laser cyclophotocoagulation: role in the management of refractory pediatric glaucomas. Ophthalmology. 2002; 109(2): 316-23.

186. Autrata R, Rehurek J. Long-term results of transscleral cyclophotocoagulation in refractory pediatric glaucoma patients. Ophthalmologica. 2003;217(6): 393-400.

187. Chen J, Cohn RA, Lin SC, et al. Endoscopic photocoagulation of the ciliary body for treatment of refractory glaucomas. Am J Ophthalmol. 1997; 124(6):787-96.

188. Plager DA, Neely DE. Intermediate-term results of endoscopic diode laser cyclophotocoagulation for pediatric glaucoma. J AAPOS. 1999;3(3):131-7.

189. Neely DE, Plager DA. Endocyclophotocoagulation for management of difficult pediatric glaucomas. J AAPOS. 2001;5(4):221-9.

190. Barkana Y, Morad Y, Ben-nun J. Endoscopic photocoagulation of the ciliary body after repeated failure of transscleral diode-laser cyclophotocoagulation. Am J Ophthalmol. 2002;133(3):405-7.

191. Kiskis AA, Markowitz. SN, Mortin JD. Corneal diameter and axial length in congenital glaucoma. Can J Ophthalmol. 1985;20(3):93-7.

192. Dominguez J, Banes MS, Alvarez MT, et al: Intraocular pressure measurements in infants under general anesthesia. Am J Ophthalmol. 1974; 78(1): 110.

193. Sampaolesi R, Caruso R. Ocular echometry in the diagnosis of congenital glaucoma. Arch Ophthalmol. 1982;100(4):S574-7.

194. Reibaldi A. Biometric ultrasound in the diagnosis and follow-up of congenital glaucoma. Ann Ophthalmol. 1982;14(8):707-8.

195. Tarkkanen A, Vusitalo R, Mianowicz J. Ultrasounographic biometry in congenital glaucoma. Acta Ophthalmol. 1983;61(4):618-23.

196. Law SK, Bui D, Caprioli J. Serial axial length measurements in congenital glaucoma. Am J Ophthalmol. 2001;132(6):926-8.

197. deLuise VP, Anderson DR. Primary infantile glaucoma (congenital glaucoma). Surv Ophthalmol. 1983;28(1):1-19.

198. Morin JD, Merin S, Sheppard RW. Primary congenital glaucoma: a survey. Can J Ophthalmol. 1974;9(1):17-28.

199. Scheie, Harold G. The management of infantile glaucoma. Arch Ophthal. 1959;62(1):35-54.

200. Biglan AW, Hiles DA. The visual results following infantile glaucoma surgery. J Pediatr Ophthalmol Strabismus. 1979;16(6):377-81.

201. Morgan KS, Black B, Ellis FD, et al. Treatment of congenital glaucoma. Am J Ophthalmol. 1981;92(6):799-803.

202. Robin AL, Quigley HA, Pollack IP, et al. An analysis of visual acuity, visual fields, and disc cupping in childhood glaucoma. Am J Ophthalmol. 1979;88(5): 847-58.

203. Meyer G, Schenn O, Pfeiffer N, et al. Trabeculotomy in congenital glaucoma. Graefes Arch Clin Exp Ophthalmol. 2000;238(3):207-13.

204. MacKinnon JR, Giubilato A, Elder JE, Craig JE, Macey DA. Primary infantile glaucoma in an Australian population. Clin Exp Ophthalmol. 2004;32(1): 14-8.

205. Gothwal VK. Management of residual vision in pediatric glaucoma. In: Mandal AK, Netland PA (Eds). The Pediatric Glaucoma.. Edinburgh, UK; Elsevier Science; 2006. Chapter 15, p. 103-6.

17

Advances in the Medical Management of Primary Open-angle Glaucoma

Rajendra K Bansal, James C Tsai

Although glaucoma is a multifactorial disease, it is widely recognized that elevated intraocular pressure (IOP) is a major risk factor for the development of glaucomatous optic neuropathy (GON). Moreover, the reduction of IOP is the only proven effective treatment for this sight-threatening disease.

In a review of epidemiological data from population in Africa, Asia and Europe, Quigley[1] estimated the number of people worldwide with primary open-angle glaucoma (POAG) by 2000 to be close to 66.8 million, with 6.7 million of them experiencing bilateral blindness. In addition, there was a distinct increase in the prevalence of glaucoma with increasing age among all of these populations, with the highest prevalence among Africans over 80 years of age.

A number of landmark studies in the last decade have firmly established the relationship between elevated IOP and an increased risk of visual loss in patients with ocular hypertension (OH), POAG and normal-pressure glaucoma (NPG).[2-5] At the present time, lowering IOP is the only proven method of slowing optic nerve damage and visual field progression.[6]

DECISION TO INITIATE MEDICAL THERAPY

The general approach is to recommend therapy whenever glaucomatous damage is documented or when the degree of IOP elevation or other risk factors is such that future damage is likely. However, the decision to initiate therapy in patients with elevated IOP but without any signs of glaucoma damage should be based on the individual's risk for developing POAG health status and life expectancy. The recently completed ocular hypertension treatment study (OHTS)[2] concluded that a reduction of IOP by at least 20%

from baseline (absolute IOP ≤ 24 mm Hg) in patients with OH resulted in a cumulative probability of developing POAG of 4.4% in the medication group vs 9.5% in the observation group, a statistically significant difference ($P < 0.0001$).

CORNEAL THICKNESS AND IOP MEASUREMENT

In another analysis from OHTS[7] the mean central corneal thickness (CCT) was 573 μm in 1,301 out of 1,636 subjects. The Caucasians had thicker cornea measurements (579 μm) as compared to African Americans (556 μm). Corneal thickness was also found to be a powerful predictor for development of POAG[8] even after adjusting for the effects of IOP, age, C/D ratio and perimetric pattern standard deviation. The risk of developing POAG was inversely correlated with CCT. Eyes with CCT <555 μm were found to be at three times more risk than with CCT >588 μm. Similarly, in established glaucoma patients, multivariate analysis demonstrated that thinner CCT was significantly associated with greater perimetric mean deviations and advanced glaucoma intervention study (AGIS) visual field scores and increased vertical and horizontal cup-disk ratios.[9]

There has been marked interest in identifying a correction factor for the Goldmann applanation tonometry based upon the CCT reading. At the present time, CCT has been found to be highly variable and no regression analysis can yet be established.[10,11] As a rough linear model estimate, for every 20 μm deviation from a mean normal CCT of 540–550 μm, the IOP should be corrected by +1.00 mm Hg. CCT also appears to have a significant effect on the clinical management of patients with glaucoma and glaucoma suspect.[12] Corneal thickness should be routinely measured in all patients with the diagnosis of glaucoma, or glaucoma suspect and documentation should be made (at a minimum) as to whether the cornea is normal, thin or thick.

PATIENT COMPLIANCE/ADHERENCE TO MEDICATION THERAPY

The major challenges in the medical treatment of glaucoma are to assure that patients fully comply with and adhere to their treatment regimen. There are multiple potential causes of noncompliance. Installation of eye drops may be problematic especially for the elderly and arthritic patients. In the setting of multiple prescribed medications, there is increased dosing frequency, more lifestyle disruption and greater risk of side effects.

Patel and Spaeth[13] found that almost 60% of patients failed to use eye drops as prescribed. According to these authors, major risk factors were frequent daily dose, forgetfulness, inconvenience and reduced affordability of the medication. Tsai and colleagues[14] described 71 unique situational obstacles to medication adherence (i.e., compliance) and grouped them into four separate categories: situational/environmental factors (49%), medication regimen (32%), patient factors (16%) and provider factors (3%); (Table 17.1).[16]

Table 17.1: Situational obstacles to medication compliance/adherence in patients with glaucoma.

Factors	Sample statements
Regimen factor	
Refill	I only forget to take my drops when I run out
Cost	When my insurance stopped paying for my medication, I didn't take my drops
Complexity	It was harder when I was taking four medications; now that I am taking three, it is better
Change	When I first started taking the drops, I had a harder time remembering
Side effects	I decided to quit taking my drops because I had a bad reaction from them
Patient factors	
Knowledge/skill	Sometimes I miss my eye when taking my drops
Memory	Sometimes I just forget to take my drops
Motivation/health beliefs	I quit taking my drops because I didn't see benefit from them and didn't think they were working
Comorbidity	It is harder to keep track of my drops because I am taking so many other medications
Provider factors	
Dissatisfaction	I quit taking my drops because I was dissatisfied with my doctor's care
Communication	I stopped taking my drops because I didn't understand initially that I need to take them forever
Situational/environmental factors	
Accountability/lack of support	Living alone, I had problems taking my drops; now I live with my daughter and have no problems
Major life events	Two years ago when my wife died, I had a hard time taking my drops
Travel/away from home	When I am on vacation, it is more difficult to take my drops
Competing activities	I miss my drops on Sunday morning when I go to church
Change in routine	Lifestyle changes that occur on weekends, such as not getting up at a normal hour, cause me to forget to take my drops

Tsai JC, McClure CA, Ramos SE. Compliance barriers in glaucoma: a systematic classification. J Glaucoma. 2003;12(5):393-8. *Used with permission from Ref. 16.*

Kass and colleagues[15] reported improved compliance just prior to a scheduled doctor's appointment. This variability in compliance resulted in documented progression of visual field loss, although examinations revealed stable and controlled IOP readings. Unless nonadherence to the glaucoma regimen is suspected, it may be difficult to determine whether disease progression is due to lack of drug efficacy, medication tachyphylaxis, or patient noncompliance.

In India, glaucoma seems to occur a decade earlier as compared to Caucasians[17] with the existing eye care services highly underutilized.[18] Medical treatment may have a very limited role for the mass population segments in India, especially in patients with poor socioeconomic status and in patients living in remote rural area.

Medications that lower IOP given topically or orally exert their action by enhancing aqueous outflow, inhibiting aqueous humor production, or via both mechanisms.

INCREASING AQUEOUS HUMOR OUTFLOW

Glaucoma results from increased resistance to aqueous outflow. Therefore, it is more physiological to use drugs that increase outflow and maintain the transport function of nutrients and toxic metabolites for avascular structures via the aqueous humor.

Aqueous outflow follows both conventional and nonconventional pathways. The conventional pathway accounts for 83–90% and is pressure-dependent, occurring through trabecular meshwork. The nonconventional (uveoscleral) outflow is pressure independent occurring through the uvea and the sclera. This pathway thought to approximate 10–15% of total outflow but has been suggested to reach as high as 40–50%.[19] Table 17.2 summarizes medications that increase aqueous humor outflow.

DECREASING AQUEOUS HUMOR PRODUCTION

The various classes of medications included in this group are β-blockers, carbonic anhydrase inhibitors (CAIs) and adrenergic agonists (Table 17.3).

β-Adrenergic agonist and carbonic anhydrase enzyme are both involved in the active secretion of aqueous humor. Thus β-adrenergic antagonists (β-blockers) and CAIs decrease aqueous humor production.[20] Since the introduction of timolol in the late 1970s, β-blockers have been the agents most widely used for lowering IOP.[21] Previously, oral CAIs played an important role in the treatment of glaucoma, but due to their high side-effect profile, more recently developed topical forms have largely replaced them.

Alpha$_2$-adrenergic–receptor agonists are thought to lower IOP by suppression of aqueous humor production. However, after chronic treatment (29 days of treatment), the resultant reduction in IOP was associated only with an increase in uveoscleral outflow (the initial decrease in aqueous inflow had reversed back to baseline levels).[22]

Beta-blockers

Timolol was the first topical β-blocker approved in late 1970s in the United States and is considered the gold standard against which all other topical

Table 17.2: Aqueous outflow enhancers.

Conventional/Trabecular

• Cholinergic agonists (parasympathomimetics):
  Pilocarpine
  Echothiophate iodide
  Carbachol

• Prostaglandin derivatives:
  Bimatoprost
  Latanoprost

• Nonspecific adrenergic agonists: Epinephrine
Nonconventional/Uveoscleral

• Prostaglandin derivatives:
  Latanoprost Bimatoprost
  Travoprost Unoprostone

• α_2-agonists: Brimonidine

Used with permission from Ref. 16.

Table 17.3: Aqueous inflow inhibitors.

β-blockers
• Timolol
• Betaxolol
• Levobunolol
• Carteolol
• Metipranolol
Carbonic anhydrase inhibitors

• Systemic:
  Acetazolamide
  Methazolamide
  Dichlorphenamide

• Topical:
  Dorzolamide
  Brinzolamide

Adrenergic agonists
• Nonspecific: Epinephrine*

• α_2-agonists:
  Brimonidine[+]
  Apraclonidine[‖]

*Also increases conventional outflow.
[+]Also increases uveoscleral outflow. *Used with permission from Ref. 16.*

Table 17.4: Beta-adrenergic antagonists used as ocular hypotensives for glaucoma.

Generic (trade) name	Concentration (%)	Cardioselectivity	Dosage
Betaxolol (Betoptic)	0.5	+	1 drop bid
Betaxolol (Betoptic S)	0.25	+	1 drop bid
Carteolol (Ocupress)	1.0	–	1 drop bid
Levobunolol (Betagan)	0.25, 0.5	–	1 drop bid
Metipranolol (OptiPranol)	0.3	–	1 drop bid
Timolol hemihydrate (Betimol)	0.25, 0.5	–	1 drop bid
Timolol maleate (Timoptic)	0.25, 0.5	–	1 drop bid
Timolol maleate gel (Timoptic-XE)	0.25 gel, 0.5 gel	–	1 drop qd

Used with permission from Ref. 16.

agents are compared. Presently, there are many noncardioselective and one cardioselective (β_1-adrenergic) receptor blocker available in the market.[20] Characteristics of currently available β-blockers are shown in Table 17.4.

Escape of IOP: Krieglestein[23] found gradual escapes from pressure-lowering effect of timolol. He documented that the IOP decrease following instillation of 0.25% timolol twice daily initially was 47% of the untreated pressure level and at the end of 3 months it was only 23% of the initial IOP level. The exact mechanism of this escape phenomenon is not known.

Side effects: The incidence of ocular side effects (such as stinging, redness, blurred vision and foreign body sensation) is low and diminishes with time. However, metipranolol has been found to cause granulomatous uveitis.[24]

A greater concern with topical β-blockers is the potential for systemic side effects, which are similar to those associated with systemic β-blockers. It is important to note that betaxolol, a cardioselective β-blocker, has less potential for causing the pulmonary adverse events but still should be dispensed with caution in patients with asthma.

The β-blockers should not be used in patients with sinus bradycardia, second or third-degree heart block, cardiogenic shock, overt cardiac failure, bronchial asthma and severe chronic obstructive pulmonary disease.

Prostaglandin Analogs

Prostaglandin (PG) analogs are the newest class of hypotensive agents, available since the release of latanoprost in 1996. Since that time, three other PG derivatives have become available and all produce significant and sustained lowering of IOP (Table 17.5).

Clinical studies have shown that all PG analogs, with the exception of unoprostone, reduce IOP to a significantly greater degree than timolol.[25-29] In December 2002, latanoprost (Xalatan) received approval for first-line usage for the treatment of OAG or OH from the US Food and Drug Administration

Table 17.5: Prostaglandin analogs used in the treatment of glaucoma.

Generic (trade) name	Concentration (%)	IOP reduction (mm Hg) (% reduction)	Dosage
Latanoprost (Xalatan)	0.005	6–8 (24–32)	1 drop qhs
Bimatoprost (Lumigan)	0.03	7–8 (27–31)	1 drop qhs
Travoprost (Travatan)	0.004	6–8 (23–32)	1 drop qhs
Unoprostone (Rescula)	0.15	3–4 (13–17)	1 drop bid

IOP: Intraocular pressure.
Used with permission from Ref. 16.

(FDA). Latanoprost also has a first-line indication in Japan and Europe. In contrast, the other three PG analogs are indicated for the treatment of OAG or OH in patients who are intolerant to other topical drugs or fail to achieve a target IOP. Pending further development, they are still to be prescribed as second-line therapy. PG analogs offer significant advantages over β-blockers.[29] PG analogs are more effective in lowering IOP than β-blockers over the diurnal cycle (both day and night), increase outflow rather than suppress aqueous production, are 100 times more potent than topical β-blockers, possess a safer systemic side-effect profile and have a simpler dosing schedule (except for Unoprostone).

Comparative clinical trials: The PG analogs have been compared with β-blockers and with each other in a number of clinical trials. Studies among the three main PG analogs (latanoprost, travoprost and bimatoprost) have been conducted to prove superior IOP lowering and/or improved tolerability of one over the other.

In a 6-month-trial, Camras[25] found that both latanoprost (0.005%) and timolol (0.5%) significantly reduced IOP from baseline levels ($P < 0.001$). Comparing 6-month with baseline diurnal IOP values (8 AM, 12 Noon, 4 PM), the mean IOP reduction achieved with latanoprost (−6.7 mm Hg) was significantly greater ($P < 0.001$) than that observed with timolol (−4.9 mm Hg). Other authors[30-32] have also concluded that latanoprost (0.005%) administered once daily is a more effective ocular hypotensive drug than timolol (0.5%) applied twice daily. Also, latanoprost (0.005%) applied once daily in the evening was statistically superior to latanoprost applied in the morning.[31]

Latanoprost vs bimatoprost vs travoprost: There have been number of studies funded by the respective pharmaceutical companies to compare IOP-lowering efficacy and/or side effects (such as conjunctival hyperemia) and the response rates based on target IOP reductions. The results have varied among studies with the specific PG analog being evaluated.[27,33-37]

In appraising the disparate results of the Parrish/XLT[33] study compared with the Noecker[36] study with regard to the IOP-lowering efficacy of latanoprost vs bimatoprost, it is important to consider the potential impact of lack of standardization of such studies. Regrettably, variables inherent in design, conduct and interpretation of results of these randomized clinical trials may lead to apparent differences in outcome when the actual discrepancies may be minimal or even nonexistent. As Kaufman[38] suggests, where the actual differences in efficacy between two drugs is slight, enormous sample sizes would be required to accurately pinpoint that difference, and divergent outcome derived from lesser sample sizes could be due to chance alone or variations in patient populations (e.g., receptor characteristic, rate of penetration in case of topical prodrugs, etc.). On the other hand, where the difference in efficacy is appreciable and clinically relevant, it is likely to be evident in nearly all studies despite the aforementioned variable factors.

Side effects: Systemic side effects are mostly rare as the concentration of any PG analogs entering the systemic circulation is considerably lower than that of circulating endogenous PGs. However, there are numerous ocular side effects like conjunctival hyperemia, increased pigmentation of the iris and periorbital tissue, eyelash growth and cystoid macular edema in high-risk patients and possible iritis. A comparative review of side effects due to various PG analogs is listed in Table 17.6.

Alpha Agonists

Currently available alpha agonists used in the treatment of POAG and OH are listed in Table 17.7.

Apraclonidine (1.0%) is approved to control or prevent post-laser spike in IOP. Apraclonidine (0.5%) was available in the market prior to brimonidine and was used in most cases for short-term adjunctive use in patients already on maximum tolerable medical therapy. This has been exclusively replaced by brimonidine (0.15%, 0.2%) for long-term use, usually as a third drug after the use of PG analogs and β-blockers. The lower dose formulation with purite (Alphagan P 0.15%) is more commonly used due to reduced incidence of allergic conjunctivitis, better satisfaction and higher-comfort rating, and similar IOP reduction when compared with the standard 0.2% concentration.[39] In comparative clinical studies, brimonidine (0.2%) was shown to be comparable to timolol (0.5%) in lowering IOP in patients with glaucoma (4–6 mm Hg for brimonidine vs 6 mm Hg for timolol).

Side effects: Alpha$_2$-agonists should not be used with monoamine oxidase (MAO) inhibitors due to its additive effect on central nervous system. They are also contraindicated in infants and young children due to increased risk of lethargy and somnolence. The common ocular and systemic side effects for apraclonidine and brimonidine are similar. However, the incidence of tachyphylaxis and side effects is higher with apraclonidine as compared to brimonidine. Ocular side effects include allergic conjunctivitis (follicular), conjunctival hyperemia and edema, eyelid erythema and edema, blepharitis and pruritis and tearing. The systemic side effects are abnormal taste, dry mouth, arrhythmias, hypertension, fatigue, drowsiness and forgetfulness.

Table 17.6: Ocular and systemic side effects of prostaglandin analogs used to treat glaucoma.

Adverse event	Latanoprost % of occurrence of side effects	Travoprost % of occurrence of side effects	Bimatoprost % of occurrence of side effects	Unoprostone % of occurrence of side effects
Ocular				
Blurred vision	5–15	1–4	3–10	5–10
Burning and/or stinging	5–15	–	3–10	10–25
Cataract	–	1–4	3–10	1–5
Conjunctivitis	<1	1–4	1–3	1–5
Cystoid macula edema	*	*	*	*
Dry eye	1–4	1–4	3–10	10–25
Eyelid skin darkening	*	*	3–10	<1
Eyelash growth/ changes	*	*	15–45	10–25
Foreign-body sensation	5–15	5–10	3–10	5–10
Hyperemia	5–15	35–50	15–45	10–25
Iris discoloration	5–15	1–4	1–3	<1
Pain	1–4	5–10	3–10	1–5
Iritis	*	*	<1	<1
Systemic				
Allergic reaction	1–2	–	–	1–5
Chest pain/ angina pectoris	1–2	1–5	–	–
Headache	–	1–5	1–5	1–5
Muscle, joint, or back pain	1–2	1–5	–	1–5
Upper respiratory infection (i.e. flu-like symptoms)	4	1–5	10	6

*Postmarketing case reports.
Used with permission from Ref. 16.

Topical Carbonic Anhydrase Inhibitors

Topical CAIs were introduced as an alternative to oral CAIs, which are associated with a wide range of serious side effects. Currently two topical CAIs are available for the treatment of elevated IOP—Dorzolamide

Table 17.7: Alpha agonists used in the treatment of glaucoma.

Generic (trade) name	Concentration (%)	IOP reduction	Dosage (mm Hg)
Apraclonidine hydrochloride (Iopidine)	0.5	5–6	1 drop tid (bid also used)
Apraclonidine hydrochloride (Iopidine)	1.0	NA	1 drop pre- and 1 drop postoperatively (laser)
Brimonidine tartrate (Alphagan P)	0.15	2.5	1 drop tid (often used bid)
Brimonidine tartrate (Alphagan)	0.2	4-6	1 drop tid (bid often used)

IOP: Intraocular pressure; NA: Not available.
Used with permission from Ref. 16.

hydrochloride (2%) and Brinzolamide (1%). They appear to reduce IOP up to 24% as monotherapy and provide an additional 15% reduction when added to timolol.[24]

Side effects: The systemic side effects of the topical CAIs are similar though considerably less than that of systemic CAIs due to the reduced systemic absorption of the topical agents. Also, ocular side effects such as corneal decompensation and hypotony have been reported with topical CAIs.

Combination Agents

Recently, fixed combination therapy (in which two topical ocular hypotensives have been combined in a single formulation) has become available. They provide simplicity of monotherapy, better efficacy and compliance. However, it is important to note that fixed combinations do not necessarily achieve the same degree of IOP-lowering efficacy as concomitant therapy with two separate medications.

Each medication in the combination may affect the bioavailability of the other. The currently available combinations are Cosopt (timolol 0.5% and dorzolamide 2%) manufactured by Merck, Inc. available in the United States and worldwide, Xalcom (timolol 0.5% and latanoprost 0.005%) manufactured by Pfizer Inc. available in Europe and Asia, not in the United States. At least three more fixed combinations are awaiting FDA approval. They include travoprost-timolol (Alcon Inc., Fort Worth, TX), bimatoprost-timolol (Allergan Inc., Irvine, CA) and brimonidine-timolol (Allergan Inc., CA).

Less Commonly Used Agents

Cholinergic agents: The two widely used agents in this class are pilocarpine and carbachol and are usually reserved for fourth- or fifth-line use due to their side effects. Due to their miotic effects, they are very useful in primary angle-closure glaucoma with or without plateau iris and OAG associated with pigmentary dispersion.

Nonspecific adrenergic agonists: Epinephrine and its prodrug Dipivefrin (Propine) were very popular at one time. But due to less effectiveness and a greater range of ocular and systemic side effects, these medications have mostly been abandoned for the treatment of glaucoma.

Oral carbonic anhydrase inhibitors: Acetazolamide (Diamox) and Methazolamide (Neptazane) are the two common drugs in this class. They are very effective in lowering IOP, but due to serious systemic side effects they are reserved for short-term use in patients with POAG.

STRATEGIES IN MEDICAL TREATMENT

The following criteria should be considered carefully in selecting a specific medical therapy:
• Efficacy in achieving target IOP reduction
• Ability to control diurnal variation in IOP
• Efficacy at trough drug concentrations
• Efficacy vs tolerability
• Comparative safety of agents
• Ease of use/dosing schedule
• Cost of medications

Setting Target IOP

Various landmark studies have clearly established that aggressive lowering of IOP either slows or aborts the progression of optic nerve damage and visual field loss in glaucoma patients. The selection of target IOP is achieved by choosing either a percentage or an actual IOP value or range. The upper boundary of this range is considered the target pressure. It will vary from patient-to-patient depending upon severity of the disease and the initial IOP.

One treatment algorithm established by the Preferred Practice Pattern Committee (Glaucoma Panel) of the American Academy of Ophthalmology calls for an initial reduction in IOP of 20–30%. When the target level is achieved but disease progression continues, the panel suggests that a further lowering of > 15% should be sought.[40]

Essentially, the more advanced the disease, the lower target IOP should be set. The AGIS found that pressures < 18 mm Hg were more effective in slowing progression of visual field loss.[3] However, the various clinical factors associated with a specific patient should drive the selection of a target IOP range rather than simple reliance on absolute IOP value(s) based on arbitrary benchmarks. More aggressive therapy should be utilized when there is greater risk of glaucomatous optic neuropathy (GON) and a subsequent field loss.

Another factor to keep in mind should be patient's age. The visual effects associated with the retinal ganglion cell (RGC) death rate (including the ability of the patient to retain useful central vision) depend to a great extent on the individual's life expectancy. Thus, young patients may need to be treated more aggressively than older patients. However, it is almost impossible to predict both the rate of RGC loss and the life expectancy for a given patient.

Controlling Diurnal Variation in IOP

Asrani and colleagues[41] have demonstrated that large diurnal fluctuations in IOP (as measured by home tonometry) create significant risk factors for disease progression in patients with open angle glaucoma. Orzalesi and co-workers[42] have shown that PG derivatives, such as latanoprost, yield a relatively flat diurnal IOP curve by providing a fairly uniform circadian reduction in IOP.

Efficacy at Trough Drug Concentrations

Usually IOP peaks in the morning (between 8 AM and 10 AM) reach a trough level at night.[42] However, this day-type IOP curve was not observed in both young (18–25 years) and older (50–69 years) volunteers who exhibited nocturnal elevation of IOP.[43] The nocturnal IOP elevation was largely explained by the shift from day time upright posture to night time supine posture. Latanoprost dosed daily has an IOP-lowering effect that is fairly constant during the 24-h circadian cycle.[42] β-blockers may offer less nocturnal protection since aqueous flow is already reduced at night and its baseline rate may not be further suppressed.

Efficacy and Tolerability

PG analogs, due to very few systemic side effects and good efficacy, have become a popular choice as the initial medication class for patients with glaucoma. However, PG agents have a few ocular and visual untoward effects like conjunctival hyperemia and iris color change. Patients with hazel or light brown irides should be warned regarding a potential change in their iris color. There has been a possible association of cystoid macular edema in patients with aphakia. For patients with advanced disease and impending risk of serious visual loss, the physician and patient may choose to tolerate a greater degree of side effects to achieve an aggressive target IOP reduction.

Unilateral Trials

Unilateral, one-eyed trials allow evaluation of a particular drug's efficacy in lowering IOP. When possible, all medications should be administered initially in one eye only. The comparison of IOP levels between the treated and control eye enables the clinician to identify and forgo the use of ineffective agents, thereby minimizing the risk of unnecessary side effects, inconvenience and financial cost to the patient.

Discontinuing a drug in one eye and then assessing the IOP effect can perform a reverse unilateral trial. This is useful to determine if adjunctive or switch therapy is required.

REDUCING SYSTEMIC ABSORPTION OF TOPICAL MEDICATIONS

Undesired systemic side effects of topical agents result from their access to lacrimal drainage system and then systemic absorption through highly vascular nasopharyngeal mucosa. Significant reduction of tear flow can be achieved by digital pressure on lacrimal sac or eyelid closure for 5 min.[44] In practice, nasolacrinal occlusion and/or eyelid closure is recommended for approximately 3 min. In rare instances, the clinician might consider a punctual plug in one or both eyes.

CHOICE OF INITIAL MEDICATION

In the PG group, latanoprost, is the only one approved by FDA for first line use. This has become most widely used as first line medication if there is no contradiction like anterior uveitis, herpes simplex keratitis or cystoid macular edema. A β-blocker is also a good alternative as an initial therapy especially in young patients as the cost is much less in comparison to PG analogs.

MAXIMUM TOLERABLE MEDICAL THERAPY

Usually three or four different classes of ocular hypotensives are used before embarking on to laser trabeculoplasty and/or filtration surgery. These classes are PG analogues, β-blockers, $alpha_2$-agonists and topical CAIs. This necessitates use of three bottles as β-blocker and CAIs can be given in a combination (Cosopt). This means that the patient ends up using five drops a day (two of Cosopt, two of Alphagan and one of PG agent). This regimen seems to be tolerable and best suited for a good compliance.

ALTERNATIVE MEDICINE

Some of the herbal drugs have attracted attention for treatment of glaucoma not by lowering IOP but by possibly increasing blood flow. Ginkgo biloba, extracted from the leaves of maiden hair tree, has been used for various neurological conditions like Alzheimer's, memory defects and dementia. Ginkgo has been shown to increase blood flow, both central and peripheral[45] and therefore may have some neuroprotective properties.

Visual field improvement has been reported in normal tension glaucoma in some patients on a short-term therapy of Gingko biloba.[46] However, problems with spontaneous bleeding (subarachnoidal hemorrhage, subdural hematoma) have occurred in patients taking this compound, and, therefore, patients who take anticoagulants or who are at risk for intracranial bleeding should take ginkgo with extreme caution.

Bilberry acts as an antioxidant[47] and may offer neuroprotection in glaucoma. Vitamin C, a ubiquitous alternative therapy, has been shown to reduce IOP when given in massive doses, based on hyperosmotic effect. Also vitamin E, though it has no effect on IOP, may offer neuroprotection by preventing platelet aggregation.

Marijuana cigarettes (2% concentration) reduce IOP by about 25% for 2 h.[48] However, smoking of marijuana is ill-advised due to its known systemic side effects (hypotension). Topical forms appear to be ineffective and cause considerable ocular irritation.

FUTURE HYPOTENSIVE AGENTS

Elevated IOP results from aqueous humor outflow resistance and is associated with increased extracellular matrix (ECM) deposition and decreased cellularity in the trabecular meshwork(TM). The ECM in TM is regularly remodeled by a balance between TM matrix metalloproteinases (MMPS) and tissue inhibitors of MMPS (TIMPS). It has been suggested that an imbalance in MMP-TIMP activity might account for increase outflow resistance.[49] PG analogs increase MMP activity in ciliary smooth muscle cells and lower IOP by enhancing the aqueous outflow through uveoscleral pathway. There is new interest in MMP activators and TIMP inhibitors.[50] Ethacrynic acid (ECA), a known chloride transport inhibitor, that increases TM cell volume and thereby conventional outflow facility, has been under study as a potential model for a better glaucoma treatment delivery system.[51]

NEUROPROTECTIVE AGENTS

So far, no medications have been approved for neuroprotection (without IOP reduction) in the treatment of glaucoma. Brimonidine, an alpha$_2$-agonist, has been shown to be neuroprotective in animal models with chronic OHT.[52]

N-methyl-D-aspartate (NMDA) antagonists block glutamate receptor activation and prevent massive influx of calcium into the neuron and subsequent apoptosis.[53] Memantine belongs to this class of agents and shows promise as a neuroprotective agent. The compound is currently undergoing multicentric phase 3 human trials in the United States.

There are many other means by which RGC apoptosis and degeneration can be prevented. Some of them include nitric oxide synthase (NOS) inhibitors, calcium channel blockers, neurotrophins, endothelin (ET) receptors antagonists and are being investigated for future study.[50]

ENHANCING OCULAR BLOOD FLOW

Compromised ocular blood flow leading to ischemia of optic nerve head may contribute to the pathogenesis of GON.[54] Dorzolamide, a topical CAI, has been shown to increase retinal artery flow velocities in normal-tension glaucoma patients,[55] and topical verapamil increased retinal artery and optic disc capillary blood flow in normal subjects.[56] However, the current methods to assess ocular blood flow and its therapeutic effects are far from satisfactory.

GLAUCOMA GENE THERAPY

Myocilin (MYOC also known as GLCIA) was discovered as the first glaucoma gene by four different laboratories. The function of myocilin is currently unknown. Its expression is induced in TM cells by glucocorticoids, transforming growth factor-β and elevated IOP.[50] Several groups are exploring the potential utility of MYOC as a therapeutic target for glaucoma.

VACCINATION FOR GLAUCOMA

Recently an innovative concept of 'protective autoimmunity,' a T-cell-based mechanism for neuroprotection, has been introduced. Vaccination with COP-1 (an FDA-approved drug for the treatment of multiple sclerosis) has been found to be neuroprotective in rat models of optic nerve crush and chronic glaucoma.[57]

REFERENCES

1. Quigley HA. Number of people with glaucoma worldwide. Br J Ophthalmol. 1996;80(5):389-93.
2. Kass MA, Heuer DK, Higginbotham EJ, et al. The ocular hypertension treatment study: a randomized trial determines that topical ocular hypotensive medication delays or prevents the onset of primary open-angle glaucoma. Arch Ophthalmol. 2002;120(6):701-13.
3. The AGIS investigators. The Advanced Glaucoma Intervention Study (AGIS) 7: the relationship between control of intraocular pressure and visual field deterioration. Am J Ophthalmol. 2000;130(4):429-40.
4. Collaborative Normal-Tension Glaucoma Study Group. Comparison of glaucomatous progression between untreated patients with normal-tension glaucoma and patients with therapeutically reduced intraocular pressures. Am J Ophthalmol. 1998;126(4):487-97.

5. Collaborative Normal-Tension Glaucoma Study Group. The effectiveness of intraocular pressure reduction in the treatment of normal-tension glaucoma. Am J Ophthalmol. 1998;126(4):498-505.

6. Wax MB, Camras CB, Fiscella RG, et al. Emerging perspectives on glaucoma: Optimizing 24-hr control of intraocular pressure. Am J Ophthalmol. 2002; 133(Supp):S1-10.

7. Brandt JD, Beiser JA, Kass MA, et al. Central corneal thickness in the ocular hypertension treatment study (OHTS). Ophthalmology. 2001;108(10): 1779-88.

8. Gordon MO, Beiser JA, Brandt JD, et al. The ocular hypertension treatment study: baseline factors that predict the onset of primary open-angle glaucoma. Arch Ophthalmol. 2002;120(6):714-20.

9. Herndon LW, Weizer JS, Stinnett SS. Central corneal thickness as a risk factor for advanced glaucoma damage. Arch Ophthalmol. 2004;122(1):17-21.

10. Feltgen N, Leifert D, Funk J. Correlation between central corneal thickness, applanation tonometry and direct intracameral IOP readings. Br J Ophthalmol. 2001;85(1):85-7.

11. Lee GA, Khaw PT, Ficker LA, et al. The corneal thickness and intraocular pressure story: Where are we now? Clin Experiment Ophthalmol. 2002;30(5): 334-7.

12. Shih CY, Graff Zivin JS, Trokel SL, et al. Clinical significance of central corneal thickness in the management of glaucoma. Arch Ophthalmol. 2004; 122(9):1270-5.

13. Patel SC, Spaeth GL. Compliance in patients prescribed eye drops for glaucoma. Ophthal Surg. 1995;26(3):233-6.

14. Tsai JC, McClure CA, Ramos SE, et al. Compliance barriers in glaucoma: A systemic classification. J Glaucoma. 2003;12(5):393-8.

15. Kass MA, Meltzer DW, Gordon M, et al. Compliance with topical pilocarpine treatment. Am J Ophthalmol. 1986;101(5):515-23.

16. Tsai JC, Forbes M. Medical Management of Glaucoma, 2nd edition. West Islip, NY: Professional Communications; 2004. pp. 100-31.

17. Das J, Bhomaj S, Chaudhuri Z, et al. Profile of glaucoma in a major eye hospital in north India. Indian J Ophthalmol. 2001;49(1):25-30.

18. Robin AL, Nirmalan PK, Krishandas R, et al. The utilization of eye care services by persons with glaucoma in rural south India. Trans Am Ophthalmol Soc. 2004;1202:47-54.

19. Brubaker RF. Measurement of uveoscleral outflow in humans. J Glaucoma. 2001;(Suppl 1):545-8.

20. Brubaker RF. The flow of aqueous humor in the human eye. Trans Am Ophthalmol Soc. 1982;80:391-474.

21. Alward WL. Medical management of glaucoma. N Engl J Med. 1998;339: 1298-307.

22. Toris CB, Camras CB, Yablonski ME. Acute versus chronic effects of brimonidine on aqueous humor dynamics in ocular hypertension patients. Am J Ophthalmol. 1999;128(1):8-14.

23. Krieglestein GK. Langzeituntersuchungen sur augendrucksenkenden wirkung von timolol-augen-tropfen. Klin Monatsbl Augenheilkd. 1979;175(5):627.

24. Schuman JS. Antiglaucoma medications: a review of safety and tolerability issues related to their use. Clin Ther. 2002;22(2):167-208.
25. Camras CB. Comparison of latanoprost and timolol in patients with ocular hypertension and glaucoma: a six-month masked, multicenter trial in the United States. The United States Latanoprost Study Group. Ophthalmology. 1996;103(1):138-47.
26. Brandt JD, VanDenburgh AM, Chen K, et al. Bimatoprost Study Group. Comparison of once- or twice-daily bimatoprost with timolol twice-daily in patients with elevated IOP: a 3-month clinical trial. Ophthalmology. 2001;108(6): 1023-32.
27. Netland PA, Landry T, Sullivan EK, et al. Travoprost compared with latanoprost and timolol in patients with open-angle glaucoma or ocular hypertension. Am J Ophthalmol. 2001;132(4):472-84.
28. Nordmann JP, Mertz B, Yannoulis NC, et al. Unoprostone Monotherapy Study Group-EU. A double-masked randomized comparison of the efficacy and safety of unoprostone with timolol and betaxolol in patients with primary open-angle glaucoma including pseudoexfoliation glaucoma or ocular hypertension 6-month data. Am J Ophthalmol. 2002;133(1):1-10.
29. Camras CB. Prostaglandins. In Ritch R, Shields MD, Krupin T (Eds). Glaucomas. (2nd edition). St Louis, Mosby Year Book; 1996. pp. 1449-61.
30. Watson PG. Latanoprost. Two years' experience of its use in the United Kingdom. Latanoprost Study Group. Ophthalmology. 1998;105(1):82-7.
31. Alm A, Stjernschantz J. Effects on intraocular pressure and side effects of 0.005% latanoprost applied once daily, evening or morning. A comparison with timolol. Scandinavian Latanoprost Study Group. Ophthalmology. 1995;102(12): 1743-52.
32. Camras CB, Hedman K. US Latanoprost Study Group. Rate of response to latanoprost or timolol in patients with ocular hypertension or glaucoma. J Glaucoma. 2003;12(6):466-9.
33. Parrish RK, Palmberg P, Sheu WP. XLT Study Group. A comparison of latanoprost, bimatoprost, and travoprost in patients with elevated intraocular pressure: A 12-week, randomized, masked-evaluator multicenter study. Am J Ophthalmol. 2003;135(5):688-703.
34. DuBiner H, Cooke D, Dirks M, et al. Efficacy and safety of bimatoprost in patients with elevated intraocular pressure: a 30-day comparison with latanoprost. Surv Ophthalmol. 2001;45(Suppl 4):S353-60.
35. Gandolfi S, Simmons ST, Sturm R, et al. Bimatoprost Study Group 3. Three-month comparison of bimatoprost and latanoprost in patients with glaucoma and ocular hypertension. Adv Ther. 2001;18(3):110-21.
36. Noecker RS, Dirks MS, Choplin NT, et al. Bimatoprost/Latanoprost Study Group. A six-month randomized clinical trial comparing the intraocular pressure-lowering efficacy of bimatoprost and latanoprost in patients with ocular hypertension or glaucoma. Am J Ophthalmol. 2003;135(1):55-63.
37. Susanna R Jr, Giampini J Jr., Borges AS, et al. A double-masked, randomized clinical trial comparing latanoprost with unoprostone in patients with open-angle glaucoma or ocular hypertension. Ophthalmology. 2001;108(2):259-63.

38. Kaufman PL. The prostaglandin wars. Am J Ophthalmol. 2003;136(4): 727-8.
39. Katz LJ. Twelve-month evaluation of brimonidine-purite versus brimonidine in patients with glaucoma or ocular hypertension. J Glaucoma. 2002; 11(2): 119-26.
40. American Academy of Ophthalmology Preferred Practice Patterns Committee Glaucoma Panel. Preferred Practice Patterns. Primary open-angle glaucoma. San Francisco, CA: American Academy of Ophthalmology; 2001. pp. 1-38.
41. Asrani S, Zeimer R, Wilensky J, et al. Large diurnal fluctuations in intraocular pressures are an independent risk factors in patients with glaucoma. J Glaucoma. 2000;9(6);134-42.
42. Orzalesi N, Rossetti L, Invernizzi T, et al. Effect of timolol, latanoprost, and dorzolamide on circadian IOP in glaucoma or ocular hypertension. Invest Ophthalmol Vis Sci. 2000;41(9):2566-73.
43. Liu JH, Kripke DF, Twa MD, et al. Twenty-four hour pattern of intraocular pressure in the aging population. Invest Ophthalmol Vis Sci. 1999;40(12):2912-7.
44. Zimmerman TJ, Kooner KS, Kandarakis AS, et al. Improving the therapeutic index of topically applied ocular drugs. Arch Ophthalmol. 1984;102(4):551-3.
45. Chung HS, Harris A, Kristinsson JK, et al. Ginkgo biloba extract increases ocular blood flow velocity. J Ocul Pharmacol Ther. 1999;15(3):233-40.
46. Quaranta L, Bettelli S, Uva MG, et al. Effect of Ginkgo biloba extract on pre-existing visual field damage in normal tension glaucoma. Ophthalmology. 2003;110(2):359-62.
47. Rhee DJ, Katz LJ, Spaeth GL, et al. Complementary and alternative medicine for glaucoma. Surv Ophthalmol. 2001;46(1):43-55.
48. Green K. Marijuana smoking vs cannabinoids for glaucoma therapy. Arch Ophthalmol. 1998;116(11):1433-7.
49. Wong TT, et al. Matrix metalloproteinases in disease and repair processes in anterior segment. Surv Ophthalmol. 2002;47(3):239-56.
50. Clark AF, Yorio T. Ophthalmic drug discovery. Nat Rev Drug Discov. 2003; 2(6):448-59.
51. Wang Y, Challa P, Epstein DL, et al. Controlled release of ethacrynic acid from poly (lactide-co-glycolide) films for glaucoma treatment. Biomaterials. 2004;25(18):4279-85.
52. Wheeler LA, Gil DW, Woldemussie M. Role of alpha-2 adrenergic receptors in neuroprotection and glaucoma. Surv Ophthalmol. 2001;45(Suppl 3): S290-4.
53. Hare W, WoldeMussie E, Lai R, et al. Efficacy and safety of memantine, an NMDA-type open-channel blocker, for reduction of retinal injury associated with experimental glaucoma in rats and monkeys. Surv Ophthalmol. 2001;45(Suppl 3):S284-9.
54. Hayreh SS. Factors influencing blood flow in the optic nerve head. J Glaucoma. 1997;6(6):412-25.
55. Harris A, Arend O, Kagemann L, et al. Dorzolamide visual function and ocular hemodynamics in normal-tension glaucoma. J Ocul Pharmacol Ther. 1999;15(3):189-97.

56. Netland PA, Feke GT, Konno S, et al. Optic nerve head circulation after topical calcium channel blocker. J Glaucoma. 1996;5(3):200-6.
57. Schwartz M. Vaccination for glaucoma: Dream or reality? Brain Res Bull. 2004;62(6):481-4.

Lasers in Glaucoma

Savleen Kaur, Sushmita Kaushik, Kiran Chandra Kedarisetti

INTRODUCTION

Lasers are an essential component in the treatment of glaucoma.[1-3] Lasers act as a double-edged sword being both advantageous and hazardous at the same time. In most of the ophthalmic applications, the laser magnitude is modulated well to minimize the side effects and increase the safety of the patient as well as the clinician. It is immensely important to understand the basic principles of each ophthalmic application of laser before we utilize the lasers for the treatment of glaucoma. A better insight of the laser equipment can help the clinician in a better and efficient operation and deployment of the laser itself.

BASICS

A laser is a device that emits light through optical amplification by stimulated emission of radiation. Laser light is generally monochromatic and has spatial and temporal coherence, which are important in some diagnostic applications but not in surgical applications. The more clinically beneficial properties of lasers are the wavelength, pulse duration and the power. Laser wavelength determines how effectively light is absorbed in the target tissue and how effectively light transmits through the media. Pulse durations can range from tens of femtoseconds (10^{-15} s) to milliseconds (ms). Power (in watts) describes the rate at which energy (in joules) is emitted from a laser or delivered to a target tissue (power = energy/time, in watts = joules/s). Spot size is the diameter of the focus beam in microns. Most commonly used lasers in glaucoma with their frequencies are given in Table 18.1.

The effects of laser on tissues are summarized in the Table 18.2.

Table 18.1: Commonly used lasers in glaucoma therapy.

Types of laser	Frequency (nm)
Argon blue green and green	488–514
Diode	810 nm
Nd YAG	1064 nm
Carbon Dioxide	10,600 nm

Table 18.2: Effect of different types of lasers on tissues.

Thermal effect		Photochemical effect		Ionising effect
Photocoagu-lation	Photovaporiza-tion	Photoablation	Photoradiation	Photodisrup-tion
Argon	Carbon Dioxide	Excimer	Diode 689 nm	Q-Switched
Krypton				Nd YAG
Frequency				Holmium YAG
doubled Nd:				
YAG				
Diode 810 nm				

HAZARDS OF LASER

Any laser used either for photocoagulation, photo disruption or ablation, if misdirected can be potentially hazardous to the biological tissues. However, in most applications these are minimal. The eye in particular is more susceptible to laser hazards than the skin. Laser safety in a clinical setting is determined by the wavelength and the duration of the pulse in cases of a pulsed laser, and power of the beam in cases of a continuous laser. In the treatment of any condition by a laser; the most important factor is its very high 'brightness' or radiance, which permits laser light to be focused on an exquisitely small spot at very high concentrations of power-per-unit-area.

The 'hazard classes' classified by safety standards worldwide include class 1 to class 4.

Class 1: Lasers pose no hazards

Class 2: Visible-wavelength laser

Class 3: Which are significant hazards to the eye and

Class 4: Which are hazardous to both skin and eye and are readily capable of cutting or photocoagulating biological tissue. Every surgical Laser can be classified into 'Class 4' in terms of laser safety.

Laser can cause following hazards to the eye:

- Ultraviolet photo-keratoconjunctivitis (also known as 'welder's flash' or simply 'photokeratitis'

Table 18.3: Ocular hazards of a particular wavelength of laser.

Wavelength (nm)	UVC (100 nm)	UVB (280 nm)	UVA (315 nm)	VISIBLE (400 nm)	IRA (760 nm)	IRB (1400 nm)	IRC (3000 nm)
Adverse effects	Photokeratitis			Retinal burns		Corneal burns	
	Erythema	Cataract		Cataract			
			Color vision/night vision				
			Thermal skin burns				

UV: ultraviolet; IR: Infrared.

- Injury to lens causing cataract
- Ultraviolet erythema
- Skin cancers arising from chronic exposure to ultraviolet light
- Thermal injury to the retina
- Blue-light photochemical injury to the retina also called as 'blue light photoretinitis,' e.g., solar retinitis and welder's maculopathy
- Thermal injury of the cornea and conjunctiva

The laser safety classes also vary with spectral band, e.g., ultraviolet (100–400 nm), visible (400–780 nm) and infrared (780 nm to 1 mm), since the biological risk varies with wavelength. The ocular hazards of laser are shown in Table 18.3.

Most surgical instruments now have black anodized or sandblasted, roughened surfaces to reduce potentially hazardous reflections. The strong curvature and surface roughening spread the reflected energy and greatly reduce the reflection hazard. Sometimes the black surface with roughening provides increased protection hence most of the equipment and wires are usually black.

Since the surgeon views the target tissue through the optics of an endoscope, operating microscope, or a slit-lamp biomicroscope, the reflections are safely attenuated within the optics, and surgeon is usually not at risk of laser exposure.

USES OF LASERS IN GLAUCOMA

Lasers can both be used for diagnostic and therapeutic purposes in glaucoma[1-3] (Fig. 18.1).

Lasers Used for Diagnosis in Glaucoma

Scanning Laser Polarimetry

Scanning laser polarimetry (SLP) is a technique for assessing retinal nerve fiber layer (RNFL) thickness in vivo on the basis of polarization changes

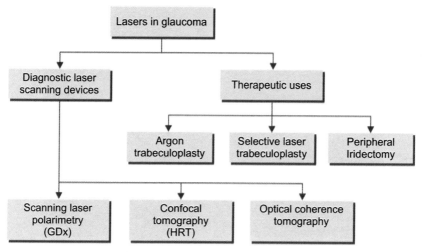

Fig. 18.1: Uses of lasers in glaucoma.

in laser light caused by the birefringent structure of the RNFL. The current instrument employs a 780-nm laser source. Measurements using the GDx, which uses scanning laser polarimetry, are reproducible and differentiate between the healthy and glaucomatous eyes with reasonable accuracy. Furthermore, serial analysis information may allow the clinician to detect changes in nerve fiber layer thickness over time in diseased eyes.

Confocal Scanning Laser Ophthalmoscopy (CSLO) and HRT

Confocal scanning laser ophthalmoscopy is a noninvasive investigation that has been used initially to receive three-dimensional images of the retinal surface in vivo. The commercial name of the device is Heidelberg Retina Tomograph (HRT). Optic nerve evaluation with confocal tomography permits the preperimetric diagnosis of glaucomatous optic disk neuropathy in its early stages when the disease is still sub-clinical. It helps in:
- Classification of the disease
- Early diagnosis of glaucoma
- Follow-up of glaucomatous patients
- Check the efficacy of therapy.

Illustrative Case

A 60-year-old female presented with bilateral pseudophakia and history of putting latanoprost OU for 1 year. Visual acuity: OD 6/9, OS: 6/6; IOP: OD 20 mmHg, OS 18 mmHg; angle is open in both eyes and CCT is 510 μm in both eyes. Figure 18.2 depicts the disk pictures of the patient at presentation and Figure. 18.3 the HRT image along with the visual fields.

The figures show that the disk is hypoplastic and visual fields are not progressive with normal HRT. Hence the treatment was stopped.

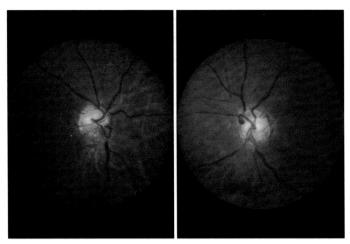

Fig. 18.2: Fundus pictures of both eyes at the time of presentation.

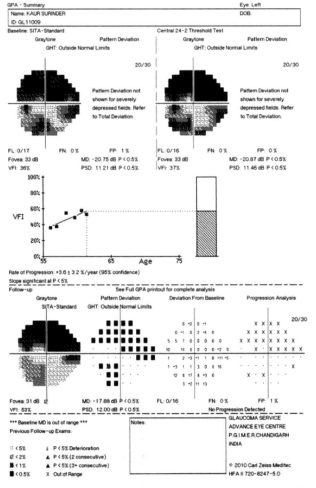

(Contd.)

(Contd.)

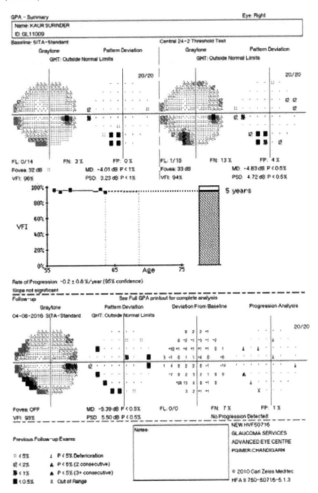

Disc size: 1.45 mm²
(small)

Disc size: 1.76 mm²
(average)

CUP
Linear Cup/Disc Ratio [ ]

0.56 ✓	Asymmetry✓ 0.00	0.56 ✓
p = 0.07	p = 0.46	p = 0.18

Cup Shape Measure [ ]

-0.19 ✓	Asymmetry✓ -0.02	-0.17 ✓
p > 0.5	p = 0.27	p > 0.5

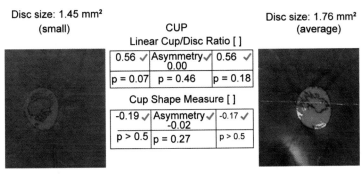

(Contd.)

(Contd.)

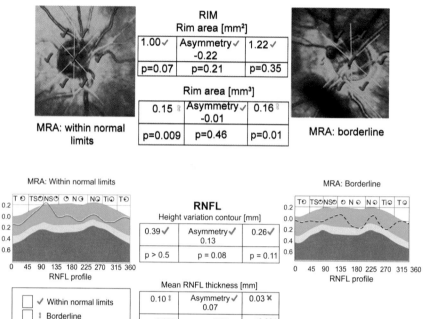

Fig. 18.3: Visual fields are stable and HRT is normal.

Optical Coherence Tomography[8]

Optical coherence tomography (OCT) is an imaging technology that performs high-resolution, cross-sectional imaging of the optic nerve head, retinal nerve fibre layer (Fig. 18.4) and macula. It uses 820 or 850 nm diode laser beam that is projected to an interferometer.

Lasers Used for Glaucoma Treatment

Therapeutic uses of lasers differ with the type of glaucoma and the treatment warranted (Fig. 18.5).

Laser Iridotomy

The term iridotomy (LI) is used to indicate laser-induced openings in the iris, whereas iridectomy indicates surgical removal of iris tissue.

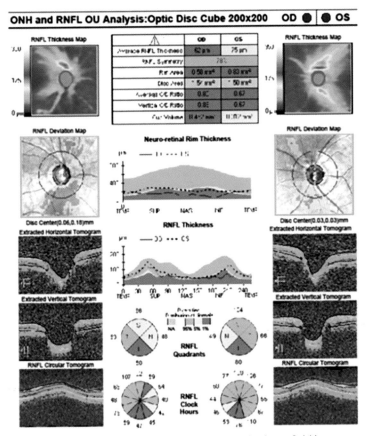

Fig. 18.4: An OCT of the RNFL with bilateral inferior field loss.

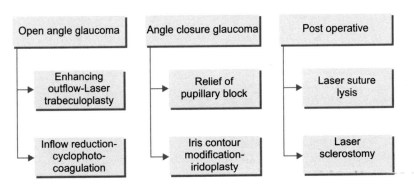

Fig. 18.5: Uses of Lasers in different types of glaucoma.

Type of laser used

LI can be done using
- Continuous wave argon laser therapy
- Pulsed argon laser therapy or
- Q-switched Nd:Yag laser

Nd:Yag laser iridotomy is the most commonly used laser due to its better efficiency and faster perforation. It has replaced argon iridotomy.

Mechanism

The mechanism is to deliver an intense amount of energy into a single spot over pico to nano seconds using high irradiance. Thus, it disrupts the tissue and produces a hole in the iris allowing aqueous to flow through.

Indications[4]

- Prophylactically in fellow eye in case of angle closure attack in the one eye
- Following termination of angle closure attack by medical therapy
- Nanophthalmos
- Pupillary block, subluxated lens, aphakic or pseudophakic eyes
- Iris bombé in seclusive pupillae
- Completion of an incomplete surgical iridectomy (when posterior pigmented epithelial layer is retained)
- Malignant glaucoma
- Positive darkroom provocative test in occludable narrow angled eyes.

Contraindications

- Hazy cornea
- Chronic inflammation and hazy anterior chamber
- It is better avoided in patients with rubeosis iridis and flat anterior chamber.

Precautions

Prior to laser, it is necessary to ensure the cornea is clear and intraocular lens (IOP) is well controlled. During an acute angle closure attack, cornea is clouded with raised IOP and LI can't be done. The procedure itself can cause sudden rise in intraocular pressures, hence high IOP prior should be controlled.

Patients shouldn't be on anticoagulants during the procedure, especially in one eyed, corneal graft or advanced glaucoma patients. If there is a resulting bleeding, the hyphema can cause acute rise in pressure or may require mechanical drainage. It is wise to stop anticoagulants 5 days prior procedure after consulting the physician concerned.

Procedure

Informed consent of the patient is taken before beginning any laser procedure. Miosis is achieved by using pilocarpine nitrate (2%) at 15 min interval starting 2 h prior to iridotomy. This is to ensure that the iris is stretched fully and is easily penetrable at its thinnest site. Syrup glycerol or hypertonic sodium

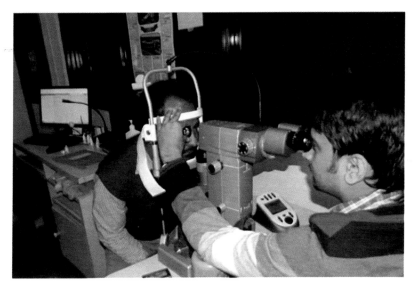

Fig. 18.6: Position of the patient during LI.

chloride (5%) may be used to get a clearer cornea. The patient is seated on a stool, head is fixed at the patient positioning frame, using a forehead strap and chin rest (Fig. 18.6). Anesthesia is gained using 1 drop topical proparacaine hydrochloride (0.5%), 4% Xylocaine eye drops or peribulbar injection of lignocaine in nystagmus or uncooperative patients. The patient is asked to look temporally or nasally during the laser procedure to avoid macular damage. An appropriate laser contact lens is used.

The lens smoothens out the corneal surface and gives pressure to prevent blood from increasing. It also avoids axial expansion of plasma, so reducing unnecessary spread of damage and increasing the density of power at the focused site.

The contact lenses used for LI are:

- Abraham iridectomy laser lens: Abraham lens has +66 D planoconvex peripheral button over a routine contact lens and increases the laser power by a factor of 2.5.
- Pollack iridotomy lens: Pollack lens has two buttons, the larger one for Iridectomy and the smaller for SLT or ALT as one can visualize the angle through it

Techniques

The techniques of performing LI include:

- Direct penetration technique: It is most commonly used. Parameters approved are 50 μm spot, 700–1200 mW over 0.1/0.2 s
- 'Hump' technique: It creates a hump on the iris, by a contraction burn caused by 200–400 mW energy, over 500 μm spot and 0.5 s exposure. The

hump so created is penetrated full thickness with 50 μm, 700–1200 MW over 0.1–0.2 s.

- 'Drumhead technique': Initially burns are placed circularly around iridotomy site with 200 μm, 200 mW at 0.2 s. This tightens the central area, which is then penetrated with 50 μmicron, 700–1200 mW over 0.1/0.2 s.

Nd:Yag laser produces 3–8 mJ per shot, and one to three shots are sufficient to complete the procedure. The axis of the focusing beam coincides with the axis of the contact lens. Higher energy levels are required in thicker iris to achieve complete penetration. Using more power per shot or more shots per burst can increase energy delivery.

Site of the iridectomy

The optimal site of iridotomy preferred is usually superonasal. Only in aphakic patients with silicon oil, an inferior iridotomy preferred. The iris should be penetrated as peripherally as possible to avoid hitting the anterior lens capsule, which lies closer in the center. Ideal point being three-fourth the distance between pupillary margin and iris periphery. Site between 10'o clock and 2 o' clock is preferred as they will be covered by the upper eye lid. At 12 o' clock position, gas bubble may collect during the LI and interfere with the procedure. The laser beam is focussed at a crypt, where it is thinnest. In the absence of crypts, wide area between pigmented freckles or radially arranged white collagen strands is targeted. In case of a small iridotomy, an additional iridotomy at a separate site or enlarging the same site is done.

The end-point is recognized by sudden outpouring of melanotic pigments, gush of aqueous into the anterior chamber, with deepening of the AC. There is also a sudden shower of pigments in the pupillary region. Retroillumination may be used after a few weeks of LI. In aphakic and pseudophakic eyes, and corneal edema or inflammatory conditions of iris, up to three iridotomies may be required for relief from aqueous entrapment.

Complications

- Uveitis: Usually pigment dispersal, and irritation of the iris.
- Pigment dispersion
- Hemorrhage: It is most common and may result in hyphema. Once there is bleeding, stop the procedure, apply pressure on the eyeball with a contact lens. If the media are clear, iridotomy can be done at a separate site. In cloudy media, the procedure is postponed.
- Corneal burn: It occurs due to poor focusing. If LI is attempted in a very shallow AC, then the endothelium may also get damaged. Since the opacity so formed is very peripheral, it doesn't cause poor vision.
- Elevated IOP: Elevated IOP is often noticed within the first 4 h (At 1 h in 75% of the cases, within 4 h in 40% of the cases with chronic angle closure

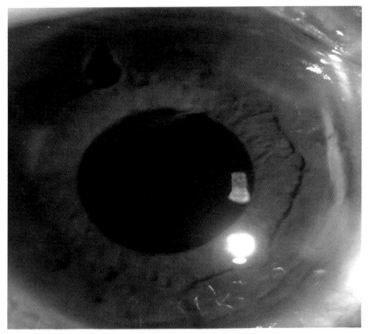

Fig. 18.7: A large LI causing uniocular diplopia to a patient.

and in 11–17% of cases in the rest of the patients. It is possibly because the collected debris may further obstruct a chronically occluded angle)

- Blurred vision
- Damage to lens and anterior capsule
- Diplopia: It occurs when the eyelid doesn't cover the iridotomy site (Fig. 18.7).
- Closure of initially patent iridotomy
- Failure to make full thickness iridotomy.

Post-Laser Management

Post laser, steroids and antiglaucoma medication should be continued for at least 3 weeks to prevent uveitis and IOP spikes. The patency of LI is checked, on the next day, 1 week post laser, 3 and 4 weeks later again. Gonioscopy shows widening of previously narrow angles. Preoperative 1% apraclonidine drops and oral acetazolamide prevent IOP spikes post laser. If at a follow-up visit iridotomy is too small create an additional iridotomy at a different site or enlarge LI with argon laser.

Nd:Yag vs Argon Laser for Iridotomy

The Nd: YAG has various advantages over the argon laser such as:
- Lower energy level
- Lower incidence of spontaneous closure

- Less inflammation
- Fewer applications are needed
- Absence of thermal injury to cornea, lens and retina
- Effective even in cases with opaque cornea.

Special Situations

Rubeosis Iridis

Argon laser pretreatment can be done followed by Nd:Yag Laser iridotomy. Argon pretreatment either in a drum head pattern or lamellar flattening is done, followed by perforation of remaining thickness of iris with 3-6 mJ of Nd: Yag laser shot. In phakic eyes, miosis is maintained with pilocarpine (2%). In pupillary block, cycloplegics are given. Cyclopentolate (1%) or tropicamide (1%) are the mydriatics commonly used.

Pearls of Iridotomy

- Keep the illumination less and the slit lamp beam wide
- Ideal iridotomy which is full thickness should be achieved by one shot
- Burst mode is not preferred
- Avoid arcus senilis and iris vessels
- End point is visibility of red reflex

Argon Laser Trabeculoplasty

A micro rupture technique was used in open angle glaucoma using ruby laser, aimed at creating an opening directly into the Schlemm's canal. Later, argon laser was used to irradiate the meshwork and this came to be called argon laser trabeculoplasty.[5-8]

Type of Laser Used

Initially, Q-switched ruby laser then argon laser and subsequently continuous wave of bichromatic blue green (454.4–528.7 nm) or monochromatic green (514.5 nm) light were used. Diode laser trabeculoplasty is a procedure similar to ALT, but it causes less disruption of the blood aqueous barrier, less PAS and less post laser pain.

Mechanism

It acts by induction of a thermal coagulation effect where collagen fibrils of trabecular meshwork are damaged and degenerate into subfibrillar fragments. The shrinkage of the collagen fibers increases the inter trabecular space and enhances aqueous outflow.

Fibrosis induced by the laser may lead to inward bowing of the trabecular meshwork and further open Schlemm's canal. Because of the induced fibrosis, macrophages enter the lasered area and engulf the extracellular matrix. The altered composition improves aqueous flow. Another theory purports that the increased phagocytic and migratory activity of surviving endothelial cells increases the transcellular flow of aqueous across the Schlemm's canal.

Indications

ALT is used in
- POAG when the IOP is uncontrolled despite maximum medication, and patient is unfit or unwilling for surgery.
- Pigmentary glaucoma
- Juvenile open-angle glaucoma and angle recession glaucoma are other conditions that may benefit from ALT.

ALT is contraindicated when
- Cornea is hazy or opaque as in angle closure glaucoma, (it is possible only when trabecular meshwork is visible)
- Congenital or developmental glaucoma
- Uveitic glaucoma
- Traumatic glaucoma
- Neovascular glaucoma and
- Aphakic glaucoma with vitreous in AC.

Procedure

The procedure involves use of a miotic agent to constrict the pupil, usually done with pilocarpine 2%. Anesthesia is gained using 1 drop topical proparacaine HCl (0.5%), 4% Xylocaine eye drops or peribulbar injection of lignocaine in nystagmus or uncooperative patients. After taking an informed consent patient is seated on a stool, head is fixed at the patient positioning frame, using a forehead strap and chin rest in a darkened or semi darkened room. An appropriate laser contact lens is used.

Contact Lens for ALT

- Ritch trabeculoplasty laser lens
- Goldmann single- or three-mirror lens
- Thorpe four-mirror gonio lens
- Latina SLT gonio lens
- Ocular magna view gonio lens
- Pollack iridotomy gonio laser lens (bigger button for iridotomy and smaller for ALT and SLT)

After choosing the preferred gonio lens, with the help of a coupling fluid, lens is fixed on the eye and entire angle is examined. The parameters recommended for ALT are energy of 400–1200 mW, a spot size of 50 μm over 0.1 s exposure. In a single session, 100 burn spots are applied over 360° area. The burns should be regularly placed.

The appropriate site of focus is at the junction of pigmented and nonpigmented trabecular meshwork. This minimizes post laser early rise of IOP and peripheral synechiae formation. A large bubble indicates high energy level. An oval spot with a blurred edge indicates that the aiming beam is not perpendicular to the laser lens.

Post laser, there may be an acute elevation of IOP. IOP is measured after 1 and 4 h of the procedure. If there is no significant rise, then patients are reviewed at 1 week, 4 weeks and 3 months. In case of satisfactory reduction in IOP, antiglaucoma medication is gradually tapered. Antiglaucoma medications used include brimonidine and apraclonidine. Topical steroids are given to control inflammation. PAS may occur in posterior placement of burns.

Complications

Worsening of POAG, iritis, corneal burns, hyphemia.

Long-term Control

The glaucoma laser treatment trial showed that 7 years after ALT, the eyes showed better IOP control, better visual fields and healthier optic nerve as opposed to those managed solely on topical medications.

Selective Laser Trabeculoplasty

Introduced in 1995, selective laser trabeculoplasty specifically targets the pigmented TM without causing any damage to the non-pigmented TM.

Laser Used

It is performed with a Q switched frequency doubled Nd: YAG laser (532 nm).

Mechanism

It acts by disrupting the melanin granules in the cells of pigmented TM, causing cell death, known as 'selective photothermolysis.' There occurs no damage to the trabecular meshwork, hence causes less scarring.[5-7]

Indications

- Similar to ALT.
- Failed ALT.

Technique

The procedure is similar to ALT. It involves use of a miotic to constrict the pupil, usually done with pilocarpine 2%. After taking an informed consent patient is seated on a stool, head is fixed at the patient positioning frame,

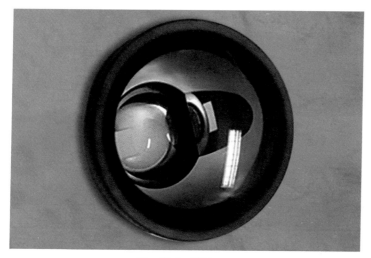

Fig. 18.8: SLT lens.

using a forehead strap and chin rest. Anaesthesia is gained using one drop of topical proparacaine HCl (0.5%), 4% Xylocaine eye drops or peribulbar injection of lignocaine in nystagmus or uncooperative patients. An appropriate laser contact lens is used (Fig. 18.8).

Lens designed for SLT with YAG bonded antireflective coating include
- Latina SLT goniolaser lens.
- Ocular magna view gonio laser lens.
- Pollack iridotomy gonio laser lens (smaller button is for SLT/ALT).

SLT laser parameters are energy of 0.6–1 mJ per pulse, to create a spot size of 400 μm. The pulse duration is of 3 ns. Fifty single short pulses are targeted to cover the entire height of trabecular meshwork spread over 180° of the TM (usually inferiorly or nasally). There is no end point of optimal energy effect, as seen in ALT. The shots should be confluent and should not overlap.

Post Laser Management

- Antiglaucoma medication is continued for at least 3 weeks.
- Topical steroids are started to control inflammation. NSAIDs can be used in their place.
- IOP is rechecked 1 and 3 h post procedure.
- Repeat SLT over the rest of the TM can be planned after reassessment.

Complications

Complications are similar to ALT such as inflammation, hyphema, discomfort and IOP spikes. However, it is preferred due to lesser tissue damage than ALT.

Peripheral Iridoplasty/Gonioplasty

First used by Karsnow, laser iridoplasty also known as gonioplasty is used to deepen the anterior chamber. The technique is to use continuous wave argon-laser burns in the peripheral iris to contract the iris and increase the space between the angle and site of burn.

Type of Laser Used

Argon laser is usually used but diode laser (810 nm) may have better penetration and can also be used.

Indications

- Plateau iris syndrome
- Angle closure attack
- Open an appositional angle closure
- Facilitate ALT/SLT in a shallow anterior chamber
- Medically uncontrolled angle closure glaucoma
- Nanophthalmos
- In topiramate-induced high myopia bilaterally with acute angle closure
- In boggy iris, causing angle closure, iridoplasty with or without a contact lens can avert the attack. Laser iridotomy can be performed at a later sitting.

Contraindications

- Flat anterior chamber
- Angle closure associated with PAS
- Corneal edema or opacity

Procedure

Informed consent is obtained. Miosis is achieved by using pilocarpine nitrate (2%) at 15 min interval starting 2 h prior. Patient is seated on a stool, head is fixed at the patient positioning frame, using a forehead strap and chin rest. A semidark or darkened room is ideal. Anaesthesia is gained using 1 drop topical proparacaine HCl (0.5%), 4% Xylocaine eye drops or peribulbar injection of lignocaine in nystagmus or uncooperative patients.

An appropriate laser contact lens is used. The laser shots are directly applied on the iris through the central area of the lens. The gonioscopic mirrors of lens are not suitable, as it leads to damage to the trabecular meshwork and scleral spur. The laser beams strike the iris tangentially and cause less stromal contraction, along with inflicting more diffuse burns.

The parameters used are energy of 200–500 mW, exposure of 0.2–0.5 s and spot size of 200–500 μm. The energy and exposure is increased if contraction doesn't occur. They are decreased in case of release of pigment, bubble formation or darker irides. In a single session, 8-12 burns are placed in each quadrant of the iris and around 180° is treated.

The end-point is contraction of iris, noticed by sudden deepening of the iris. If deepening doesn't occur, one should change the spot size or increase the power. If there are peripheral anterior synechiae at the site, 100 iridoplasties are unlikely to help.

Post laser steroids and antiglaucoma medication are advised for a week. Complications include transient IOP rise, corneal burn, iris atrophy, mild uveitis and pupillary distortion.

Cyclodestructive Procedures

Cyclophotocoagulation is a laser destructive procedure of the ciliary body, a surgical method used to reduce intractable IOP. It is advised in refractory glaucoma, unresponsive to glaucoma filtration surgeries and valve implants.

Types of cyclophotocoagulation

- Transpupillary cyclophotocoagulation
- Endo cyclophotocoagulation (destruction by trans vitreal route)
- Transscleral cyclophotocoagulation (most commonly used). Can be diode or Nd:YAG

The mechanism of cyclophotocoagulation involves irreversible destruction of the ciliary body. There may be associated visual loss due to inflammation incited or cystoid macular edema.

Indications

- Failure of outflow enhancing surgeries
- Painful blind eye
- Aphakic glaucoma
- Neovascular glaucoma
- Glaucoma due to endothelial ingrowth

Contraindications

- Associated active uveitis
- Thin sclera

Modes of Delivery

- Contact method: Nd:YAG laser with sapphire contact probe is used (Fig. 18.9).
- Noncontact method: Nd:YAG laser free running or continuous wave mode is used.

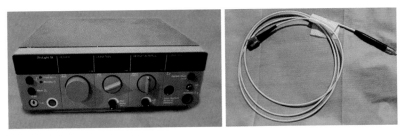

Fig. 18.9: Diode laser cyclophotocoagulation machine with probe (G-probe).

Transscleral Diode Laser Cyclophotocoagulation

Indications

- Eyes with refractory glaucoma as the last resort after failure of other surgeries and palliative treatment.
- As a primary management in eyes with low visual acuity.

Procedure

It requires a retrobulbar or peribulbar block. A 810 nm diode laser with a G probe is used, at power of 1750–2000 mW for 2.0 s and increasing it at 250 mW until an audible pop is heard. At this point, power is reduced by 250 mW and further proceeded. At 270° the ciliary body is lasered through the sclera leaving sites of previous filtering surgery or tube implants.

Post-laser Management

Post laser steroids and antibiotics are necessary. Antiglaucoma is gradually tapered over a month depending on the response. Pressure lowering is evident by around a month.

Complications

Complications seen are hypotony, loss of visual acuity and breakdown of blood brain barrier. Rarer complications observed are retinal detachment, scleral thinning and even sympathetic ophthalmia.

Transpupillary Cyclophotocoagulation

It can be done in situations where ciliary processes are directly visualized, e.g., in aphakic eyes or aniridia. Goldmann 3 mirror lens is applied with a coupling agent after topical anesthesia. Argon laser with 1000 mW, with a 50-μm spot size is focused on the ciliary body for 0.1 s. For hemostasis 200-μm spot size with a lower power can be used. One to 3 quadrants can be treated as per visibility.

Transvitreal Cyclophotocoagulation

It is indicated in neovascular glaucoma (when retinal laser is also planned) and silicone oil-induced glaucoma. The technique involves a three ports pars plana vitrectomy, with infusion in the infratemporal quadrant. Through a superior port endo-laser probe is introduced, the other two ports are closed. Low infusion pressure is required. External depression of the ciliary body is done with a muscle hook or a bud. The ciliary processes are visualized and a continuous mode power is applied. It is started at 150 mW and slowly increased till whitening and shrinking of ciliary processes takes place. An area of 270° to 300° is lasered in a session.

Argon Laser Pupilloplasty

It is a technique to alter the shape, size or location of an eccentric or irregular pupil. Photomydriasis is a variation where a miotic pupil is enlarged.

In glaucoma, it is used to relieve pupillary block in aphakia or pseudophakia, especially in cloudy cornea, as an alternative to laser iridotomy.

- Active uveitis
- Corneal edema

The initial procedure is similar to that of LI. It involves informed consent; mydriasis obtained by 1% tropicamide, 10% phenylephrine, at 15 min interval, starting 2 h prior to laser in a darkened or semi-darkened room. Anesthesia is gained using one drop of topical proparacaine HCl (0.5%), 4% Xylocaine eye drops or peribulbar injection of lignocaine in nystagmus or uncooperative patients. Patient is asked to look temporally or nasally during the procedure.

Technique

The technique is to place 360° continuous, concentric small argon laser burns just adjacent to the pupillary margin. The parameters used are 200–400 mW power of 0.2 s duration over an area of 200 μm. Following this, larger argon laser burns are shot concentrically just outside the initial laser shots in a double or single row. Here power of 400–500 mW of 0.2 to 0.5 second duration is used over an area of 500 microns.

Post laser steroids and antiglaucoma medication is advised. Miotics are discontinued. Complications include transient IOP rise, iris atrophy and iritis.

Other Uses of Lasers in Glaucoma Management

Laser Synechiolysis

Argon laser can be used to pull lightly adherent anterior synechiae away from the angle similar to iridoplasty. The usual parameters are 400–800 MW, 0.1–0.2 s, 50–100 μm spot size.

Control of a Large Bleb

Large bleb that causes discomfort, inadequate eye closure and exposure keratitis, can be lasered to flatten it. A dye such as gentian violet is used to stain the bleb, after topical anesthesia. A coagulative laser like argon, double frequency YAG, or diode is used (similar to gonioplasty) to create a large spot of 500 μm over 15 s with a power of 0.2 to 0.4 W. The dye absorbs the laser and the bleb is flattened out.

SUMMARY

Laser is used in some equipments for diagnostic purpose. The laser therapy has become the method of choice for treating many forms of glaucoma, especially when medical modalities prove inadequate or patient compliance with medical regimens is poor.[9] In open-angle glaucoma laser treatment can reduce the intraocular pressure by increasing outflow of aqueous from the eye (laser trabeculoplasty), or decrease the formation of aqueous (cyclophotocoagulation). In narrow angle glaucoma, aqueous outflow is improved via laser iridotomy where a small hole is made in the iris, or via iridoplasty where the angle is opened. Hence, lasers in glaucoma are an integral part of patient diagnosis as well as management.

REFERENCES

1. Kumar S. Lasers in glaucoma. Nepal J Ophthalmol. 2010;2(1):51-8.
2. Thomas R, Sekhar GC, Kumar RS. Glaucoma management in developing countries: Medical, laser, and surgical options for glaucoma management in countries with limited resources. Curr Opin Ophthalmol. 2004;15(2):127-31.
3. Detry-Morel M. Current place of laser in the management of glaucomas. J Fr Ophtalmol. 2002;25(8):843-55.
4. He M, Friedman DS, Ge J, et al. Laser peripheral iridotomy in primary angle-closure suspects: biometric and gonioscopic outcomes: the Liwan Eye Study. Ophthalmology. 2007;114(3):494-500.
5. Damji KF, Shah KC, Rock WJ, et al. Selective laser trabeculoplasty v argon laser trabeculoplasty: a prospective randomised clinical trial. Br J Ophthalmol. 1999;83(6):718-22.
6. Gulati V, Fan S, Gardner BJ, et al. Mechanism of action of selective laser trabeculoplasty and predictors of response. Invest Ophthalmol Vis Sci. 2017;58(3):1462-8.
7. Matos AG, Asrani SG, Paula JS. Feasibility of laser trabeculoplasty in angle closure glaucoma: a review of favourable histopathological findings in narrow angles. Clin Exp Ophthalmol. 2017 Feb 28.
8. Tsang S, Cheng J, Lee JW. Developments in laser trabeculoplasty. Br J Ophthalmol. 2016;100(1):94-7.
9. Ekici F, Waisbourd M, Katz LJ. Current and future of laser therapy in the management of glaucoma. Open Ophthalmol J. 2016;10:56-67.

Glaucoma Surgery

Ramakrishnan R, Sindhushree R

INTRODUCTION

Though the discovery of disease called glaucoma dates back to 17th century and association between glaucoma and intraocular pressure (IOP) was first suggested by Richard Bannister in 1962, surgical attempt to lower the IOP for treatment of glaucoma was developed only in 19th century.[1]

Albrecht Von Graefe in 1856 was the one who performed the first glaucoma surgery called iridectomy to treat glaucoma.[2] However in 1867, Louis De Wecker performed anterior sclerotomy (full-thickness scleral incision 1 mm posterior to the limbus), thereby becoming the first one to suggest the concept of filtration of aqueous from anterior chamber to the subconjunctival space as a means of lowering the IOP and has been regarded as 'father of glaucoma surgery.'

Flowchart 19.1 shows classification of glaucoma surgery.

FULL THICKNESS FILTRATION SURGERIES

The first one to perform full thickness filtering surgery as mentioned was Louis De Wecker in 1867 who performed anterior sclerotomy. Holth[3] in 1908 introduced iridencleisis, which involved incarceration of iris tissue between the lips of scleral tissue, which lowered the IOP. But because of risk of sympathetic ophthalmia the procedure was abandoned by many surgeons. Later in 1909, Elliot[4] introduced the technique of limbal trephination. In 1958,[5] Scheie described thermal sclerostomy wherein he observed that application of an electric cautery for hemostasis of posterior lip of sclerectomy incision produced inadvertent filtering blebs. Since then Scheie's procedure was the most frequently performed filtering surgery in early 1970s and 1980s. However, because of uncontrolled transscleral outflow there was increased risk

Flowchart 19.1: Classification of glaucoma surgery.

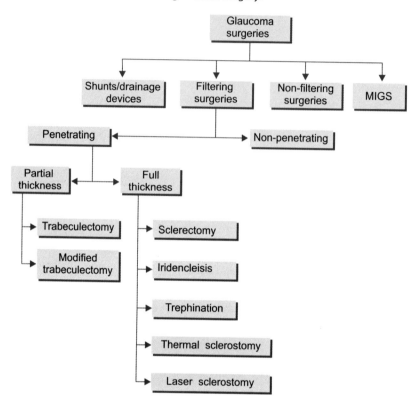

of hypotony and its associated complications, which led many surgeons to switch over to partial thickness filtering procedure.

Disadvantages of full thickness procedure are as follows:
- Hypotony and shallow anterior chamber
- Increased incidence of cataract
- Increased risk of endophthalmitis

PARTIAL THICKNESS FILTERING SURGERY

Trabeculectomy is regarded as gold standard for surgical treatment of glaucoma. It was first described by Sugar in 1962 and later popularized by Cairns[6] in 1968. This technique provided satisfactory IOP control with fewer postoperative complications when compared to full thickness procedure.

Mechanism of Aqueous Drainage

- Cut ends of Schlemm's canal
- Suprachoroidal space
- Scleral vessels

- Thin scleral flap
- Scleral flap borders

TECHNIQUE

Surgical Exposure

After adequate anesthesia and akinesia, the eye to be operated is painted and draped. Appropriate speculum preferably one with adjustable screw is applied in order to avoid undue pressure over the globe.

Superior rectus bridle suture is applied in order to expose the superior bulbar conjunctiva. However, it is associated with risk of conjunctival button holing, globe perforation, superior rectus hematoma and also risk of postoperative ptosis.

Hence most of the surgeons prefer corneal traction suture with 8-0 silk/nylon suture 1 mm anterior to the limbus. Care should be taken not to apply too deep or too superficial suture, which may result in full thickness corneal perforation or cheesewiring of cornea respectively.

Conjunctival Flap

Either limbal-based or fornix-based conjunctival flap is created.

Limbal Based

At around 8 mm away and parallel to limbus, small opening is made through conjunctiva and extended. Care should be taken to avoid superior rectus tendon injury.

Fornix Based

Conjunctiva is grasped close to the limbus using nontraumatic forceps and conjunctiva and tenon's are cut together using Wescott scissors leaving around 1–2 mm of conjunctiva near the limbus (Fig. 19.1).

The advantages and disadvantages between fornix- and limbal-based flaps are given in Table 19.1.

Hemostasis

Unipolar or bipolar wet field cautery is preferably used. Excess cautery over flap site and flap bed should be avoided.

Scleral Flap

A partial thickness scleral flap is made. It can be fashioned in different shapes like triangular, rectangular or quadrangular. Most surgeons prefer triangular

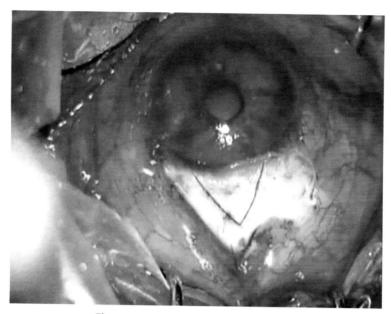

Fig. 19.1: Fornix-based conjunctival flap.

Table 19.1: Advantages and disadvantages of fornix-based and limbal-based flaps.

Fornix -based flap	Limbal-based flap
Advantages	*Advantages*
– Easier to make	– Decreased risk of bleb leak
– Helps in forming a more diffuse bleb	– Safe when antimetabolites are used
– Less time consuming	
Disadvantages	*Disadvantages*
– Increased risk of bleb leak	– Cumbersome and time-consuming
	– Increased risk of posterior limitation of bleb leading to formation of localized bleb

flap. A 4 × 4 mm triangular scleral flap is made with base at the limbus. Flap outline is made using sharp blade like Bard Parker blade no. 11 placed perpendicular to the globe. The flap is then dissected using crescent blade or Bard Parker no. 15 blade by holding the apex of the flap using Castrovejo corneal suture forceps and with constant traction toward cornea a lamellar uniform dissection is made. The dissection is carried till blue gray zone but should never extend beyond that zone. Use high magnification to dissect flap accurately and safely avoiding flap related complications (Fig. 19.2).

Paracentesis

Paracentesis is made at 3 or 9 o'clock position using side port or micro vitreo retinal (MVR) blade. Entry should be made tangential to limbus and parallel to iris plane in order to avoid inadvertent damage to the iris or lens. It helps

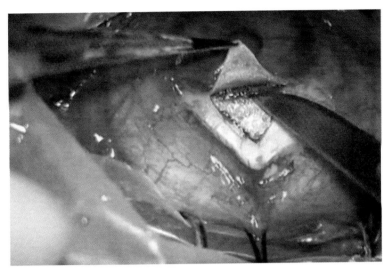

Fig. 19.2: Triangular scleral flap.

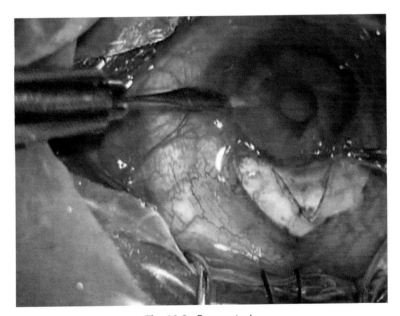

Fig. 19.3: Paracentesis.

in controlled decompression of globe, allows titration of bleb at the end of surgery and also facilitates the formation of anterior chamber if it becomes shallow during the surgery (Fig. 19.3).

Stoma/Ostium Creation

Using 1 mm V-shaped lancet blade anterior chamber is entered through clear cornea under partial thickness scleral flap. Using Kelly's punch, an internal block of tissue (2 × 1 mm) containing trabecular meshwork is excised in five

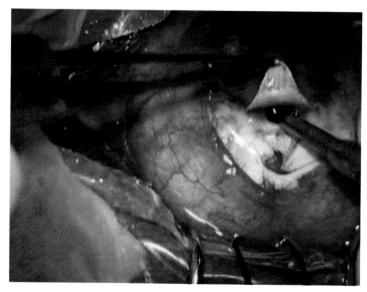

Fig. 19.4: Stoma/ostium creation using Kelly's Descemet punch.

to six bites from posterior lip of incision. At least 1 mm of scleral bed is left on either side of the scleral flap so that when flap is sutured the sclerostomy margins are not exposed. Care should be taken not to punch too posteriorly to avoid scleral spur and underlying ciliary body (Fig.19.4).

Peripheral Iridectomy

Broadbased peripheral iridectomy is done using Collibri forceps and De Wecker's scissors or vannas scissors. This is done to prevent blocking of the ostium due to iris incarceration (Fig.19.5).

Scleral Flap Suturing

The scleral flap is sutured using three 10-0 nylon sutures. In case of triangular flap, one apical suture and one suture on either side of scleral flap is applied. The knot is tightened by 3-2-1 or 2-1-1 throws. Knot is pulled away from the scleral flap and buried. The tightness of sutures should be titrated such that it is neither too loose that may cause postoperative hypotony or too tight that may lead to high IOP postoperatively.

Anterior Chamber Reformation

Using blunt 30-gauge cannula, the chamber is reformed with balanced salt solution through the paracentesis to determine if there is a controlled leak through the scleral flap. If flow is excessive and chamber shallows, knots are tightened. If there is inadequate leakage then the surgeon may loosen the knots.

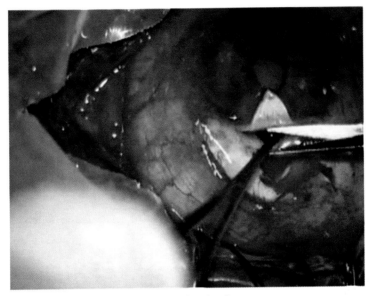

Fig. 19.5: Peripheral iridectomy.

Conjunctival Flap Closure

The conjunctival flap is closed using either interrupted or continuous suture. With fornix based conjunctival flap wing shaped closure using 8-0 vicryl is done. In this technique, the free conjunctival edge is made taut against the limbus to prevent leak through the edge. The knot is tied using 2-1-1 throws and tightened. The conjunctival closure should be water tight.

Bleb Titration

At the end of surgery, balanced salt solution is injected through the side port. There should be mild to moderate elevation of the bleb with no conjunctival leak.

MOORFIELD'S SAFE SURGERY SYSTEM[7]

In order to minimize the postoperative complications like hypotony, shallow anterior chamber and other bleb-related complications (mainly bleb failure) and to improve surgical outcomes the following recommendations have been given by Moorfields Eye Hospital, London.

- *Choosing site for surgery*
  Usually the superior quadrant is preferred site as there is less chances of inflammation, dysthesia and endophthalmitis. Since the upper lid covers the iridectomy there is less chance of diplopia.
- *Surgical exposure*
  Corneal traction suture is preferred over superior rectus bridle suture, thereby reducing risk of superior rectus hematoma and failure of bleb.

- *Conjunctival flap*
  Fornix-based flap is preferred over the limbal based flap to minimize the risk of posterior limitation of bleb (ring of steel phenomenon) and cystic overhanging bleb.
- *Conjunctival pocket*
  A wide conjunctival pocket is created for applying antimetabolite. A special conjunctival T-clamp is designed to hold back conjunctiva to prevent exposing cut edge of conjunctiva to the antimetabolite. Three circular medical grade polyvinyl alcohol sponges, which are usually used for LASIK as corneal shields are used. It is cut into half or whole and folded like lens to pass underneath conjunctival pocket making sure it doesn't come into contact with conjunctival edge.
- *Scleral flap*
  A rectangular scleral flap is fashioned by cutting a horizontal incision parallel to the limbus. A partial thickness scleral pocket is created and finally it is cut by two side incisions but not upto the limbus so that the aqueous is directed more posteriorly forming diffuse posterior bleb.
- *Paracentesis*
  It is usually made obliquely and parallel to limbus and preferred slightly inferiorly, which will allow access to the anterior chamber if necessary in the outpatient clinic. An anterior segment infusion cannula is usually used to maintain chamber pressure and globe integrity throughout the surgery.
- *Sclerostomy*
  A special punch named Khaw small Descemet's membrane punch No. 7 made of titanium is used to create ostium of around 0.5 mm. It allows anterior access and thereby minimizes chance of bleeding due to ciliary body injury. The punch is aligned perpendicular to the eye to create clean nonshelved sclerostomy.
- *Peripheral iridectomy*
  A peripheral iridectomy is done by cutting it with scissors parallel to limbus.
- *Scleral flap closure*
  The scleral flap sutures are preplaced but not tied. Once trabecular meshwork punch and iridectomy is done, the sutures are tightened one by one so as to allow adequate flow through the flap. Safer and releasable sutures are preferred.
- *Conjunctival closure*
  Using round bodied needle conjunctival closure is done with continuous nylon suture and knots are buried in shallow corneal grooves. This helps to reduce conjunctival leaks and suture discomfort in patients.

ANTIMETABOLITES AND FILTERING SURGERY

Indications

Antimetabolites are indicated in eyes with increased risk of scarring such as:
- Young age

- African race
- Long-term use of topical antiglaucoma medications
- Previous conjunctival surgeries/failed trabeculectomies
- Secondary glaucomas

The commonly used antimetabolites are the following.

5-Fluorouracil (5-FU)

Mechanism of Action

- Inhibits thymidylate synthase enzyme that catalyzes rate limiting step in DNA synthesis, thereby resulting in death of rapidly growing cells.

  Dosage

  Intraoperative use: Sponge soaked in 25 or 50 mg/ml solution placed for 3–5 min

  Post-operative use: 5 mg injection (0.1 ml of 50 mg/ml) adjacent to bleb/180° away from the bleb.

Mitomycin-C[8,9]

Antitumor antibiotic isolated from *Streptomyces caespitosus.*

Mechanism of Action

- Causes cross-linking and inhibition of DNA synthesis
- Cell cycle nonspecific
- More potent than 5 FU

  Drug availability: available as powder in strengths 2, 10, 40 mg

  Intraoperative use: Decided on case to case basis

- 0.1–0.5mg/ml soaked sponges
- Duration: 1–5 min
- *Post-operative use:*
- 0.02 mg/ml as injection adjacent to bleb or 180°away from bleb

COLLAGEN IMPLANTS IN FILTERING SURGERY

Ologen Collagen Matrix (Fig. 19.6)

- Collagen matrix (ologen) is a biodegradable and implantable extracellular matrix, which helps in modulating wound repair.
- It is highly porous scaffold made up of cross linked lyophilized porcine type 1 atelocollagen ($\geq$90%) and glycosaminoglycans (<10%) that encourages random growth of fibroblast, through its pores and secretes connective tissue in the form of nonscarring loose matrix. This was introduced mainly to overcome certain issues associated with use of antimetabolites like Mitomycin-C, which is associated with serious complications like hypotony, blebitis and endophthalmitis. In addition, dangers of handling

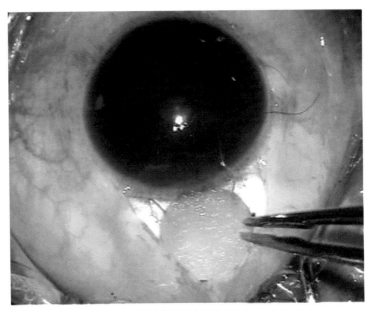

Fig. 19.6: Collagen implant (ologen).

MMC are avoided. It also acts as space maintainer, reducing chances of fibrosis and enhancing formation of an ideal bleb with minimal scarring. It is available in various shapes and dimensions.

ROLE OF RELEASABLE SUTURE IN FILTERING SURGERY

This technique minimizes the incidence of shallow anterior chamber and hypotony in the early postoperative period. It has an advantage over laser suturolysis wherein sutures cannot be cutoff in the presence of thick Tenon's or blood due to presence of subconjunctival hemorrhage due to poor visibility. There are various techniques of applying releasable suture. The most popular one is that introduced by Cohen and Oscher.

Technique (Figs. 19.7 to 19.10)

The first bite is taken 1–2 mm anterior and parallel to the limbus through partial thickness of the cornea for a length of about 3–4 mm (Fig. 19.7) and taken out on the right or the left side depending on whether surgeon is right or left handed. A second short vertical bite is taken in line with the apex of the flap 1–2 mm anterior to the limbus (Fig. 19.8) through partial corneal thickness and comes out at the limbus. The third bite is taken through the apex of the flap and out through the sclera posterior to the flap (Fig.19.9). Using tying forceps four throws are taken and tied to the suture segment lying over the sclera flap to make a slip knot (Fig.19.10). The tightness of the suture is adjusted based on the approximation of the flap edges and amount of fluid egress. The corneal end of the suture is cut flush with the surface

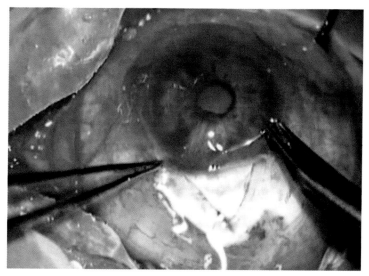

Fig. 19.7: Bite taken 1–2 mm anterior and parallel to the limbus through partial thickness of the cornea for a length of about 3–4 mm.

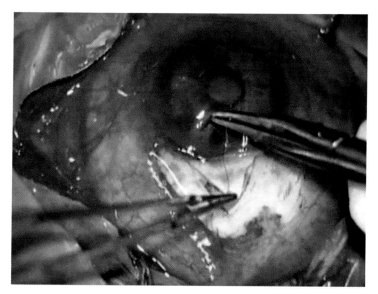

Fig. 19.8: Vertical bite taken in line with the apex of the flap 1–2 mm anterior to the limbus.

of cornea to avoid leaving suture end from protruding through the corneal surface.

COMPLICATIONS

Complications can be divided into the following.

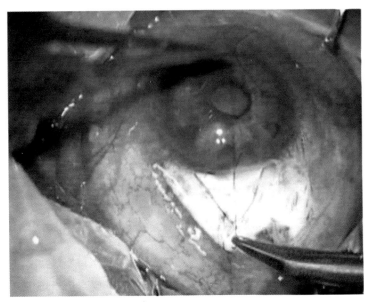

Fig. 19.9: Bite taken through the apex of the flap and out through the sclera posterior to the flap.

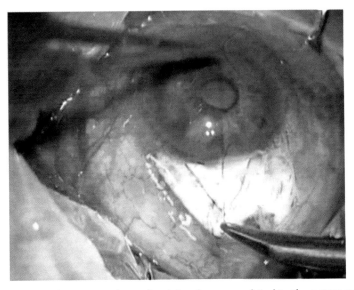

Fig. 19.10: Four throws are taken using tying forceps and tied to the suture segment lying over the sclera flap to make a slip knot.

Preoperative

They are mainly anesthesia related. The main issue will be when excess of local anesthetic is injected or in case of acute retrobulbar hemorrhage, the elevated IOP may damage the already compromised optic nerve in advanced glaucoma. Always stop anticoagulants preoperatively to minimize chance of bleeding.

Intraoperative

Superior Rectus Hematoma

While applying superior rectus (SR) bridle suture, one must be careful not to inadvertently produce globe puncture and SR hematoma, which may increase the chance of postoperative bleb failure due to increased fibrosis.

Conjunctival Button Hole

One must be very careful while handling the conjunctiva. Always use non-toothed forceps and handle the conjunctiva gently. The risk of creating button holes is highest in previously operated eyes that have extensive sub-conjunctival scarring. Once button hole occurs it is difficult to treat and may be responsible for failure of surgery.

If the tear is very large and if closure seems to be very difficult, choose a new surgical site. Small button holes may be repaired by direct closure using 10-0 nylon. One must ensure water-tight conjunctival closure. At the end of the surgery, one must apply fluorescein dye to conjunctival surface to aid detection of any unrecognized button hole defects or wound leaks.

Scleral Flap Related Complications

Scleral flap should be dissected with utmost caution. The flap should neither be too thick nor too thin. If it is too thick we might end up in premature entry as underlying scleral tissue is very thin. If it is too thin it results in button hole of flap and amputation of flap. If recognized early, the flap may be dissected either superficially or deep if it is too thick or thin respectively. However, if the scleral flap is amputated another site should be chosen.

Intraoperative Bleeding

There is increased risk of bleeding in patients who are on oral anticoagulants and uncontrolled systemic hypertension. Always stop the oral anticoagulants well ahead before planning surgery after getting fitness from the physician. Gentle cautery has to be applied as excess cautery can lead on to increased fibrosis and risk of bleb failure. Never apply cautery at the scleral flap bed or its sides as this may cause scleral shrinkage and difficulty in closure of the flap.

Suprachoroidal Hemorrhage

Suprachoroidal hemorrhage can occur in rare cases. Patients who are at particularly risk are those with aphakia, postvitrectomized eyes, congenital glaucoma, pathological myopia, prolonged hypotony and patients on oral anticoagulants. In high risk patients, it is advisable to do slow decompression of eye and preplacing scleral flap sutures for rapid closure, thereby reducing significant duration of hypotony. In high-risk eyes like Sturge-Weber syndrome, preventive sclerotomies should be done.

Iridectomy-related Complications

These include a large iridectomy, iridodialysis, excessive bleeding or inadvertent cyclodialysis cleft.

Vitreous Loss and Lens Injury

These can occur when lens zonular complex is inadvertently damaged during iridectomy. Adequate anterior vitrectomy should be done to prevent ostium blockage with vitreous. Vitreous loss is more common with angle closure glaucoma and congenital glaucoma.

Early Postoperative Complications

Early postoperative complications are shown in Flowchart 19.2.

Normal AC with Increased IOP

Blockage of Internal Ostium

Internal ostium may be blocked with blood,fibrin,vitreous or membranes. Gonioscopy is mandatory to assess the patency of ostium and should be performed with lens whose diameter is smaller than cornea to avoid accidental bleb injury. If blockage is noted laser procedure may be required to free the ostium.

Tight Scleral Flap Sutures

Laser suturolysis can be done with as little conjunctival manipulation and laser energy as possible. Only one suture should be lysed at a time to minimize the risk of hypotony. Suturolysis is effective only if it is done within 2–3 weeks of trabeculectomy without antifibrotic; however, window period is longer if antifibrotic agnet is used.

Flowchart 19.2: Early postoperative complications

	Preoperative (anesthesia related)
	Intraoperative
	Postoperative

Table 19.2: Differential diagnosis of shallow AC with elevated IOP and treatment.

Mechanism	Pupillary block	Suprachoroidal hemorrhage	Aqueous misdirection
IOP	Normal to high	Normal to high	Normal to high
Nature of AC shallowing	Iris bombé with shallow peripheral AC	Uniformly shallow	Uniformly shallow
Seidel test	Negative	Negative	Negative
Fundus	Normal	Choroidal elevation	Normal
Treatment	Laser iridotomy	Observation, if large needs drainage when echography shows liquefaction of blood	Mydriatic- cycloplegic drugs Aqueous suppressants, Yag hyaloidotomy, vitreous tap or vitrectomy

II. Shallow AC with Elevated IOP

Differential diagnosis of shallow AC with elevated IOP and management are summarized in Table 19.2.

Shallow AC with Low IOP

Shallow AC with low IOP may occur due to:
• Bleb leak
• Overfiltration
• Ciliochoroidal detachment

Bleb Leak (Fig. 19.11)

Small conjunctival leaks may be managed conservatively with 8 mm pressure patch, Simmon's tamponade shells, symble pharon rings or by using contact lens of appropriate size.

When there is wound dehiscence in case of limbal-based flap or retraction of flap in case of fornix-based flap or scleral flap edge is exposed, early surgical intervention with closure of conjunctival wound should be done with nonabsorbable suture.

• *Overfiltration*: Large diffuse bleb with low IOP and absence of wound leak (Seidel's sign negative) suggest overfiltration. Treatment may be done conservatively producing tamponade with Simmon's shell or symblepharon ring. Other techniques to decrease filtration include compression sutures (Fig.19.12), autologous blood injection into bleb (Fig.19.13), cryo or laser application. AC reformation can be done using BSS, air and viscoelastic agents.

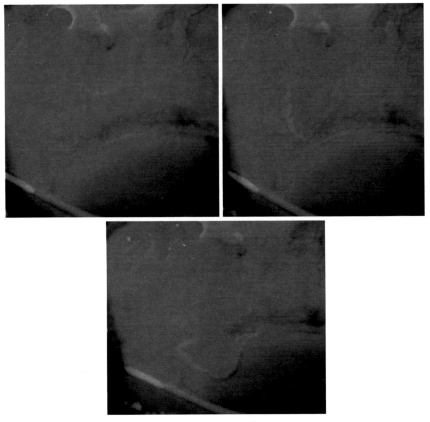

Fig. 19.11: Bleb leak.

- *Ciliochoroidal detachment:* It is more common after full thickness procedures. Small choroidal detachments can be conservatively managed with administration of topical and systemic steroids and cycloplegics. Surgical intervention is required in the following cases.
- Kissing choroidals
- Flat AC with risk of corneal decompensation secondary to lens endothelial touch.

Wipe Out/Snuff Out Phenomenon

The phenomenon of severe visual loss after surgery, with no obvious cause is known as wipe out or snuff out phenomenon. It is believed to occur in patients with advanced glaucoma with visual fields demonstrating the presence of macular split. The reason may be attributed to the fact that the already damaged optic nerve may not tolerate even slight fluctuations of intraocular pressure. The severe loss of central vision following trabeculectomy with mitomycin C occurred in 6% of patients who had glaucoma with marked visual field loss. However, controversy still exists regarding the exact incidence of this phenomenon.

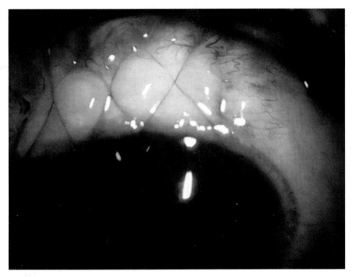

Fig. 19.12: Bleb compression sutures.

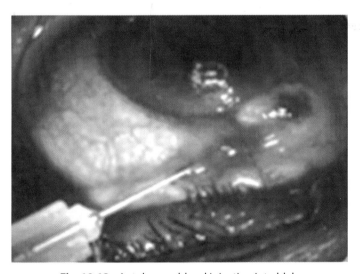

Fig. 19.13: Autologous blood injection into bleb.

Decompression Retinopathy

Due to sudden decompression of globe with drastic fall in IOP, there may be transient increase in retinal and choroidal blood flow resulting in retinal or subretinal hemorrhage. The clinical picture may resemble with that of central retinal vein occlusion (CRVO).

Hypotony Maculopathy

Overfiltration may result in hypotony with IOP being less than 6 mm. Severe hypotony may lead to disc edema, choroidal folds in macular area and increase in macular thickness. Patient may have fluctuating refraction. The risk factors include young age, male patient, use of antimetabolites like MMC, myopes, pigmentary glaucoma, and so on.

LATE POSTOPERATIVE COMPLICATIONS

Filtration failure is the most common late postoperative complication. It can be due to excessive wound healing response secondary to significant subconjunctival fibroblast proliferation.

One must pay attention to appearance of bleb. Presence of congestion and increased vascularization of the bleb may indicate early signs of late bleb failure. Causes of bleb failure are the following:

Blockage of Internal Ostium

Late blockage of internal ostium may be produced by fibrovascular membrane in neovascular glaucoma, fibrous tissue in fibrous ingrowth, epithelium in epithelial downgrowth or corneal endothelium and Descemet's membrane in iridocorneal endothelial syndrome.

Episcleral Fibrosis

Episcleral fibrosis is a major cause of failure of filtration surgery. In the initial postoperative period if aqueous flow is not established through the fistula either due to the tight scleral flap sutures or aqueous hyposecretion, the conjunctiva remains in contact with the episclera leading to subsequent vascularization, leucocytic infiltration, connective tissue proliferation and formation of granulation tissue.

Treatment

Bleb needling can be done either under slit lamp or operating microscope. A 27-gauge needle bent at 60° is introduced into subconjunctival space 5–10 mm distal to the scleral flap area with the bevel facing anteriorly. To and fro motions are made through the scar tissue formed between scleral flap and overlying conjunctiva. If this maneuver is not successful, attempts are made to cut scleral flap edge. Needle has to be advanced under the flap through the ostium into AC. Antimetabolites like MMC/5-FU can be injected away from the site of the bleb.

Encapsulated Bleb/Tenon Cyst (Fig.19.14)

Typically, it occurs during the first eight postoperative weeks. The appearance of bleb will be dome-shaped, vascularized and firm with overlapping conjunctiva being mobile. The IOP is raised.

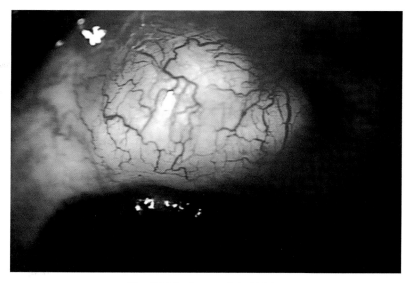

Fig. 19.14: Encapsulated bleb.

Risk factors include:
- Young age
- Prior ALT
- Prolonged use of topical antiglaucoma medications
- Tendency for keloid formation
- Secondary glaucoma, repeat filtering procedure etc.

Most of the cases may be managed conservatively using topical aqueous suppressants. The subsequent decrease in aqueous production allows for remodeling of cyst wall and eventually improves aqueous flow across it.

Treatment

- Topical aqueous suppressants
- Digital compression to elevate the bleb
- Needling of bleb
- Surgical revision

If final pressure is not low enough to permit preservation of visual field or if medical therapy is insufficient to control IOP elevation then surgical revision of bleb may be required. Sometime excision of tenon's cyst into to is required.

Cataract

There is increased risk for the formation of cataract. The causes may be intra-operative inadvertent trauma to the lens, postoperative hypotony, inflammation, and lens corneal touch.

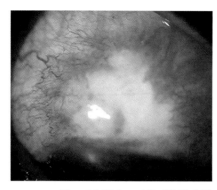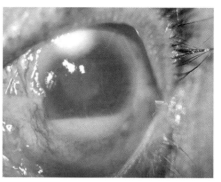

Figs. 19.15A and B: (A) Blebitis. (B) Bleb-related endophthalmitis.

Bleb-related Endophthalmitis

The incidence of bleb-related endophthalmitis has increased in recent years due to use of antifibrotic agents. The infection is due to migration of bacteria through the bleb wall. This is in contrast to early postoperative endophthalmitis, which is due to entry of organism into the eye at the time of surgery.

Endophthalmitis may have following stages:

Stage 1: Only limited to the bleb. A milky white injected bleb is seen (Fig.19.15A).

Stage 2: The injected bleb may be associated with anterior chamber involvement with presence of hypopyon (Fig. 19.15B).

Stage 3: Organism may spread to the vitreous causing a full blown endophthalmitis.

Streptococcus viridans and *Staphylococcus epidermidis* are frequently isolated.

Treatment

If infection is limited to the anterior segment, topical and periocular injection of antibiotics may suffice. Vitreous tap is indicated in presence of hypopyon or vitreous involvement. After 12–24 h following administration of antibiotics, topical steroids should be started to prevent scarring.

Overhanging Bleb (Fig.19.16)

Sometimes there may be migration of bleb over the cornea causing discomfort to the patient (bleb dysesthesia). It may also result in tear film abnormalities with secondary dellen formation, ocular surface abnormalities and irregular astigmatism. The corneal portion of the bleb can be easily excised. The conjunctival edge is then closed with 10-0 nylon.

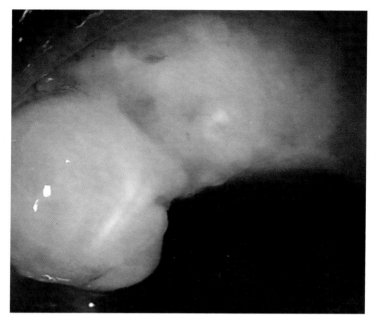

Fig. 19.16: Large cystic overhanging bleb.

Corneal Complications

- *Wind shield wiper keratopathy:* It occurs due to rubbing of suture end over the cornea with lid movements during blinking. This happens when the releasable suture is not trimmed or not removed after surgery.
- Corneal epithelial and endothelial toxicity can occur secondary to the use of antimetabolites like 5 FU and MMC.

NONPENETRATING GLAUCOMA SURGERIES

Trabeculectomy, the gold standard for filtering surgery, is associated with serious early and late postoperative complications. In order to overcome these complications and improve the safety of conventional filtering procedures, nonpenetrating glaucoma surgeries have been introduced. Nonpenetrating glaucoma surgeries evolved during the late 1950s and early 1960s by Epstein and Krasnov.

Principle

The main aim of nonpenetrating glaucoma surgeries is to facilitate the passage of aqueous humor through the trabeculum and Schlemm's canal, bypassing the juxtacanalicular meshwork, which is the site of highest resistance to aqueous outflow, without opening the anterior chamber and decompressing the eye. The aqueous passes through trabeculo-Descement's membrane creating subscleral lake without bleb formation.

Indications

- POAG
- Pseudoexfoliation glaucoma
- Pigmentary glaucoma
- Glaucoma in aphakia
- Uveitic glaucoma without extensive PAS
- Congenital glaucoma

Contraindications

- Angle closure glaucoma
- Neovascular glaucoma
- Posttraumatic angle recession glaucoma

Nonpenetrating glaucoma surgeries include:
- Deep sclerectomy
- Viscocanalostomy
- Viscocanaloplasty

Deep Sclerectomy

Fornix-based conjunctival flap is made. A 5 × 5 mm superficial scleral flap of one-third thickness is created (Fig. 19.17). Second deep scleral flap 4 × 4

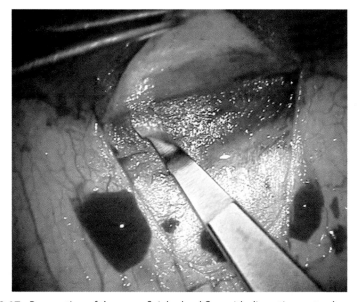

Fig. 19.17: Preparation of the superficial scleral flap with dissection upto clear cornea.

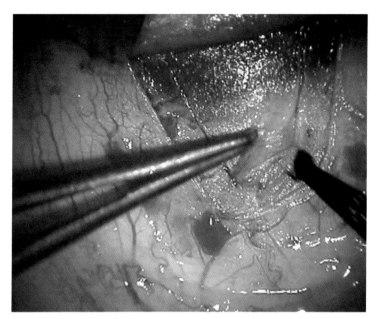

Fig. 19.18: Preparation of the deeper scleral flap using a mini crescent knife, note the smaller size of the deeper scleral flap.

mm is made beneath the superficial one (Fig. 19.18) with remaining sclera being as thin as 50–100 μm. Once anterior dissection is completed, the deep scleral flap is removed. The innerwall of Schlemm's canal and juxtacanalicular meshwork are then peeled off (Fig. 19.19). To avoid secondary collapse of the superficial flap, high-density viscoelastic material like Healon GV or a space maintainer implant (T-flux, Aquaflow, Sk gel, Esnoper clip) is placed in scleral bed (Figs. 19.20 and 19.21).

Viscocanalostomy

Viscocanalostomy was first introduced by Robert Stegman. He emphasized the importance of injecting high-viscosity sodium hyaluronate into Schlemm's canal thereby dilating Schlemm's canal and collector channels (Fig. 19.22). It causes focal disruption of inner wall endothelium of the canal and disorganization of juxtacanalicular zone resulting in direct communication of juxtacanalicular extracellular spaces with lumen of Schlemm's canal.

Viscocanaloplasty (Figs. 19.23 to 19.26)

A 250 μm flexible microcatheter with lighted beacon tip is passed through the canal 360° after injecting viscoelastic. A 9-0 or 10-0 polypropylene suture is introduced into the canal using microcatheter and suture is retrieved through the other end and tightened. It maintains inward radial force on TM and acts as a stent.

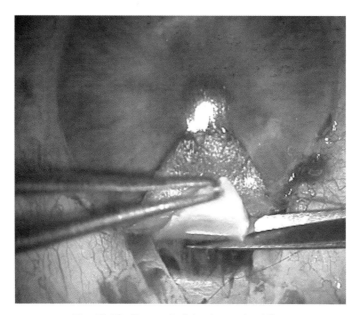

Fig. 19.19: Removal of the deep scleral flap.

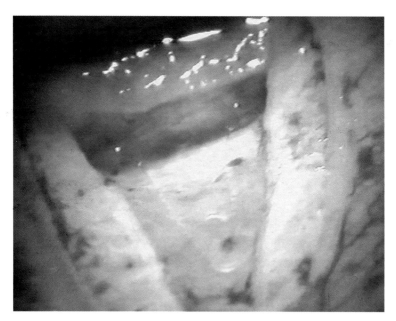

Fig. 19.20: T-Flux positioned in scleral bed, note both arms are implanted in the surgical ostia of Schlemm's canal.

Several studies have been done comparing trabeculectomy and nonpenetrating glaucoma surgeries. According to these studies, trabeculectomy seems to be most effective in IOP control though complication rates are higher compared to nonpenetrating glaucoma surgeries.[10]

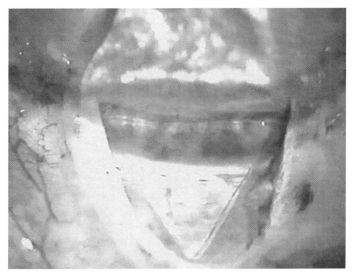

Fig. 19.21: SK-Gel in deep sclerectomy placed in the scleral bed.

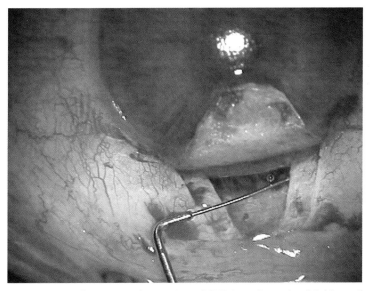

Fig. 19.22: Viscocanalostomy with injection of OVD into the ostia of Schlemm´s canal with a special canula.

GLAUCOMA DRAINAGE DEVICES (GDDS)

Glaucoma drainage devices act as an alternate channel for aqueous to drain from the anterior chamber into the subconjunctival space forming bleb. They are classified into three groups:

- Shunts
- Setons
- Valves

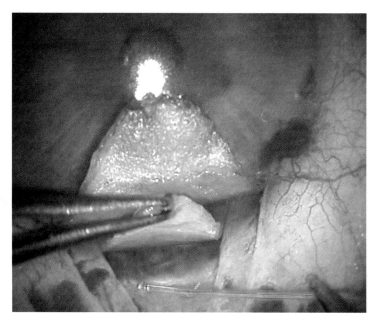

Fig. 19.23: Microcatheter before insertion into the Schlemm's canal.

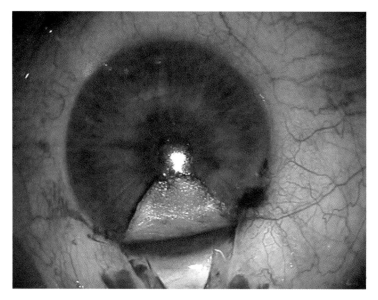

Fig. 19.24: Red spot indicating the position of the microcatheter at 5 o´clock position in the Schlemm's canal.

Mechanism of Action

GDDs usually consist of end plates made of either silicon or polypropylene which in turn is connected to with a tube made of silicon which is placed into the anterior chamber. A fibrous capsule is formed over the surface of

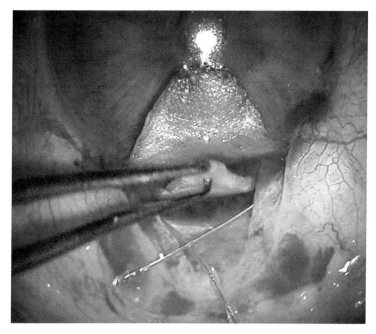

Fig. 19.25: After complete 360° cannulation of the Schlemm´s canal, 10x0 Prolene tensioning suture is fixed to the microcatheter.

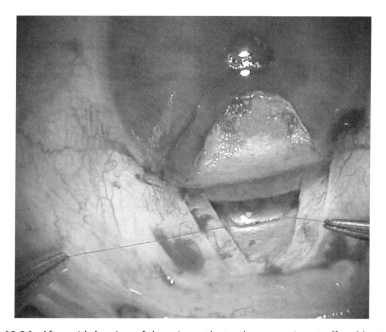

Fig. 19.26: After withdrawing of the microcatheter the suture is cut off and knotted under tension to pull the inner wall of Schlemm´s canal and the descemets window towards the anterior chamber to prevent failure of the surgery due to collapse of these structures.

the endplate. Aqueous drains from the anterior chamber and pools into the space between the plate and the surrounding fibrous capsule. The aqueous then diffuses passively through the capsule.

Indications

- Refractory glaucoma
- High risk of failure of trabeculectomy
- Neovascular glaucoma
- Iridocorneal endothelial syndrome
- Aniridia
- Posttraumatic glaucoma
- Glaucoma in aphakia
- Glaucoma in pseudophakia
- Uveitic glaucoma
- Glaucoma following penetrating keratoplasty and vitroretinal surgery
- Previously failed glaucoma surgery
- Eyes with scleral thinning
- Refractory pediatric glaucoma
- Severe conjunctival scarring as in cases of ocular surface disorders, multiple surgeries, chemical burns, Steven-Johnson's syndrome, cicatricial pemphigoid,
  Common types of glaucoma drainage devices are shown in Table 19.3.

Aurolab Aqueous Drainage Implant (Fig. 19.27)

Aurolab Aqueous Drainage Implant (AADI), prototype developed by Aurolab, Aravind Eye Care System, Madurai, India is a nonvalved aqueous shunt

Table 19.3: Common types of glaucoma drainage devices.

Type	Endplate material	Size	Valved/Nonvalved	Number of plates
Molteno	Silicon	134mm^2	Nonvalved	Single
		268mm^2		Double
Baerveldt's	Silicon	250mm^2	Nonvalved	
		350mm^2		
Krupin	Sialistic	183mm^2	Valved	
Ahmed	Polypropylene	184mm^2(S2)	Valved	Single
		364mm^2(B1)		Double
		96mm^2(S3)		Pediatric
	Silicon	184mm^2(FP7)		Single
		364mm^2(FX1)		Double
		96mm^2(FP8)		Pediatric
AADI	Silicon	350mm^2	Nonvalved	Single

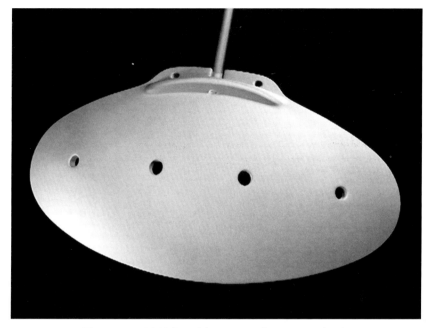

Fig. 19.27: AADI (Aurolab aqueous drainage implant).

made up of Nusil permanent implant silicone elastomer, which has passed tissue culture cytotoxicity testing. Its design is similar to the original Baerveldt glaucoma implant 350. It has a surface area of 350 mm² with plate and tube length of 32 mm and 35 mm respectively. The end plate is provided with four fenestrations.

Complications of Drainage Implant Surgery

- Hypotony
- Elevated IOP
- Tube migration/extrusion/erosion
- Endophthalmitis
- Corneal decompensation
- Tube malposition
- Cataract
- Diplopia

MINIMALLY INVASIVE GLAUCOMA SURGERY(MIGS)

Recently, newer implants and devices have been introduced to attain lower IOP with minimal surgical risk when compared to the previously established antiglaucoma surgeries such as trabeculectomy, nonpenetrating glaucoma surgery and glaucoma drainage devices.

MIGS has the following characteristics:
- *Ab interno* microincisional approach

- Minimally traumatic to the target tissue
- High safety profile
- Rapid recovery with minimal impact on the patient's quality of life
- Typically indicated for mild to moderate POAG
- Frequently combined with cataract surgery.
  MIGS can be classified as follows.
- *Trabecular meshwork based*
  - Glaukos iStent
  - Glaukos iStent inject
  - Ivantis Hydrus
  - GATT
  - Neomedix Trabectome
- *Suprachoroidal*
  - Cypass-Transcend
  - iStent Supra-Glaukos
  - *Subconjuctival*
  - XEN implant

CONCLUSION

The choice of surgery depends on the patient need, merits and demerits of surgery, cost factor and more than that the surgical skill and experience of the surgeon.

REFERENCES

1. Kronfeld PC. The rise of the filtering operations. Surv Ophthalmol. 1972;17(3):168-79.
2. Razeghinejad MR, Spaeth GL. A history of the surgical management of glaucoma. Optometry Vision Sci. 2011;88(1):E39-47.
3. Holth S. Iridencleisis antiglaucomatous. Ann Oculist. 1908;137: 345-6.
4. Elliot RH. A preliminary note on a new operative procedure for the establishment of a filtering cicatrix in the treatment of glaucoma. Ophthalmoscope. 1909;7:804.
5. Scheie HG. Retraction of scleral wound edges as a fistulizing procedure for glaucoma. Am J Ophthalmol. 1958;45:20-9.
6. Cairns JE. Trabeculectomy: preliminary report of a new method. Am J Ophthalmol. 1968;66(4):673-9.
7. Khaw PT, Dahlmann-Noor A, Mireskandari K. Trabeculectomy technique. Glaucoma Today. 2005:22-9.
8. Ramakrishnan R, Michon J, Robin AL, et al. Safety and efficacy of mitomycin C trabeculectomy in Southern India: a short-term pilot study. Ophthalmology. 1993;100(11):1619-23.

9. Robin AL, Ramakrishnan R, Krishnadas R, et al. A long-term dose-response study of mitomycin in glaucoma filtration surgery. Arch Ophthalmol. 1997;115(8): 969-74.
10. Rulli E, Biagioli E, Riva I, et al. Efficacy and safety of trabeculectomy vs non-penetrating surgical procedures: a systematic review and meta-analysis. JAMA Ophthalmol. 2013;131(12):1573-82.

20

Nonpenetrating Glaucoma Surgery

Shaarawy T, Mermoud A

INTRODUCTION

The first suggestion of a disease associated with a rise in intraocular pressure (IOP) and thus corresponding to what is now known as glaucoma seems to occur in the Arabian writings of Shams-ad-Deen of Cairo, the 13th-century Egyptian ophthalmologist, who described a 'headache of the pupil, an illness associated with pain in the eye, hemicrania and dullness of the humors, and followed by dilatation of the pupil and cataract; if it becomes chronic, tenseness of the eye and blindness supervened.' Ever since, the mainstay of glaucoma therapy remained a battle to lower IOP, medically or surgically. Trabeculectomy has been the gold standard of glaucoma surgery ever since Sugar and Cairns[1-3] suggested in 1961 a shift from the then widely practiced full thickness glaucoma filtering procedures. The use of a superficial flap was of paramount importance in creating a resistance to aqueous outflow, lowering the incidence of postoperative hypotony as well as offering a protection against the catastrophic occurrence of endophthalmitis. Throughout the years, evidence mounted, showing that trabeculectomy is perhaps not the holy grail of the quest for an ideal surgery for glaucoma. Most surgeons prefer to delay surgery because of the potential vision-threatening complications of classical trabeculectomy, with or without antimetabolites. Complications include hypotony, hyphema, flat anterior chamber, choroidal effusion or hemorrhage, surgery induced cataract, and bleb failure. In spite of the tendency to delay surgery, it remains a very effective way of lowering IOP. Some authors hypothesize that if the safety margin of glaucoma surgery could be increased significantly without sacrificing efficacy, surgical intervention for glaucoma might be considered earlier. Mikhail Leonidovich Krasnov,[4,5] of the former USSR, paved the ground for nonpenetrating filtering surgery, when he published his pioneer work on what he called sinusotomy. Several techniques have since evolved, probably the most popular of which are deep sclerectomy with collagen implant (DSCI)[6-15] and viscocanalostomy.[16-21]

Principles of Nonpenetrating Filtering Surgery

The main idea behind nonpenetrating filtering surgery is to somehow surgically enhance the natural aqueous outflow channels, rather than to create a new and possibly overly effective drainage site. The avoidance of penetration into the anterior chamber should allow the anterior segment to recover more quickly with less risk of hypotony and its sequelae. In primary and in most cases of secondary open-angle glaucoma, the main aqueous outflow resistance is thought to be located at the level of the juxtacanalicular trabeculum and the inner wall of Schlemm's canal. These two anatomic structures can be removed. This technique was first proposed by Zimmermann,[22,23] and he used the term *ab-externo trabeculectomy to describe it. Another way to increase the aqueous outflow in a patient with restricted posterior trabeculum outflow is to remove the corneal stroma behind the anterior trabeculum and Descemet's membrane. This has been called deep sclerectomy and was first described by Fyodorov*[24] *and Kozlov.*[25] After deep sclerectomy, the main aqueous outflow occurs at the level of the anterior trabeculum and Descemet's membrane. The so-called trabeculo-Descemet's membrane (TDM). In viscocanalostomy, described by Stegmann,[18] the aqueous filters through the TDM to the scleral space, as in deep sclerectomy, but it does not form a subconjunctival filtering bleb because the superficial scleral flap is tightly closed. From the scleral space, the aqueous reaches the Schlemm's canal ostia, which are surgically opened, and dilated with a viscoelastic substance.

SURGICAL TECHNIQUE OF NONPENETRATING GLAUCOMA SURGERY

Deep Sclerectomy

Three to four milliliters of a solution of bupivacaine 0.75 percent, xylocaine 4 percent and hyaluronidase 50 U are usually sufficient for a successful local anesthesia. Topical and subconjunctival anesthesia are also possible and have been performed successfully in selected cases. A superior rectus muscle traction suture is placed and the eyeball is rotated to expose the site of the DS (usually the superior quadrant). To avoid superior rectus muscle bleeding, a superior intracorneal suture may be placed, not too near to the limbus so that anterior dissection of DS is not harmed. The conjunctiva is opened either at the limbus or in the fornix. The limbal incision offers a better scleral exposition but needs a more careful closure, especially when antimetabolites are used.

The sclera is exposed and moderate hemostasis is performed. To facilitate the scleral dissection, all Tendon's capsule residue should be removed with a hockey stick. Sites with large aqueous drainage veins have to be avoided, to preserve as much as possible the aqueous humor physiological outflow pathways. A superficial scleral flap measuring 5 × 5 cm is dissected including one-third of the scleral thickness (about 300 μm). The initial incision is done with a No. 11 stainless steel blade. The horizontal dissection is done with a crescent ruby blade (Fig. 20.1). In order to later be able to dissect the corneal stroma down to Descemet's membrane, the scleral flap is dissected 1–1.5 mm into clear cornea. In patients with high risk of scleroconjunctival scar formation (young, secondary glaucoma, and blacks), a sponge soaked in mitomycin-C 0.02 percent may be placed for 45 s in the scleral bed and between the sclera and the Tenon's capsule. Deep sclero-keratectomy is done by performing a second deep scleral flap (4 × 4 mm) (Fig. 20.2). The two lateral and the posterior deep scleral incisions are made using a 15° diamond blade. The deep flap is smaller than the superficial one leaving a step of sclera on the three sides. This will allow a tighter closure of the superficial flap in case of an intraoperative perforation of the TDM. The deep scleral flap is then dissected horizontally using the ruby blade (Fig. 20.3). The remaining scleral layer should be as thin as possible (50–100 μm). Deep sclerectomy is preferably started first in the posterior part of the deep scleral flap. Reaching the anterior part of the dissection, Schlemm's canal is unroofed. Schlemm's canal is located anterior to the scleral spur where the scleral fibers are regularly oriented, parallel to the limbus. In patients with congenital glaucoma, Schlemm's canal localization is more difficult, because it is often more posteriorly situated. Schlemm's canal is opened and the sclerocorneal dissection is prolonged anteriorly for 1–1.5 mm in order to remove the sclerocorneal tissue behind the anterior trabeculum and Descemet's membrane. This step of the surgery is quite challenging because there is high risk of perforation

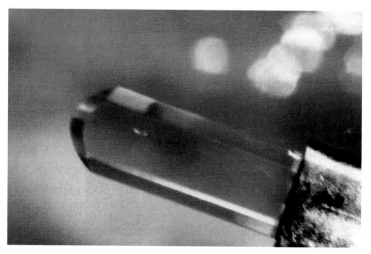

Fig. 20.1: Mermoud's ruby crescent knife.
Courtesy: HUCO, Switzerland

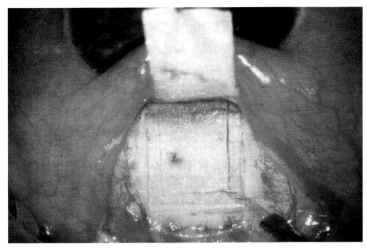

Fig. 20.2: Deep scleral flap incision with diamond knife.

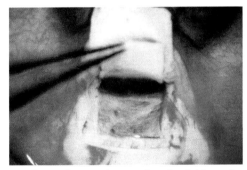

Fig. 20.3: Deep scleral flap is dissected, unroofing the Schlemm's canal and advanced anteriorly into corneal stroma detaching the Descemet's membrane.

of the anterior chamber. The best way to perform this last dissection is to do two radial corneal cuts without touching the anterior trabeculum or the Descemet's membrane. This is performed with the 15° diamond knife. When the anterior dissection between corneal stroma and Descemet's membrane is completed, the deep scleral flap is cut anteriorly using the diamond knife. At this stage, there should be a diffuse percolation of aqueous through the remaining TDM. The juxtacanalicular trabeculum and Schlemm's endothelium are then removed using small blunt forceps. The superficial scleral flap is then closed and secured with two loose 10/0 nylon sutures (Fig. 20.4). So, in fact, the procedure has evolved into combining deep sclerectomy and ab externo trabeculectomy.

Use of Implants

To avoid a secondary collapse of the superficial flap over the TDM and the remaining scleral layer, a collagen implant is placed in the scleral bed and

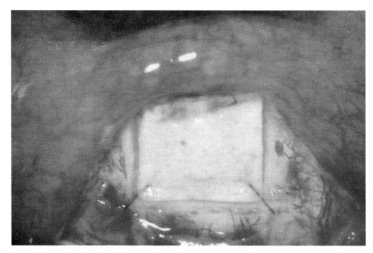

Fig. 20.4: Superficial scleral flap is loosely repositioned with two 10.0 nylon sutures.

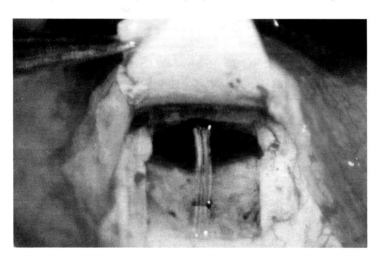

Fig. 20.5: Collagen implant is sutured into the thin scleral remnant.

secured with a single 10/0 nylon suture[25,26,27] (Fig. 20.5). The implant is processed from porcine scleral collagen. It increases in volume after contact with aqueous and is slowly resorbed within 6 to 9 months leaving a scleral space for aqueous filtration. Other implants may be used to fill the sclerocorneal space left after DS dissection; reticulated hyaluronic acid[28] implant resorbing in about 3 months or T-shaped hydrophilic acrylic implant, which is nonabsorbable. The role of implants in nonpenetrating surgery is still controversial, but the bulk of studies comparing deep sclerectomy with an implant versus without seems to show higher success rates with the use of an implant.

Viscocanalostomy

In the case of viscocanalostomy, high-viscosity hyaluronic acid is injected into the two surgically created ostia of Schlemm's canal, aiming at dilating both the ostia and the canal. It is also placed in the scleral bed. The material is resorbed in 4–5 days. The superficial scleral flap has to be tightly sutured in order to keep the viscoelastic substance in situ, and to force the aqueous percolating through the TDM into the two ostia.

Nd-YAG Laser Goniopuncture after Deep Sclerectomy

When filtration through TDM is considered to be insufficient because of elevated IOP, Nd:YAG goniopuncture can be done.[29] Using a gonioscopy contact lens, the aiming beam is focused on the semitransparent TDM. Using the free running Q-switched mode, with a power of 4–5 mJ, 2–15 shots are applied. This should result in the formation of microscopic holes through the TDM allowing a direct passage of aqueous from the anterior chamber to the subconjunctival space. The success rate of Nd:YAG laser goniopuncture is satisfactory, with an immediate reduction in IOP of about 50 percent. The success of goniopuncture depends mainly on the thickness of the TDM, hence the importance of sufficiently deep intraoperative dissection. By opening the TDM, however, goniopuncture transformed a nonperforating filtration procedure into a perforating one. Although the potential risk of late bleb-related endophthalmitis may be increased after goniopuncture, no such case was ever reported.

Mechanisms of Filtration after Nonpenetrating Surgeries for Glaucoma

There are two sites of interest when studying the mechanisms of function of nonpenetrating surgeries.
1. The aqueous humor flow through the trabeculo-Descemet's membrane.
2. The aqueous resorption after its passage through the trabeculo-Descemet's membrane.

Flow through the Trabeculo-Descemet's Membrane

The trabeculo-Descemet's membrane offers a resistance to aqueous outflow. This resistance will provide a slow decrease in IOP during surgery and will count for the reliable and reproducible IOP on the first postoperative day. Thus, the main advantage of the trabeculo-Descemet's membrane is to reduce the immediate postoperative complication such as hypotony, flat anterior chamber, choroidal detachments and induced cataract. In an experimental model, the gradual decrease in IOP was studied and the resistance of the trabeculo-Descemet's membrane calculated.[30] Experiments were performed on enucleated human eyes unsuitable for keratoplasty. The mean IOP decrease speed was 2.7 + 0.6 mm Hg/min. The trabeculo-Descemet's membrane resistance dropped from a mean of 5.34 + 0.19 ml/min/mm Hg to a mean of 0.41 + 0.16 ml/min/mm Hg. The trabeculo-Descemet's membrane resistance is apparently low enough to ensure a low IOP and high enough to maintain the anterior chamber depth and avoid the postoperative complications in relation to hypotony. In the same study, the authors histologically examined the surgical site using ocular perfusion with ferritin. They were able to demonstrate that the main outflow through the trabeculo-Descemet's membrane occurred at the level of the anterior trabeculum. There was, however, some degree of outflow through the posterior trabeculum and Descemet's membrane.

Aqueous Humor Resorption

After aqueous humor passage through the trabeculo-Descemet's membrane, four hypothetical mechanisms of aqueous resorption may occur:

1. *Subconjunctival bleb: As after trabeculectomy, patients undergoing non-*penetrating filtering surgeries have, in almost 100 percent of the cases, a diffuse, subconjunctival bleb in the first postoperative day. Years after the operation, using ultrasound biomicroscopy (UBM) assessment, all successful cases still showed a low profile and diffuse subconjunctival filtering bleb. This bleb is, however, usually smaller than the one seen after trabeculectomy.

2. *Intrascleral bleb: When the deep sclerectomy is performed, a certain volume of sclera is removed ranging between 5 and 8 mm³.* If the superficial scleral flap does not collapse, this scleral volume may be transformed into an intrascleral filtering bleb. In order to keep this intrascleral volume, different implants may be used such as the collagen implant. Hyaluronic acid or nonresorbable HEMA implants have also been used. Using the UBM method, an intrascleral bleb was observed in more than 90 percent of the cases. The mean volume of the intrascleral bleb was 1.8 mm³ (Kazakova et al., Ultrasound biomicroscopic study: long-term results after deep sclerectomy, unpublished data). In the intrascleral filtering bleb the aqueous resorption may be different than that occurring in the subconjunctival bleb. The aqueous is probably resorbed by new aqueous drainage vessels as demonstrated in the study of Delarive et al. (Delarivet T, Rossier A, Uffer S, Ravinet E, Mermoud A. Deep sclerectomy with collagen implant: an animal model, unpublished data). In this study performed on rabbits, Delarive et al. showed that in the scleral space created after the deep sclerectomy, regardless of the use of a collagen implant, new aqueous humor drainage vessels were growing and resorbing the aqueous flowing through the trabeculo-Descemet's membrane. Similar results were obtained by Nguyen and coworkers using the same model and performing anterior segment fluorescein and indocyanine green angiography (Nguyen C, Roy S, Shaarawy T, Boldea R, Mermoud A. Aqueous drainage veins formation after deep sclerectomy with and without collagen implant using fluorescein and indocyanine green anterior segment angiography, unpublished data).

3. *Subchoroidal space:* Since the remaining layer of sclera over the ciliary
    body and peripheral choroid after deep sclerectomy is very thin, there may
    be drainage of aqueous humor into the suprachoroidal space. *Using UBM,*
    it is possible to observe the fluid between the ciliary body and the remaining
    sclera in 45 percent of the patients studied years after the deep sclerectomy
    (Kazakova et al., unpublished data). Aqueous in the choroidal space may
    reach the uveoscleral outflow and increase this outflow pathway. It could
    also induce a chronic ciliary body detachment and reduce the aqueous
    production. Aqueous dynamics study in patients who underwent non-
    penetrating filtering surgery may be of interest to better understand the
    mechanism of action of this operation.

4. *Schlemm's canal:* When performing the deep sclerectomy dissection,
    Schlemm's canal is opened and unroofed. On either side of the deep
    sclerectomy the two ostia of Schlemm's canal may drain the aqueous
    humor into the episcleral veins. This mechanism may be more import-
    ant after viscocanalostomy since the Schlemm's canal is dilated with
    high-viscosity hyaluronic acid during the surgery. It may also play a role
    when a HEMA implant is used since this implant has two arms inserted
    into the two ostia of Schlemm's canal. More evidence is required to estab-
    lish the importance of this mechanism.

DO NONPENETRATING GLAUCOMA SURGERIES LOWER IOP?

In a prospective nonrandomized trial comparing 44 patients with medically
uncontrolled primary open-angle glaucoma who underwent deep sclerectomy
with collagen implant with a matched group of 44 patients who underwent trabeculectomy complete success rate, defined as an IOP lower than 21 mm Hg
without medication, was 69 per cent 24 months postoperatively in the deep
sclerectomy group versus 57 percent in the trabeculectomy group.[8] When considering the patients needing laser goniopuncture as failed cases, the complete
success rate of deep sclerectomy with collagen implant was 66 per cent at 24
months. In another nonrandomized prospective trial, 100 eyes of 100 consecutive patients with medically uncontrolled primary and secondary open-angle glaucoma underwent deep sclerectomy with collagen implant.[9] Complete
success rate, defined as an IOP lower than 21 mm Hg without medication, was
44.6 per cent at 36 months. Qualified success rate, defined as an IOP lower
than 21 mm Hg with and without medication, was 97.7 per cent at 36 months.
When comparing the different types of open-angle glaucoma, no difference
was found in terms of reduction in IOP, number of patients requiring anti-glaucoma medications, or success rate. There was, however, a tendency for lower
success rate in patients with pseudoexfoliative and pseudophakic glaucoma.
In a recent study, Shaarawy et al. reported that after five years, the mean IOP
of 105 patients who underwent deep sclerectomy with collagen implant was

11.8 mm Hg.[31] Complete success rate was 63 per cent and qualified success was 95.1 per cent. Other authors reported favorable results of nonpenetrating surgery. Zimmerman[22,23] reported good results of nonpenetrating trabeculectomy in phakic and aphakic patients. Stegmann[18] described a similar technique, in which the scleral space was filled with a viscoelastic substance, and reported complete success in 61 per cent of patients and qualified success in 77 per cent at 25 months follow-up. Performing deep sclerectomy with collagen implant, Kozlov[25] reported 85 per cent success rate, but no information regarding success criteria or follow-up is available. Demaily et al.[32] reported a mean decrease in IOP of $9.1 + 7.1$ mm Hg 219 cases after deep sclerectomy with collagen implant procedures. Using Kaplan-Meier survival analysis, they reported a success rate without glaucoma medication of 89 per cent at 6 months, and 75.6 per cent at 16 months; with glaucoma medication, their success rate increased to 97 per cent at 6 months, and 79 per cent at 16 months.

CONCLUSION

Nonpenetrating filtering surgeries performed by several investigators offer a significant drop in IOP and satisfactory success rate after several years of follow-up for all types of open-angle glaucoma. The immediate postoperative complication rates are low, and visual acuity is almost unaffected. This is mainly due to the presence of the TDM, which allows a progressive drop in IOP and offers enough resistance to prevent the immediate postoperative complications. When comparing trabeculectomy, the golden standard, with non-penetrating filtering surgery, the new corner, it is perhaps desirable to remember the words of Hiraclitus, uttered thousands of years ago: 'Nothing endures but change.'

REFERENCES

1. Cairns JE. Trabeculectomy: Preliminary report of a new method. Am J Ophthalmol. 1958;66(4):673-79.
2. Cairns JE. Trabeculectomy: asurgical method of reducing intraocular pressure in chronic simple glaucoma without subconjunctival drainage of aqueous humour. Trans Ophthalmol Soc UK. 1969;88:231-3.
3. Cairns JE. Trabeculectomy for chronic simple open-angle glaucoma. Trans Ophthalmol Soc UK.1970;89:481-90.
4. Krasnov MM. The technic of sinusotomy and its variants. Vestn Ophthalmol. 1968;81(3):3-9.
5. Krasnov MM. Externalization of Schlemm's canal (sinusotomy) in glaucoma. Br J Ophthalmol. 1968;(52):157-61.
6. Sanchez E. Deep sclerectomy: results with and without collagen implant. Int Ophthalmol. 1996;20(1-3):157-62.
7. Sanchez E, Schnyder CC, Mermoud A. Comparative results of deep sclerectomy transformed to trabeculectomy and classical trabeculectomy. Klin Monatsbl Augenheilkd. 1997;210(5):261-4.

8. Mermoud A. Comparison of deep sclerectomy with collagen implant and trabeculectomy in open-angle glaucoma. J Cataract Refract Surg. 1999;25(3): 323-31.

9. Karlen ME, Sanchez E, Schnyder CC, et al. Deep sclerectomy with collagen implant: medium term results. Br J Ophthalmol. 1999;83(1):6-11.

10. Mermoud A. Deep sclerectomy: surgical technique. J Fr Ophthalmol. 1999;22(7): 781-6.

11. Szaflik J et al. Deep sclerectomy ab externo with implant: description of surgery technique. Klin Oczna. 1999;101(4):261-6.

12. Bylsma S, Nonpenetrating deep sclerectomy: collagen implant and viscocanalostomy procedures. Int Ophthalmol Clin. 1999;39(3):103-9.

13. Dahan E, Drusedau MU. Nonpenetrating filtration surgery for glaucoma: control by surgery only. J Cataract Refract Surg. 2000;26(5):695-701.

14. El Sayyad F, Helal M, El-Kholify M, et al. Nonpenetrating deep sclerectomy versus trabeculectomy in bilateral primary open-angle glaucoma. Ophthalmology. 2000;107(9):1671-4.

15. Mermoud A. Sinusotomy and deep sclerectomy. Eye. 2000, 14(Pt3B) (2): 531-5.

16. Carassa RG, Bettin P, Fiori M, et al. Viscocanalostomy: a pilot study. Eur J Ophthalmol. 1998;8(2):57-61.

17. Carassa RG, Bettin P, Brancato R. Viscocanalostomy: apilot study. Acta Ophthalmol Scand Suppl. 1998;25(227):51-2.

18. Stegmann R, Pienaar A, Miller D. Viscocanalostomy for open-angle glaucoma in Black African patients. J Cataract Refract Surg. 1999;25(3):316-22.

19. Crandall AS. Nonpenetrating filtering procedures: viscocanalostomy and collagen wick. Semin Ophthalmol. 1999;14(3):189-95.

20. Drusedau MU, von Wholff K, Bull H, et al. Viscocanalostomy for primary open-angle glaucoma: the gross Pankow experience. J Cataract Refract Surg. 2000;26(9):1367-73.

21. Jonescu-Cuypers CP, Jacobi P, Konen W, et al. Primary viscocanalostomy versus trabeculectomy in white patients with open-angle glaucoma: arandomized clinical trial. Ophthalmology. 2001;108:254-8.

22. Zimmerman TJ et al. Trabeculectomy vs. nonpenetrating trabeculectomy: aretrospective study of two procedures in phakic patients with glaucoma. Ophthalmic Surg. 1984;15(9):734-40.

23. Zimmerman TJ, Kooner KS, Ford VJ, et al: Effectiveness of nonpenetrating trabeculectomy in aphakic patients with glaucoma. Ophthalmic Surg. 1984;15(1): 44-50.

24. Fedorov SN, Lofee DI, Ronkina TI. Glaucoma surgery—deep sclerectomy. Vestn Ophthalmol. 1982;(4):6-10.

25. Kozlov V et al. Non-penetrating deep sclerectomy with collagen. Eye Microsurgery (in Russian).1990;3:157-62.

26. Mermoud A, Schnyder CC, Sikenberg M, et al. Comparison of deep sclerectomy with collagen implant and trabeculectomy in open-angle glaucoma (see comments). J Cataract Refract Surg. 1999;25(3):323-31.

27. Sourdille P, Santiago PY, Villain F, et al. Reticulated hyaluronic acid implant in non-perforating trabecular surgery (see comments). J Cataract Refract Surg. 1999;25(3):332-9.

28. Mermoud A, Karlen ME, Schnyder CC,et al. Nd:YAG Goniopuncture after deep sclerectomy with collagen implant. Ophthalmic Surg Lasers. 1999;30(2):120-5.
29. Rossier A, Uffer S, Mermoud A. Aqueous dynamics in experimental ab externo trabeculectomy. Ophthalmic Res. 2000;32(4):165-71.
30. Shaarawy T, Mansouri, K, Schnyder C, et al. Long-term results of deep sclerectomy with collagen implant. J Cataract Refract Surg. 2004;30(6):1225-31.
31. Demailly P, Jeanteur-Lunel MN, Berkani M, et al. Non-penetrating deep sclerectomy combined with a collagen implant in primary open-angle glaucoma. Medium-term retrospective results. J Fr Ophthalmol. 1996;19(11): 659-6.

21

Management of Coexistent Cataract and Glaucoma

Bhartiya S, Bhagat PR, Deshpande KV, Albis-Donado O

INTRODUCTION

Cataract and glaucoma are often found to coexist since both affect the elderly. The incidence of angle-closure glaucoma, open-angle glaucoma and cataract increases with age.[1,2] The presence of cataract can confound the evaluation of glaucoma, and glaucoma can impact the visual results of cataract surgery. It is therefore essential to have a treatment plan for these patients, especially since clear-cut guidelines are not available for this subgroup of patients.

The therapeutic approach for each patient thus will need to be individualized, keeping in mind the following important points.

Coexistence may be primary or it may be secondary to each other as in phacomorphic glaucoma, phacolytic glaucoma, cataract after glaucoma surgery, antiglaucoma drug-induced cataract or iatrogenic. They may even coexist in other conditions like pseudoexfoliation syndrome, ectopia lentis syndromes, congenital anomalies, chronic steroid use, following trauma or inflammation.[3]

The presence of a cataract can affect the ability to detect glaucoma (Figs. 21.1A and B), while cataract surgery can affect both intraocular pressure (IOP) control and the effectiveness of a previously performed glaucoma surgery. On the other hand, a trabeculectomy accelerates cataractogenesis (Fig. 21.2).

Although guidelines exist for the indications for cataract surgery in the otherwise healthy eye and for glaucoma surgery in eyes with glaucoma, there is controversy regarding the management when both conditions coexist in a single patient. The aim of managing these two conditions is to avoid postoperative spikes in IOP, long-term control of IOP and to achieve visual rehabilitation.

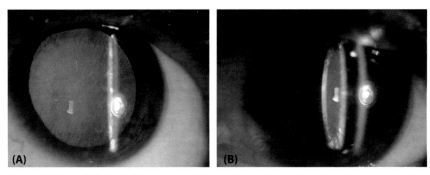

Figs. 21.1A and B: Anterior and posterior subcapsular cataract causing glare, halos, reduced best-corrected visual acuity, diffuse generalized sensitivity loss in the visual field and difficulty in performing imaging.

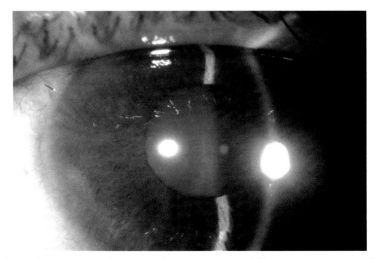

Fig. 21.2: Cataract appearing 1 month after a successful filtering surgery that will now need additional surgical management.

The idea of combining surgery is an old one but several gray zones exist regarding the timing, technique and choice of procedure. With developments in phacoemulsification, refinements in trabeculectomy and introduction of nonpenetrating surgeries plus minimally invasive glaucoma surgery (MIGS), combined surgery is emerging as the favored trend.

The risks and benefits of staged and combined surgery, short and long-term effects on IOP, use of antimetabolites, type of antiglaucoma surgery, and postoperative management are some of the concerns which shall be addressed in this chapter.

IMPACT OF CATARACT ON GLAUCOMA EVALUATION

- Intumescent cataract causes shallowing of the anterior chamber mimicking primary-angle closure disease.[4]

- Cataract prevents proper visualization of the optic nerve head.[4]
- It worsens the mean deviation/defect across all tests including standard automated perimetry, frequency doubling perimetry and short wavelength perimetry. It affects the glaucoma progression indices as well. It also produces artifacts in visual fields (VF). Development of cataract in a glaucoma patient resulting in generalized reduction of sensitivity may sometimes be mistaken as progression, urging the ophthalmologist to step up glaucoma therapy and hence interpretation of VF should always be done considering the severity of glaucoma as well as the type and location of the lenticular opacity.[4,5]
- Optical coherence tomography (OCT) may show false underestimation of the retinal nerve fiber layer (RNFL) due to cataract.[6]
- Even scanning laser polarimetry (SLP) may give erroneous results primarily due to reduced signal-to-noise ratio. SLP measurements tend to change significantly after cataract surgery especially in posterior subcapsular cataracts.[7]
- In pseudophakics, the type of intraocular lens implanted and IOL glistening can also affect RNFL measurement.[8]
- Posterior capsular opacification, contrary to cataract, causes overestimation of RNFL thickness.[9]
- More advanced cataract would mean that the patient would be unable to perform VF, making both diagnosis and monitoring more difficult. In case of increased media haze, optic nerve visualization and even RNFL imaging may not possible due to poor visibility.
- In case of angle closure disease with significant cataract, a laser peripheral iridotomy may be avoided, and the cataract removal maybe planned in order to eliminate pupillary block.
- Hence it is suggested that a new baseline be established after cataract surgery to assess the RNFL thinning and visual field defects.

IMPACT OF GLAUCOMA ON CATARACT

- Elevated IOP increases risk of nuclear cataract.
- Miotics like pilocarpine would be contraindicated in patients with posterior subcapsular cataracts, since they would result in a significant drop in vision. Miotics have also been implicated in hastening of cataractogenesis.
- Trabeculectomy can result in formation of cataract with a higher risk in eyes, which have a postoperative shallow anterior chamber and/or persistent inflammatory reaction (Fig. 21.2).
- Glaucoma also impacts the visual prognosis of cataract surgery and necessitates several modifications of cataract surgery technique.
- Patients of glaucoma per se, and especially those after trabeculectomy, have a significantly reduced endothelial count.

- Mutifocal IOLs should be avoided in patients with moderate to severe glaucoma.

CATARACT AND IOP: IMPACT OF CATARACT SURGERY ON IOP

Mechanisms of IOP reduction are different in open and closed angle glaucomas.

Cataract Surgery in Angle Closure Glaucoma (ACG)

- Outflow obstruction is a macroscopic problem in ACG typically precipitated by mechanical blockage at the pupil or the angle.
- Removal of the lens relieves the risk of pupillary block and posterior forces crowding the angle.
- Width and depth of the anterior chamber angle expand significantly following cataract extraction and IOL implantation, making the anatomy of the ACG eye appear almost similar to those without it.[10]
- Cataract surgery can remove any preexisting pupillary block, obviating the need for laser iridotomy in angle closure and mixed mechanism glaucomas. It can also open the angle in nonpupillary block mechanisms of angle closure such as iris plateau.
- Cataract surgery is also known to result in a long-term, significant decrease in IOP. This better IOP control means several patients may be off glaucoma medications, or may at least have a decrease in the number of drops, depending on disease severity. Glaucoma surgery may even be deferred in certain patients due to better eye pressure control.

Cataract Surgery in Primary Open Angle Glaucoma (POAG)

The main site of resistance in POAG is the juxtacanalicular trabecular meshwork. Some mechanisms postulated are the following:
- Higher fluid flow rates reducing glycosaminogly can deposition in the trabecular meshwork[11]
- Inflammation-induced changes in the trabecular meshwork similar to the effects of trabeculoplasty[12]
- Alterations in the blood–aqueous barrier[13]
- Increased posterior zonular traction due to cataract surgery has been postulated to improve patency of the trabecular meshwork and result in lower IOP changes in anterior chamber architecture are thus important in reducing IOP in POAG as well.[14]

It has also been shown that the ultrasonic energy of phacoemulsification results in the secretion of certain proteins that can modulate the trabecular cells and lead to a stress-responsive IOP lowering.[15]

In eyes that have undergone filtration surgery, subsequent cataract surgery is known to have an adverse effect on the bleb, even though the area of bleb may have been untouched.[1] This may require subsequent modification of glaucoma therapy. It is important to always avoid the site of the bleb, and perform phacoemulsification through a temporal clear corneal incision.

PREOPERATIVE EVALUATION[17]

- Information about the number of antiglaucoma medications being used by the patient will help to decide the type of surgical option best suited for the patient.
- Conjunctiva should be assessed to select the site for filtering surgery.
- Anterior chamber (AC) depth: Rule out microphthalmos, relative anterior microphthalmos and nanophthalmos. Shallow AC may necessitate use of highly retentive viscoelastics. Relative anterior microphthalmos may further be associated with pseudoexfoliation, guttate changes and poorly dilating pupils. Cilio-lenticular block is common postoperatively in these cases. IOL power calculation should be done in these short eyes using specific formulae (e.g., Haigis, Holladay II).
- Adequacy of pupillary dilatation: Patients on miotic therapy and those with posterior synechiae dilate poorly. The need for pupil expanders should be kept in mind.
- Type, size and location of lens opacities as in any cataract case: It also helps to identify field defects mimicking glaucoma.
- Pseudoexfoliation (PXF): Presence of typical powder-like pseudoexfoliative material on the pupil edge, endothelium and lens capsule aids in the diagnosis. Examination of the eye after dilation is mandatory, as sometimes PXF can be missed in the undilated state. It is often associated with poor corneal endothelium, rigid nondilating pupil, zonular instability and postoperative capsular contractures. In view of the pupillary and zonular status, early cataract surgery maybe recommended.
- Assessment of zonular integrity with dilated pupils: Weakness of zonules may warrant the use of capsular rings/segments and special IOLs.
- IOP: Target IOP and diurnal variation using the Goldmann applanation tonometer.
- Gonioscopy: It is mandatory preoperatively especially to identify the presence and site of synechiae to plan the incision sites. Large areas of synechiae also suggest that cataract surgery alone would not help to significantly lower the IOP.
- Compression gonioscopy: It will indicate if the lens is a confounding factor for the narrow angle configuration.
- When planning angular surgery such as ab-internal trabeculotomy with the Kahook dualblade (KDB, New World Medical, CA) or the iStent (Glaukos Corporation), it is very important to identify the nasal trabecular

meshwork (Fig. 21.3) with indentation gonioscopy because the presence of synechiae or an impossibility to open the angle preoperatively may hallmark a difficult or impossible angle surgery.

- Dilated stereoscopic optic nerve assessment with +78D/+90D lens: It is also mandatory. If optic nerve photographs have been previously taken, a careful comparison can be made. A pale disk may appear pink due to nuclear sclerosis, so attention should be paid to the contour to determine the extent of cupping rather than color.
- Imaging of the RNFL: Poor quality images and false low RNFL thickness values in presence of cataract limit their use preoperatively.
- Anterior segment imaging for angle and lens status: The lens vault can be measured using Scheimpflug topography (Fig. 21.4) as well as ultrasound biomicroscopy and a phacomorphic component of angle closure can be documented.

Visual Fields Analysis

- Standard threshold perimetry preoperatively helps in preventing postoperative surprises due to extensive glaucomatous disk damage.
- It is also an important tool to counsel the patient regarding the prognosis.
- The total deviation probability plot crudely correlates to the extent of cataract and the pattern deviation plot to the extent of glaucoma damage, except in very advanced glaucoma.
- Presence of split fixation in macular programs may necessitate appropriate counseling and consent due to the risk of Snuff-out effect/Washout phenomenon.[18]
- Specular microscopy for all glaucoma cases, in particular those with shallow anterior chamber or visible corneal guttae.

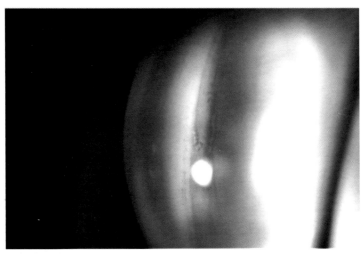

Fig. 21.3: Location of a nasal iStent in a right eye after combined phaco-iStent procedure.

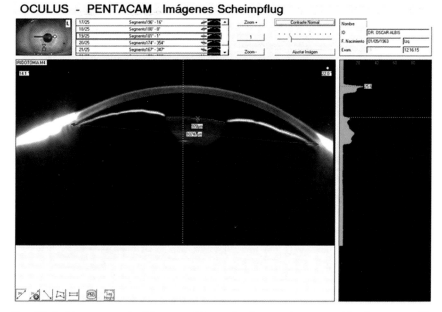

Fig. 21.4: Measurement of lens vault in angle closure phacomorphic glaucoma with Scheimpflug imaging: a line is traced between the nasal and temporal scleral spur using the image at 180°, and the distance from that line to the most prominent part of the anterior capsule is measured. Values above 600 μm are compatible with a significant phacomorphic mechanism[28].

- B-scan ultrasonography to document optic nerve head cupping in cases of dense cataracts. Such cataracts when present in an eye with elevated IOP or more than two antiglaucoma medications warrant a combined procedure.
- The potential acuity meter (PAM) to indicate macular potential in cases of dense cataracts.
- Syndromes associated with ectopia lentis and glaucoma (homocystinuria, Marfan's), microspherophakia (Weill-Marchesani), congenital anomalies (iridocorneal dysgenesis syndromes), and so on, should be looked for.
- General medical history.
- Preoperative counselling for prognosis and need for long-term follow-up.
- Inquire also about access to healthcare, compliance to treatment and follow-up, socioeconomic status.

OPTIONS OF MANAGEMENT

No strict guidelines regarding preferred procedure exist. Patient and surgeon preferences have to be considered among several other factors.

The various surgical options include the following:
- Cataract surgery only
- Simultaneous cataract and glaucoma surgery

- Filtering surgery followed by cataract surgery
- Laser trabeculoplasty followed by cataract surgery
- Cataract surgery followed by filtering surgery
- Combination of newer antiglaucoma surgeries and cataract surgery

SEQUENCE OF SURGERY

In case the patient has advanced cataract with early glaucoma, the cataract should be tackled first. In case of advanced glaucoma with early cataract, the former should be managed first. In case where both diseases are significant, most specialists prefer to do cataract surgery first, and then assess the need for subsequent glaucoma surgery. A combined procedure may also be planned for this subgroup of patients. It is important to remember that a combined surgery has a higher incidence of failure and is less efficacious than sequential surgery. Two-site surgery is probably better than single site surgery in terms of IOP control. On the other hand, an additional goal to try to reduce glaucoma medication dependence might justify the use of one of the newer MIGS, such as an iStent or KDB trabeculotomy, if affordable.

Broad guidelines are enumerated in Tables 21.1 to 21.3.

Table 21.1: Sequence of surgery in case of coexistent cataract and glaucoma.

Cataract first	Significant cataract in patients with:
	Early glaucoma
	Ocular hypertension
	Medically controlled glaucoma
	Media haze precluding evaluation of glaucoma
	Early cataract in patients with:
	Pupillary block and/or angle closure
Trabeculectomy first	Advanced glaucoma
	IOP not controlled on maximal medical therapy
	Poor prognosis for trabeculectomy
	Pseudoexfoliation or a subluxated lens with anticipated vitreous loss
Combined surgery	Patients with early-moderate glaucoma, and significant cataract and:
	IOP not controlled on maximal medical therapy
	Patients with persistent angle closure and elevated IOP with advanced glaucomatous damage and despite patent iridotomy
	Noncompliant patient, despite counseling
	Economic reasons: patient can't afford two surgeries, or cannot come back for surgery/subsequent checkups

Table 21.2: Advantages and disadvantages of combined cataract and trabeculectomy.

Advantages	Disadvantages
Faster visual rehabilitation	Longer surgical time
Single procedure, more cost-effective in terms of direct and indirect costs	Increased intraoperative and postoperative complications
Better short- and long-term intraocular pressure control	Intensive postoperative care needed unlike for simple cataract surgery

Table 21.3: Single site versus two-site combined procedure.

Single-site combined surgery	Two sites surgery
Relatively simpler, and faster	More time-consuming
Manipulation of filtering site during cataract surgery	Minimal manipulation of conjunctiva and scleral flap
Requires longer time for skill transfer	Easier when combined with temporal phacoemulsification
Potentially higher chances of postoperative astigmatism	Lesser incidence of post-operative astigmatism

GENERAL PRINCIPLES: PRE- AND PERIOPERATIVE MODIFICATIONS

- Always operate with the IOP as low as possible using as many antiglaucoma medications as needed. Surgery in an eye with uncontrolled pressures can be disastrous.
- Stop prostaglandin analogs and miotics 1–4 weeks prior to surgery, shift to oral acetazolamide if necessary.
- Preoperative soft steroids or nonsteroidal anti-inflammatory drugs (NSAIDs) may be started if the ocular surface appears inflamed.
- Perform biometry cautiously as extremes of IOP may influence the readings leading to postoperative refractive surprises.[19] Immersion ultrasound is the most accurate.[20]
- Any anesthesia according to patient's convenience and surgeon's preference may be used.
- Avoid large volumes of local anesthesia and local massage as this may jeopardize the optic nerve health further.
- Consider topical anesthesia plus sedation in cases of advanced glaucoma to reduce the risk of snuff-out due to large volumes of retrobulbar or peribulbar agents.
- Expect poor pupillary dilation, use hooks or rings when necessary.

- Expect a poor endothelial count, use a dispersive viscoelastic, a soft-shell technique also helps. Meticulously remove any viscoelastic at the end of surgery.
- Chilled BSS plus with glutathione may be used.
- Perform cataract surgery in a closed chamber as far as possible and keep the phacodynamics low.
- Anticipate increased postoperative inflammation and IOP spikes.
- Consider increased incidence of steroid responsiveness.

Cataract Surgery Only

Indications

- Tolerating topical medication well
- Well controlled on low dose/single drug
- Minimal optic nerve damage
- Lens-induced glaucomas, e.g., phacomorphic glaucoma, spherophakia
- Ocular hypertension
- Typical candidate is an elderly patient with narrow angles

Surgical Pearls

- Clear corneal temporal phacoemulsification is the preferred procedure. Extracapsular extraction and superior scleral tunnels are avoided to preserve superior conjunctiva.
- Adequate control of IOP in the perioperative period is essential so that postoperative spikes occurring due to inflammation/retained viscoelastic/steroid response do not accelerate optic nerve damage.
- Poor pupillary dilatation:
  - Special devices such as iris hooks/rings may be needed. Use of pupil expanders may lead to pigment dispersion, additional incisions and more inflammation, which can have an effect on the postoperative IOP.
  - Mechanical dilatation by hooks or sphincterotomies causes loss of sphincter tone resulting in floppy iris and predisposing to synechiae-formation.
  - Viscodilatation by a highly cohesive viscoelastic may be effective after posterior synechiae are broken.
  - It may be advisable to stop Pilocarpine drops one week preoperatively as its continued use may prevent mydriasis and may also exacerbate or prolong inflammation.
- Role of viscoelastic devices:
  - Cohesive: Space maintaining properties help to deepen shallow anterior chambers, viscomydriasis cleaves adhesions.
  - Dispersive: Coat the endothelium, sequester areas of zonular dialysis and prevent vitreous prolapse.
  - Viscoadaptive: Combine cohesive and dispersive properties. (2.3% sodium hyaluronate)

- PXF: Complication rates in PXF are 5–10 times more than in normal eyes.[19] The aspects of concern are PXF keratopathy, poor endothelial count, nondilating pupil, zonular instability, more IOP fluctuations and rapid glaucoma progression. Capsular phimosis and contractures are more common; hence silicone lenses are not recommended. Acrylic IOLs open slowly in the bag and minimize zonular stress. Adequate haptic to haptic distance and capsular tension rings prevent IOL decentration in cases of compromised zonules. Pseudophakodonesis may occur as a late-stage complication. Insufficient capsular support or severe generalized zonular weakness may need iris supported or scleral fixated IOLs. Angle supported lenses are to be avoided.
- Shallow anterior chambers in angle closure or narrow angle patients are also a problem for surgery and frequently predispose to many of the same complications as in PXF eyes. Remember that the two conditions may coexist, so one should plan accordingly.
- Viscoelastic wash should be thorough.
- Special situations like nanophthalmosare associated with serious retinal detachment and choroidal detachment. Dissection of partial thickness scleral windows near vortex veins helps in preventing development of such effusions.
- All due measures should be taken to prevent/delay posterior capsular opacification and incidence of Nd:YAG capsulotomy (and associated IOP spike >5 mm Hg).
- Goniosynechiolysis can be attempted carefully in cases of synechial angle closure.

Advantages

- Easiest and fastest to perform with lesser perioperative complications compared to other surgical options.
- Rapid recovery.
- It is possible to manage astigmatism in a more reliable way using toric IOLs, and for mild glaucoma or narrow angle eyes multifocal or extended-range IOLs might be considered.
- IOP reduction may reduce the future need of glaucoma surgery and medications.
- Aids proper postoperative evaluation of the optic nerve.
- Imaging becomes more reliable.
- Conjunctiva and superior sclerocorneal junction remain undisturbed in temporal phaco, should the need for subsequent trabeculectomy arise.

Disadvantages

- Early postoperative IOP spikes common.
- Prostaglandin analogs might need to be stopped, at least temporarily, during the early postoperative period due to increased inflammation

from complicated procedures, which might be exacerbated by the medication.
- Need for antiglaucoma surgery in the future cannot be excluded.
- Long-term effects on IOP show less reduction than combined procedure hence monitoring needs to be more frequent.
- Surgical complications of cataract like damage to trabecular meshwork, iris manipulation and pigment dispersion, posterior capsular rupture and vitreous disturbance reduce the chances of success of future trabeculectomy.
- Does not overcome diurnal variations of IOP.

Simultaneous Cataract and Glaucoma Surgery

Indications

- Moderate glaucomatous damage and poor control in spite of multiple medications.
- Advanced glaucoma that is poorly controlled with three or four topical medications along with significant cataract.
- Poor compliance/noncompliance.
- Inability to follow-up frequently.
- Intolerance to medications.
- Nonaffordability.
- If lens instability is encountered before surgery, a temporal corneal incision might be used to perform a lens extraction, so the filtering surgery can be performed superiorly (Fig. 21.5).
- If lens instability is found during surgery and phacoemulsification cannot be performed in an eye with elevated IOP, one should consider the implantation of an Ahmed valve (Fig. 21.6) in another quadrant, since the sclera, conjunctiva and cornea might be so manipulated as to preclude a trabeculectomy or nonpenetrating deep sclerectomy (NPDS).
- Special situations where separate/staged surgeries cannot be performed e.g., high-risk anesthesia, multiple health issues, and difficulties in returning to control visits.
- Presence of other risk factors like PXF, angle recession and monocular status.[20]

Surgical Pearls

One site Surgery

Option 1

- Fornix-based (for better visualization) superior conjunctival flap.
- Mitomycin C or 5-fluorouracil generally used as chances of bleb fibrosis are more.
- Mitomycin C in a dose of 0.2–0.4 mg/ml applied for about 2 min followed by a thorough wash.

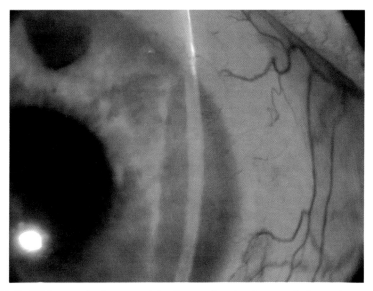

Fig. 21.5: Mild corneal edema persists after performing temporal phaco plus superior trabeculectomy with MMC, IOP is 7 mm Hg.

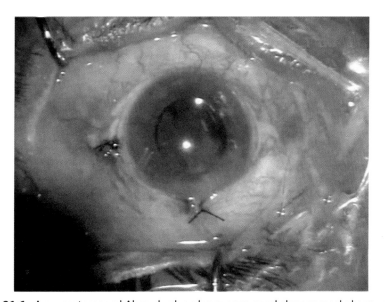

Fig. 21.6: A superotemporal Ahmed valve plus supero-nasal clear corneal phaco were performed simultaneously in a patient with zonular weakness due to pseudoexfoliation glaucoma.

- Scleral tunnel at 12 o'clock position.
- Phaco with IOL implantation through the scleral tunnel.
- Scleral tunnel converted to partial thickness scleral flap.
- Trabeculectomy performed.
- Peripheral iridectomy done.
- Scleral flap closed with 10-0 nylon.

- Meticulous conjunctival closure.
- If over filtering is suspected, viscoelastic might be left in the anterior chamber.

Option 2

- The scleral tunnel is not converted into a flap, but the floor of the tunnel is cut using Kelly's Descemet punch to form a trabeculectomy window.
- Tunnel may or may not be sutured.
- Conjunctiva is sutured.

Two-site Surgery

- Fornix-based superior conjunctival flap.
- Regular scleral flap prepared and left.
- Routine phacoemulsification with IOL implantation performed through temporal clear corneal incision.
- Trabeculectomy, iridectomy and wound suturing completed superiorly.
- Alternatively, a nonpenetrating deep sclerectomy (NPDS) can be performed (Fig. 21.7).

Advantages

- Prevents postoperative IOP elevations which can be detrimental in cases of advanced glaucoma.
- Elimination of need for glaucoma medications.

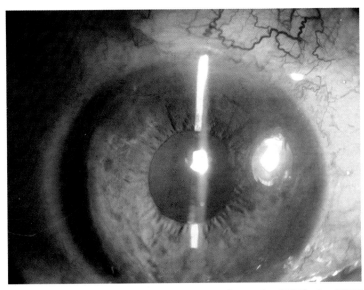

Fig. 21.7: One month of combined clear-cornea phaco plus NPDS plus MMC in the superior quadrant.

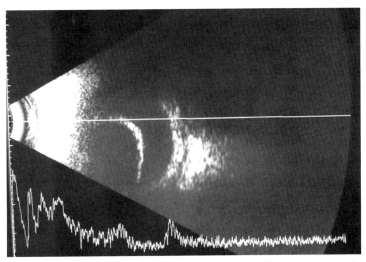

Fig. 21.8: Choroidal detachment in a patient with an overfiltering phaco-trabeculectomy. Medical management solved the issue in 2 weeks.

- Reduces overall long-term cost.
- Additional advantages of a two-site surgery: less manipulation of sclera and conjunctiva, less risk of excessive coagulation which can cause significant tissue shrinking leading to greater, unpredictable astigmatism and difficult closure, less risk of antimetabolite entering into the anterior chamber and postoperative suture modification will not affect the cataract incision.

Disadvantages

Complications: They are more common in combined surgery as compared to trabeculectomy or cataract surgery alone and mainly arise as the two procedures have contrasting end points; trabeculectomy requires the inner ostium to be patent with aqueous leaking subconjunctivally. Cataract surgery on the other hand requires all incisions to seal in a water-tight manner.

The common complications are:

- Hypotony, choroidal detachment (Fig. 21.8)
- Suprachoroidal hemorrhage
- Hyphema
- Infection
- Bleb-related complications: Failure, thin walled bleb, cystic bleb, bleb migration onto cornea (Fig. 21.9)
- Uveitis
- Maculopathy secondary to hypotony
- Blebitis, endophthalmitis (more common with use of antimetabolites)
- Unpredictable refractive outcomes.

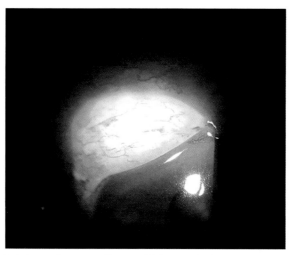

Fig. 21.9: A slightly overhanging filtering bleb in a phakic eye that had uncontrolled glaucoma and no visually significant cataract.

The procedure takes longer surgical time and requires more intensive postoperative care.

Filtering Surgery Followed by Cataract Surgery

Indications

- Need for very low target IOP.
- Advanced glaucomatous optic neuropathy—unlikely to tolerate postoperative IOP spikes.
- Very high IOP not controlled medically.
- High risk cases with poor prognosis, e.g., uveitic or neovascular glaucomas, scarred ocular surface, etc.
- Mild visually insignificant cataract with any of the above.
- Corneal edema due to elevated IOP precluding a safe visualization for cataract surgery.
- IOP reduction after trabeculectomy is rapid, sustained and greater as compared to phacotrabeculectomy.[21]
- In uncontrolled glaucoma, it is preferable to reduce the IOP by filtering surgery first, then plan cataract surgery after 4–6 months. This allows the IOP to stabilize.
- Keratometry, anterior chamber depth, and lens position are altered as a result of trabeculectomy. So fresh biometry is essential before cataract surgery.
- During cataract surgery in presence of a preexisting bleb:
  - Care should be taken not to inadvertently damage the bleb during peribulbar anesthesia.
  - Massage should be avoided because IOP may reduce significantly and result in hypotony.

- Temporal clear corneal phacoemulsification is preferred to avoid disturbing the superior bleb.
- A subconjunctival injection of antimetabolite 5-FU (5 mg/0.1 ml) may be given away from the bleb, taking care that it does not enter the anterior chamber, or escape over the corneal epithelium to avoid inflammation, corneal toxicity and fibrosis-related bleb failure.
- Needling of the bleb can be performed if bleb function is poor.
- The inner ostium of the trabeculectomy site can be opened if needed using a needle from across the anterior chamber or subconjunctivally.

Laser Trabeculoplasty Followed by Cataract Surgery

- Argon laser trabeculoplasty (ALT) or selective laser trabeculoplasty (SLT) can precede cataract surgery by minimum one month.

ALT
- Argon laser 488 or 514.5 nm
- Applied over 180° to 360° of trabecular meshwork.
- Spot size: 50 μm
- Power: 100 mW
- Duration: 0.1 s

SLT
- Q-switched frequency doubled Nd:YAG laser (532 nm)
- Spot size: 400 μm
- Small 'champagne' bubbles should appear with a proper energy setting (Fig. 21.10).

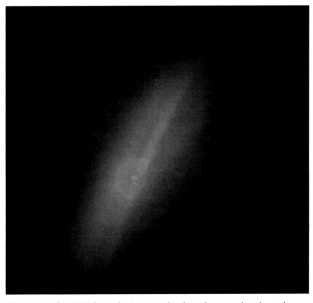

Fig. 21.10: The spot of an SLT laser being applied to the nasal trabecular meshwork has a diameter of 400 μm. Small 'champagne' bubbles should appear with a proper energy setting.

Complications of Laser Treatments

- IOP rise, synechiae formation, hyphema, and uveitis
- Will not blunt the early post-operative IOP spike occurring after cataract surgery

Cataract Surgery Followed by Filtering Surgery

Reserved only for medically uncontrolled IOP following cataract surgery in early or late postoperative period. It is also the solution to eyes that have an unexpected rise in IOP after cataract surgery, despite the fact that the surgery went well.

Combination of Newer Antiglaucoma Surgeries and Cataract Surgery

Filtering surgery, although being the gold standard, is not free of complications, majority of which are bleb related.

Tubes, valved or nonvalved are gradually replacing conventional trabeculectomies. In such surgeries, the valve is secured initially, then phaco is completed in a regular manner and lastly the tube is inserted into the anterior chamber followed by tube fixation and closure (Figs. 21.11A to C).

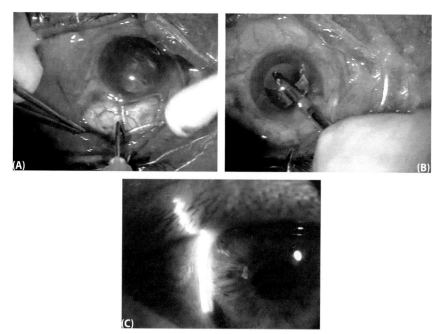

Figs. 21.11A to C: (A) A long needle-generated tunnel is made before phaco is started when the Ahmed valve is fixed in place. (B) Viscoelastic material under the IOL is aspirated, but it is left over the IOL in the anterior chamber to reduce chances of hypotony. (C) Final postoperative outcome; the tube is directed tangential to the limbus, away from the pupil to reduce chances of endothelial trauma in the visual axis.

Additional newer surgical options such as MIGS, are also available, which can be combined with cataract surgery.[22] Most of them are preferable in mild to moderate glaucoma cases, although Xen might be an exception.

Types of Procedures

- Deep sclerectomy: Procedure is initiated. Just before cleaving the sclera-Descemetic membrane, tunnel is prepared, phaco with IOL implantation is completed followed by cleavage of the membrane and completion of the surgery (Fig. 21.12).
- Viscocanalostomy
- Canaloplasty (Figs. 21.13A and B)

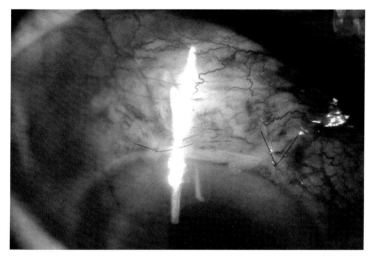

Fig. 21.12: First day after successful phaco cum nonpenetrating deep sclerectomy. The anterior chamber is well formed, a diffuse bleb without leaks can be seen.

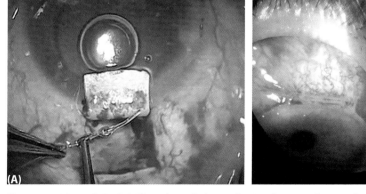

Figs. 21.13A and B: (A) The glaucolight probe is about to be used to cannulate Schlemm's canal after the phaco has been made. (B) First postoperative day of phaco cum canaloplasty procedure. The anterior chamber is well formed, no bleb is formed, the prolene suture inside Schlemm's canal is tensioning the trabecular meshwork, which lowers IOP by increasing outflow through the conventional pathway.

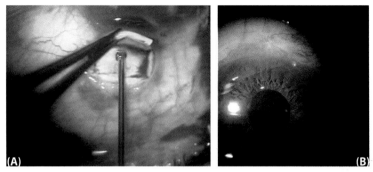

Figs. 21.14A and B: (A) Ex-Press shunt is implanted under a previously constructed superonasal scleral flap after a hypermature cataract removal through a temporal self-sealing small incision cataract surgery. (B) One month after surgery vision improved from light perception to 20/60 and IOP was 11 mm Hg without medications.

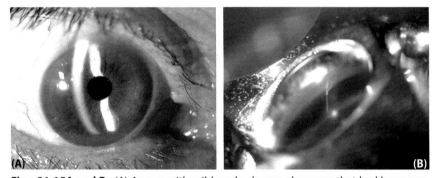

Figs. 21.15A and B: (A) An eye with mild angle closure glaucoma that had been controlled on two topical medications and a patent iridotomy 8 days after an uneventful clear-corneal phaco with a multifocal IOL plus inferonasal iStent is now medication-free. (B) Gonioscopic view through a four-mirror lens of the iStent of the case.

- Ex-PRESS shunt (Figs. 21.14A and B)
- iStent (Figs. 21.15A and B)
- *Xen:* Xen is a new gel stent for surgical intervention in refractory glaucoma.
- *Trabectome:* Phacoemulsification can be done through same incision as that of the trabectome.
- Kahook Dual Blade (KDB) ab-internal trabeculotomy (Figs. 21.16A and B)
- Endocyclophotocoagulation (ECP): Variable and irreversible response.[23]

Indications and Advantages of Newer Procedures

- Mild to moderate reduction in IOP desired
- Mild tomoderate glaucomatous neuropathy

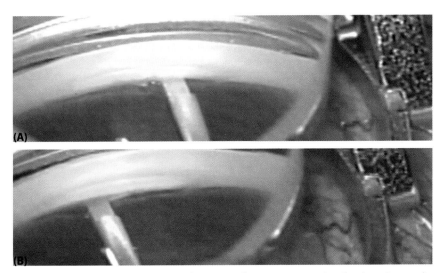

Figs. 21.16A and B: (A) The KDB is being used to remove a strip of trabecular mesh-work from the nasal angle. Some bleeding is expected from the canal due to reflux. (B) A pigmented strip of trabecular meshwork is being removed with the tip of the KDB, and a white portion of visible Schlemm's canal can be seen on the opposite side of the KDB.

- Reduce drug requirement
- Avoid blebs
- Safety profile and complication rates better than conventional glaucoma surgeries
- Do not preclude conventional filtration surgery at a later date as they are conjunctiva independent
- Those performed through the same phaco incision induce no additional astigmatism e.g., Xen, iStent, KDB, ECP. Trabectome and might permit the use of toric IOLs for a lower final residual distance refraction, or monovision planning in patients with moderate to advanced glaucoma.

Disadvantages

- Frequent patient follow-up is crucial
- Surgeon expertise required
- Inadvertententry into the anterior chamber is common with the nonpenetrating surgeries
- Limited evidence about efficacy of procedures

General guidelines for management have been shown in a Flowchart 21.1 below as described by Brown et al.[24] .

Comparison of the different surgical options has been highlighted in Table 21.4.

Flowchart 21.1: Empirical guidelines for management of coexistent cataract and glaucoma.

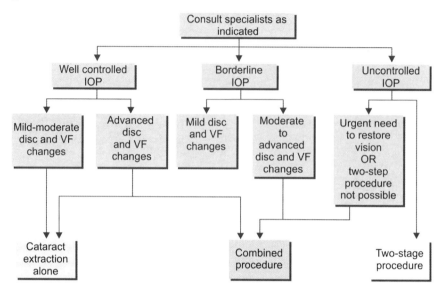

Table 21.4: Comparison of different surgical options for management of coexistent cataract and glaucoma.

	Cataract surgery only	Trabeculectomy only	Combined surgery	Phaco and MIGS
Visual rehabilitation	Faster	Slower, hastens cataract progression	Slower	Faster
Postoperative course	Shorter	Longer	Much Longer	Shorter
IOP reduction	Transient, Occasional IOP spikes	Significant	Moderate	Moderate
Need for glaucoma drugs	Usually needed	Usually not needed	Not often needed	Usually not needed
Complications	Few	Moderate	More	Few

IOL Considerations in a Glaucoma Patient

- Aspheric and blue light filtering IOLs maybe considered as they improve the contrast sensitivity.[25]
- Toric IOLs have limitations considering the refractive changes that may possibly be induced by a filtering surgery and the resultant bleb.[25]
- Multifocal (MF) IOLs may augment the photic phenomenon and contrast sensitivity problems in glaucomatous eyes.[26]
- Visual field and imaging results may be inaccurate in eyes with MF IOLs.[17]

All these problems are seen more with refractive MF IOLs than diffractive types.[27]

Diffractive types, which are pupil independent, can be considered in miotic pupils.[27]

Overall, MF IOLs are contraindicated in moderate and advanced disease and should be used with extreme caution in other glaucoma cases which under all circumstances should be well controlled and stable.[27]

- All premium IOLs should be used cautiously in PXF where decentration is a common phenomenon.
- Extended-range IOLs might become a better option since, in contrast to MF IOLs, they seem to improve contrast sensitivity.

Postoperative Care

- Frequent steroid (prednisolone 1%) and antibiotic drops. IOP should be monitored especially in steroid responders, especially in eyes where only cataract surgery is performed.
- Atropine topically to prevent malignant glaucoma, especially in angle closure cases.
- Steroids tapered slowly over 8–10 weeks.
- Systemic steroids may be needed to counter uveitis or choroidal effusions.
- If IOP lowering agents needed, avoid prostaglandin analogs and pilocarpine.
- Digital massage maybe advised in cases of combined surgery, only after confirming the complete healing of the cataract wound, which should always be closed with a single suture to reduce the risk of wound reopening following hypotony or massage.
- Reevaluate glaucoma after IOP and refraction stabilize. Reset a new baseline and modify treatment accordingly.

SUMMARY

Though there is no rule of thumb concerning which procedure best suits an eye with coexistent cataract and glaucoma. Combined surgery is an effective approach in managing the two conditions together providing the benefit of rapid visual rehabilitation and IOP reduction in one surgery. Treatment, however, has to be individualized based on surgeon's comfort, patient's expectations and patient's ocular, systemic and socio-economic status. Meticulous planning and vigilant follow-up yield gratifying results in these eyes, which are at risk of preventable blindness due to cataract and glaucoma.

Key points in management are summarized below:
- Individualize management for each glaucoma patient and each eye. Decision making about the management of coexisting cataract and glaucoma involves a careful consideration of multiple factors as discussed above.

- Whenever possible, first perform the cataract surgery, reevaluate the severity of glaucoma, baseline IOP and target IOP. Rethink about your decision regarding the need of glaucoma surgery.
- In case performing combined surgery, remember it is less efficacious than trabeculectomy alone.
- Two-site procedure is more effective than single site combined surgery.
- Keep in mind the impact of cataract extraction on filtering bleb, and aggressively manage any signs of bleb failure.
- Reiterate that glaucoma is a lifetime disease and cataract surgery may improve vision, but does not cure the vision loss due to glaucoma. The importance of a lifelong follow-up despite better vision following surgery cannot be over emphasized.

REFERENCES

1. Friedman DS, Jampel HD, Lubomski LH, et al. Surgical strategies for coexisting glaucoma and cataract: an evidence-based update. Ophthalmology. 2002;109(10):1902-13.
2. Lee RK, Gedde SJ. Surgical management of coexisting cataract and glaucoma. Int Ophthalmol Clin. 2004;44(2):151-66.
3. Eid TM, Spaeth GLS. Glaucoma associated with lens disorders. The Glaucomas: Concepts and Fundamentals. Philadelphia, PA: Lippincott Williams & Wilkins;2000. p. 160.
4. Chung HJ, Choi JH, Lee YC, et al. Effect of cataract opacity type and glaucoma severity on visual field index. Optom Vis Sci. 2016;93(6):575-8.
5. Rao HL, Jonnadula GB, Addepalli UK, et al. Effect of cataract extraction on Visual Field Index in glaucoma. J Glaucoma. 2013;22(2):164-8.
6. Holló G, Naghizadeh F, Hsu S, et al. Comparison of the current and a new RTVue OCT software version for detection of ganglion cell complex changes due to cataract surgery. Int Ophthalmol. 2015;35(6):861-7.
7. Gazzard G, Foster PJ, Devereux JG, et al. Effect of cataract extraction and intraocular lens implantation on nerve fibre layer thickness measurements by scanning laser polarimeter (GDx) in glaucoma patients. Eye (Lond). 2004;18(2):163-8.
8. Park RJ, Chen PP, Karyampudi P, et al. Effects of cataract extraction with intraocular lens placement on scanning laser polarimetry of the peripapillary nerve fiber layer. Am J Ophthalmol. 2001;132(4):507-11.
9. García-Medina JJ, García-Medina M, Dorta SG, et al. Effect of posterior capsular opacification removal on scanning laser polarimetry measurements. Graefes Arch Clin Exp Ophthalmol. 2006;244(11):1398-405.
10. Hayashi K, Hayashi H, Nakao F, et al. Changes in anterior chamber angle width and depth after intraocular lens implantation in eyes with glaucoma. Ophthalmology. 2000;107(4):698-703.
11. Kim DD, Doyle JW, Smith MF. Intraocular pressure reduction following phacoemulsification cataract extraction with posterior chamber lens implantation in glaucoma patients. Ophthalmic Surg Lasers. 1999;30(1):37-40.

12. Tong JT, Miller KM. Intraocular pressure change after sutureless phacoemulsi-
    fication and foldable posterior chamber lens implantation. J Cataract Refract
    Surg. 1998;24(2):256-62.
13. Miyake K, Asakura M, Kobayashi H. Effect of intraocular lens fixation on the
    blood-aqueous barrier. Am J Ophthalmol. 1984;98(4):451-5.
14. Johnstone MA. The aqueous outflow system as a mechanical pump: evidence
    from examination of tissue and aqueous movement in human and non-human
    primates. J Glaucoma. 2004;13(5):421-38.
15. Wang N, Chintala SK, Fini ME, et al. Ultrasound activates the TM ELAM-1/IL-1/
    NF-kappaB response: A potential mechanism for intraocular pressure reduc-
    tion after phacoemulsification. Invest Ophthalmol Vis Sci. 2003;44(5):1977-81.
16. Dada T, Bhartiya S, Begum Baig N. Cataract surgery in eyes with previous glau-
    coma surgery: pearls and pitfalls. J Current Glaucoma Practice. 2013;7(3):99-
    105.
17. Murthy GJ. Challenges in the management of glaucoma coexistent with cata-
    ract. Kerala J Ophthalmol. 2010; 22(4):325-9.
18. Costa VP, Smith M, Spaeth GL, et al. Loss of visual acuity after trabeculectomy.
    Ophthalmology. 1993;100(5):599-612.
19. Lumme P, Laatikainen L. Exfoliation syndrome and cataract extraction. Am J
    Ophthalmol. 1993;116(1):51-5.
20. Swain S, Das S, Subudhi BNR, et al. Decision making in surgical management—
    coexisting cataract and primary open angle glaucoma. Odisha J Ophthal.
    2015;88-90.
21. Park HJ, Weitzman M, Caprioli J. Temporal corneal phacoemulsification com-
    bined with superior trabeculectomy; a retrospective case-control study. Arch
    Ophthalmol. 1997;115(3):318-23.
22. Budenz, DL, Gedde SJ. New options for combined cataract and glaucoma sur-
    gery. Current Opin Ophthalmol. 2014;25(2):141-7.
23. Kahook MY, Schuman JS, editors. Chandler and Grant's Glaucoma. 5th edition.
    Thorofare, NJ: Slack Inc.; 2013.Vol. 2, p. 575.
24. Brown R, Zhong L, Lynch M. Lens-based glaucoma surgery: using cata-
    ract surgery to reduce intraocular pressure. Cataract Refract Surg. 2014;40:
    1255-62.
25. Eid TM. Primary lens extraction for glaucoma management: are review article.
    Saudi J Ophthalmol. 2011;25(4):337-45.
26. Teichman JC, Ahmed IK. Intraocular lens choices for patients with glaucoma.
    Curr Opin Ophthalmol. 2010;21(2):135-43.
27. Ichhpujani P, Bhartiya S, Sharma A. Premium IOLs in glaucoma. J Current Glau
    Prac. 2013;7(2):54-57.
28. Nongpiur ME, He M, Amerasinghe N, et al. Thickness, and position in Chinese
    subjects with angle closure. Ophthalmology. 2011;118(3):474-9.

22

Progression of Optic Disk and Visual Field Changes in Glaucoma

Murali Ariga

INTRODUCTION

Glaucoma is defined as a progressive optic neuropathy and therefore optic disk examination and visual field evaluation are of fundamental importance.

HOW TO EXAMINE AND DOCUMENT CHANGES IN THE OPTIC NERVE HEAD?

Clinical examination of the optic nerve head (ONH) can be done with direct and indirect ophthalmoscopes but is best performed in a dilated pupil on a slit-lamp biomicroscope using either 78 or 90 D handheld lenses. The advantages of this examination include the magnification provided by the slit-lamp and stereoscopic view provided by these lenses. Certain characteristic optic disk features are typical of glaucoma.

NEURAL RIM

Uniform pink color, contour and thickness of the neural rim are generally found in the normal eye (Fig. 22.1). The disk obeys 'ISNT' rule, which means that usually the inferior rim is the thickest followed by superior, nasal and temporal rim. Glaucomatous changes noted are rim loss, notches in superior, inferior rim or both. Concentric enlargement of the cup with concentric rim thinning may also occur.

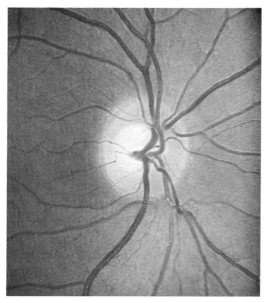

Fig. 22.1: Normal optic disc with healthy uniform neural rim.

RETINAL NERVE FIBER LAYER

The retinal nerve fiber layer (RNFL) may show slit- or wedge-shaped defects. They are seen as dark areas in an arcuate pattern wider than the retinal vessels.

BLOOD VESSEL CHANGES

When neural rim loss occurs, the overlying circumlinear vessel may be 'bared.'

PERIPAPILLARY ATROPHY

Peripapillary atrophy (PPA) or a temporal crescent of chorioretinal and retinal pigment epithelial (RPE) layer atrophy is noted in two zones, namely outer alpha and inner beta zones. The area of atrophy may correspond to the area of neural thinning. Beta zone atrophy occurs more often in glaucoma patients than in normal individuals and enlargement may indicate a progressive glaucoma.

CUP–DISK RATIO

An increase in cup-disk ratio (CDR) and asymmetry of CDR of 0.2 or greater between the two eyes have been considered as important signs of primary open-angle glaucoma. However, an assessment of optic disk size is important because smaller disks will have smaller cups. It has been noted that there is a tendency to overdiagnose glaucoma in larger disks with larger cups and miss the diagnosis of glaucoma in smaller disks in which the rim changes may be subtle. A classical glaucomatous optic disk will usually present a rim loss, inferior notch, peripapillary atrophy and disk hemorrhage (Fig. 22.2).

The European Glaucoma Society[1] has suggested schematic guidelines for the glaucomatous changes in the optic nerve head (Fig. 22.3).

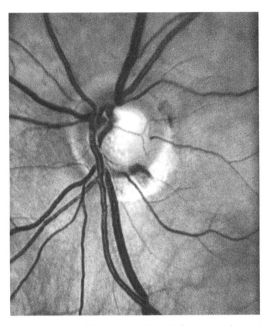

Fig. 22.2: Glaucomatous optic disk with rim loss, inferior notch, peripapillary atrophy and disk hemorrhage.

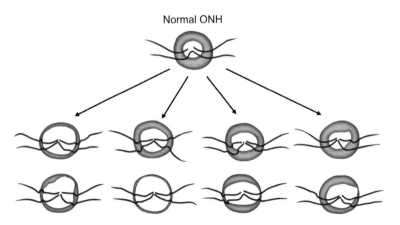

Fig. 22.3: Schematic changes in ONH (adapted from European Glaucoma Society guidelines).

DOCUMENTATION

Documentation of the ONH changes in glaucoma can be done by the following procedures:

- Changes can be documented in the form of a diagram in the patient's chart.
- Fundus photography/stereophotography/red-free photography can provide details.
- Imaging of the optic disk and RNFL using imaging devices like GDx, HRT or optical coherence tomography (OCT).

DETECTING CHANGE OR PROGRESSION IN GLAUCOMA

- Objective (structural) changes seen in ONH/RNFL/Disc hemorrhages
- Subjective (functional) changes seen in visual fields
- Changes noted on serial testing with imaging devices (OCT, Heidelberg retinal tomography (HRT) and GDx VCC)

SIGNIFICANCE OF OPTIC DISK HEMORRHAGES (DRANCE HEMORRHAGES)

The prevalence of these hemorrhages is about 0.2% in the normal population. However, a larger proportion of glaucoma patients have these hemorrhages which are thought to be RNFL infarction. They are intermittent and tend to disappear over time. Very often they are missed on clinical examination and seen only in photographs. Recent publications have confirmed that the appearance of disk hemorrhages is associated with glaucoma progression.[6]

DETECTION PROGRESSION IN VISUAL FIELDS

Detecting progression in a chronic and slowly progressive disease like glaucoma is difficult. Monitoring visual fields is only one means of assessing progression. In following visual fields in glaucoma patients, it is often difficult to differentiate between normal short-term and long-term fluctuations and true disease progression. Due to variability, a new change on a visual field needs to be confirmed on repeat testing.

FLUCTUATION VERSUS PROGRESSION

The main problem in deciding whether or not a glaucoma patient's visual field loss is progressing is to separate true progression from changes due to variability or fluctuation between tests. Fluctuation[2] is defined as the variability in the response to the same stimulus that is not due to true disease progression. As visual fields testing is a subjective examination, variable responses may be obtained each time the test is performed (intertest or long-term fluctuations) or during the same test (intratest or short-term fluctuations). Fluctuation varies among patients and among sectors in the same visual field, and increases with severity of disease. To detect true progression, one has to evaluate whether the observed change exceeds the expected fluctuation in the tested area.

Visual field progression in glaucoma may be seen as

- Development of a new defect
- Deepening or enlargement of a preexisting defect
- Diffuse loss of sensitivity (less common).

Most often progression is identified as a deepening of a preexisting scotoma (as shown by various research studies), along with enlargement of the scotoma. In a study[3] evaluating visual field progression in glaucoma, most cases showed deepening (86%) or enlargement (23%) of a previous scotoma, while none of the eyes developed new visual field defects in previously normal areas. This highlights the importance of evaluating areas adjacent to existing scotomas when searching for visual field progression. However, these adjacent areas are also known to exhibit larger degrees of fluctuation, which makes identification of true progression more difficult. Diffuse sensitivity loss may also represent glaucoma progression, although it is usually accompanied by new defects or worsening of previous focal defects. Progressive diffuse loss should raise the suspicion of cataract progression and must be correlated with clinical examination.

The Humphrey field analyzer (HFA) has statistical software, STATPAC, which is capable of analyzing a single visual field for abnormalities or a series of fields for progression. The single field analysis provides a printout of a single visual field with most detailed information about that test. In the Overview printout, several visual fields are arranged chronologically on the same page for the ease of comparison. The Change Analysis printout provides a chronologic box plot analysis, the time course of the four global indices (only MD and PSD in SITA) and the linear regression analysis of MD.

HOW FREQUENTLY SHOULD VISUAL FIELDS BE DONE TO ASSESS GLAUCOMA PROGRESSION?[2]

Most glaucoma patients under treatment will have slow rate of progression over the years, but there are those few who will have rapid progression rates. Published rates for mean deviation (MD) deterioration in glaucoma patients have varied and depends on individual susceptibility, severity of disease and treatment strategies.[4] One should perform enough visual fields at the beginning of follow-up in order to detect cases that present with fast progression rates. It has been suggested that six visual field examinations be done in the first 2 years, in order to rule out aggressive disease and to establish a consistent baseline. Subsequently, the frequency of testing may be reduced to once or twice yearly as long as no change is detected. At any time during follow-up that a change is identified on the visual field, one should not wait another year to proceed with a confirmatory test, but instead the frequency of examinations should again be increased in order to confirm or exclude progression.

EVENT- AND TREND-BASED ANALYSES

There are two main approaches to analyze progression: event-based and trend-based analyses. The first approach compares the current examination with a previous one (usually the baseline test). If the results are significantly worse on the follow-up examination, progression is indicated. This is called *event-based analysis*. In the second approach, instead of only comparing a few tests, one looks for progressive change by analyzing all the tests available in a specific period of time. This is called *trend-based analysis*, as a trend in the values is plotted over time, and significant deterioration can be assessed by observing the slope or decline of the regression line. Besides evaluating whether progression has occurred, trend-based analysis also allows an estimation of the rate of progression. It is well known that some patients deteriorate faster than others, and estimating each individual's rate of progression may help decide aggressiveness of treatment and the response to treatment.

The older software version is the Glaucoma Change Probability (GCP) software. The GCP performs individual comparisons of each visual field point on follow-up examinations with a set of baseline fields. Progression is flagged if two or more adjacent points within adjacent to an existing scotoma show significant deterioration confirmed on two consecutive tests. The GCP performs individualized analysis of the sectors in the visual field; however, as it is based on the total deviation plot, it is affected by diffuse media opacities such as cataract.

The new Guided Progression Analysis (GPA) software was developed to overcome the limitations mentioned above. Both the GCP and the GPA are event-based analyses, but the GPA has following advantages when compared with the GCP.

- The GPA is based on the pattern deviation plot, as opposed to the total deviation plot used by the GCP. Therefore, the GPA evaluates progression adjusted for diffuse effects.
- The GPA runs not only on SITA tests, but also accepts full-threshold tests for the baseline pair (the GCP did not), which is convenient as some patients with long-term follow-up have been tested with the full-threshold strategy during early follow-ups.

As detection of new or progressing visual field defects is performed by comparison to the baseline, it is imperative to have reliable baseline examinations. The software automatically selects the first two available examinations as the baseline tests. However, one can override this automatic selection to a more suitable time-point (e.g., change in therapy after progression), or to reject fields that are unreliable due to initial learning effects (which could reduce the sensitivity to detect progression). The GPA software then compares each follow-up test to the average of the baseline tests. It identifies points that show change greater than the expected variability (at the 95% significance level), as determined by previous studies with stable glaucoma patients (Fig. 22.4). If significant change is detected in at least three points

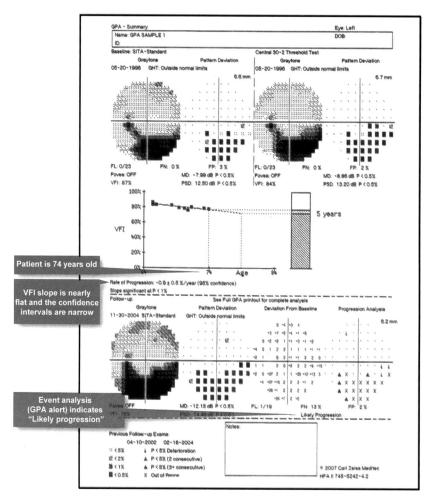

Fig. 22.4: Visual field loss progression using the GPA in sample analysis .
Courtesy: Carl Zeiss Meditec brochure 2008.

and is repeated in the same points over two consecutive follow-up tests, then the GPA software will flag the last examination as *Possible Progression*. If the same three or more points have significant change detected and repeated in three consecutive follow-up tests, the GPA software will flag the last examination as *Likely Progression*.

The latest version of the Humphrey field analyzer provides the visual field index (VFI) and VFI progression plot.[5] The VFI is a newly developed index that is proposed to evaluate the rate of progression. The aim of this analysis is not to detect progression, which can be done with the GPA, but to provide valuable information on the rate of deterioration. The VFI is calculated as the percentage of normal visual field, after adjustment for age. Therefore, a VFI of 100% represents a completely normal visual field, while a VFI of 0% represents a perimetrically blind visual field. The VFI is shown on the GPA printout both as a percent value for each individual examination and as a trend analysis, plotted against age. While the MD is based only on the total deviation map, and thus is largely affected by cataract, the VFI is based both on the pattern deviation and the total deviation probability maps. The former (pattern deviation) helps in the identification of possibly progressing points and the latter (total deviation) is used for the actual calculation of change of the total deviation value. In addition, the VFI algorithm gives weightage for different locations, giving more weight to the central points. The final VFI score is the mean of all weighted scores. For glaucoma patients with worsening cataract, however, the VFI showed a slower rate of progression than the MD, which would be a more accurate representation of the actual rate of glaucoma progression. Conversely, for glaucoma patients who had cataract surgery during follow-up, improvement in media clarity masked glaucoma progression when assessed by the MD. It did not happen when assessment was performed with the VFI. The VFI also provides an estimate of the visual field loss that will occur in the next 5 years, assuming that the same rate of progression is maintained. This is valuable for the treating ophthalmologist as it estimates the number of years that a patient has before advancing to blindness. A summary of the progression of visual field loss analysis is presented in Table 22.1.

Table 22.1: Summary of progression analyses available in HFA.

Tool used	Index used for analysis	Analysis	Progression
Mean deviation (MD) plotted against time	Mean deviation	Plots MD values over time	Decrease in MD over time
Glaucoma change probability	Total deviation	Compares individual field points at follow-up to baseline	Two or more adjacent points in or next to an existing scotoma show a significant deterioration on two consecutive tests
Guided progression analysis	Pattern deviation	Compares each follow-up tests to the average of the two baseline tests; identifies points that show change at the 95% significance level	Possible progression = significant change in at least three points that is repeated over two consecutive tests; likely progression = significant change in a least three points that is repeated over three consecutive tests.
Visual field index	Mean deviation and pattern deviation	Provides information on the rate of progression; gives more weight to central visual field points	Provides an estimate of additional field loss that will occur over the next 5 years given a steady rate of deterioration

PROGRESSION ANALYSIS USING OCTOPUS EYE SUITE PERIMETRY

The Octopus Eye suite software provides a number of useful analyses such as:
- The overview analysis provides an overview of all previous examinations to show and look for changes (Fig. 22.5).
- It can also provide bilateral viewing as a two on one report.
- Trend analysis of the mean defect (MD) helps to calculate the rate of progression per year including the probability level and fluctuations (Fig. 22.6).
- The trend graph also shows areas for normal range (gray band), impaired (15 dB) and legal blindness (25 dB).
- A red icon arrow will be displayed when significant worsening is noted (Fig. 22.7).
- Trends can also be shown for sLV, DD, Cluster analysis and Polar graphs.

MONITORING PROGRESSION WITH PHOTOGRAPHY AND IMAGING DEVICES

- Optic disk and RNFL documentation using a fundus camera is an established method. This method has the advantage of being objective, simple and easy to interpret by a clinician. Changes in the rim, cup–disk ratio, vessel changes, RNFL loss and progressive enlargement and development of new disk hemorrhages can be well documented. However, the disadvantages of photography include possible disagreement in diagnosis even between experts and also that change cannot be quantified. Data from the

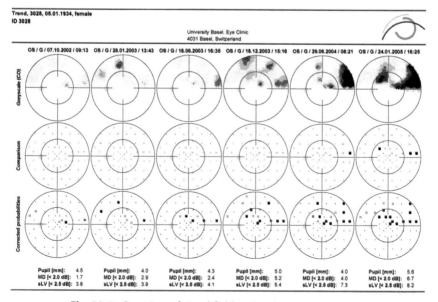

Fig. 22.5: Overview of visual fields using Octopus perimeter.

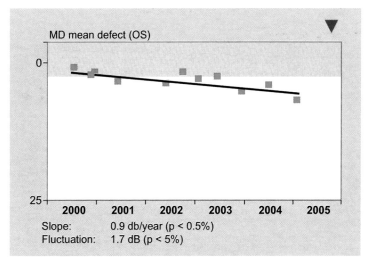

Fig. 22.6: Trend for MD indicates worsening of the field over time (red downward arrow).

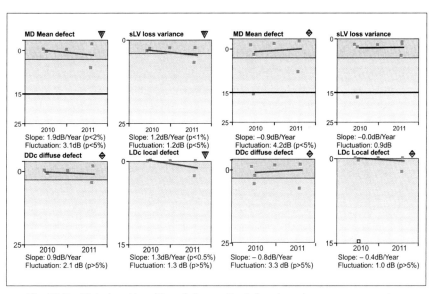

Fig. 22.7: Global and local Trends in a patient showing glaucoma progression.

Ocular Hypertension Study (OHTS) show that in many cases glaucoma progression and optic disk hemorrhages were detected on photographs by trained observers and not on routine clinical examinations.[6]

- Imaging devices: Imaging devices are in widespread use now and these include the GDx nerve fiber analyzer, which is a scanning laser polarimeter that quantifies RNFL thickness by providing a map of the retardation of polarized light in the parapapillary retina. The recent GDx VCC has a variable corneal compensator to provide patient-specific neutralization of corneal light retardation. The more recent GDx ECC provides accurate assessment in eyes with pale fundus and myopia. The HRT is a confocal scanning laser ophthalmoscope and gives quantitative measurements of the optic disk, rim and cup size along with three-dimensional height map. New software (glaucoma probability score) developed for HRT III gives ONH measurement without the need to draw a contour line. OCT is available as spectral domain and time domain techniques. Although both give quantitative measurements of RNFL thickness (sector wise and overall average), the spectral domain is capable of 3-D imaging and provides higher resolution.

These imaging based technologies for quantitative assessment are continuously evolving (software and hardware) and there are currently no clear-cut guidelines (which technology should be used and how often?) to monitor progression using these devices. HRT has been the instrument with the longest track record and published data are available on progression detection using HRT.

THE FUTURE

GDX Glaucoma Progression Analysis (GPA)

It can help identify progressive RNFL loss, using terminology that is similar to what is used by GPA on the Humphrey Field Analyzer determine the rate of progression, in terms of microns per year and the confidence interval help assess treatment efficacy by comparing progression before and after treatment.

Progression Monitoring using OCT

Currently, one can use the Stratus OCT's Serial Analysis function to follow patients. Basically, it is an overlay of the RNFL thickness at each of the 256 points along the scan. A different color represents each visit date. A new version of the software, GPA Advanced Serial Analysis, will be available soon, which takes into account measurement variability, scan quality and the patient's age. It displays an overlay of multiple thickness profiles and provides progression analysis of average RNFL thickness by quadrants and o'clock hours. It also provides trend (regression), event analysis and reports slope of change.

In studies evaluating the ability of imaging instruments to detect glaucoma progression, it is observed that a large proportion of patients show progression by imaging instruments only, but the clinical relevance of progression detected only by imaging instruments is still unclear. Several studies have evaluated the ability of optical imaging technologies to detect glaucomatous change over time. Although the clinical predictive value of longitudinal progression detected by imaging instruments has yet to be established, there is some evidence that abnormal results obtained on these tests are associated with future worse outcomes in glaucoma patients and that baseline measurements may be predictive of future development of visual field loss.

REFERENCES

1. Terminology and Guidelines for Glaucoma. 3rd edition. European Glaucoma Society, 2008.
2. Kim J, Dally LG, Ederer F, et al.; AGIS Investigators. The advanced Glaucoma Intervention Study (AGIS). Distinguishing progression of glaucoma from visual field fluctuations. Ophthalmology. 2004;111(11):2109-16.
3. Boden,C, Blumenthal EZ, Pascual J, et al. Patterns of glaucomatous visual field progression identified by three progression criteria. Am J Ophthalmol. 2004;138(6):1029-36.
4. Chauhan BC, Garway-Heath DF, Goñi FJ, et al. Practical recommendations for measuring rates of visual field change in glaucoma. Br J Ophthalmol. 2008;92(4):569-73.
5. Bengtsson B, Heijl A. A visual field index for calculation of glaucoma rate of progression. Am J Ophthalmol. 2008;145(2):343-53.
6. Prata TS, De Moraes CG, Teng CC, et al. Factors affecting rates of visual field progression in glaucoma patients with optic disc hemorrhage. Ophthalmology. 2010;117(1):24-9.
7. Keltner JL, Johnson CA, Quigg JM, et al. for the Ocular Hypertension Treatment Study Group. Confirmation of visual field abnormalities in the Ocular Hypertension Treatment Study. Arch Ophthalmol. 2000 118: 1187-94.

23

Refractory Glaucoma: Management

Marshall DH, Perkins TW

INTRODUCTION

For the purposes of this chapter, refractory glaucoma will be defined as any glaucoma with intraocular pressure (IOP) inadequately controlled with maximally tolerated medical therapy or laser trabeculoplasty. Pressure-lowering efforts are then directed toward incisional surgical interventions or cyclodestructive procedures. The situation of angle-closure glaucoma unresponsive to standard therapy is also discussed.

NEOVASCULAR GLAUCOMA

Neovascular glaucoma (NVG) occurs when an abnormal fibrovascular membrane grows into the drainage angle and obstructs aqueous outflow. In the early stages, the angle may remain open but is covered by the neovascular membrane. As the membrane organizes, it can pull the angle closed with synechia formation. Urgent therapy should be instituted at the first sign of new vessel growth on the iris. If the angle is uninvolved or if the neovascular membrane has covered the angle but not closed it with synechia, then the process can often be reversed by prompt panretinal photocoagulation (PRP). Medical therapy may hold the patient's pressure in an acceptable range until the laser takes effect. If retinal visualization is inadequate due to cataract or posterior synechia, then consideration should be given to removing the cataract in conjunction with PRP. An additional procedure to control IOP such as trabeculectomy, tube shunt or endolaser could be performed at the same time. If this is not possible, then retinal cryoablation can be used instead of PRP.

Commonly, NVG is not diagnosed until synechial angle closure has compromised part or all of the angle. In this situation, PRP should still be urgently performed, but is unlikely to reopen the angle and the IOP may not be

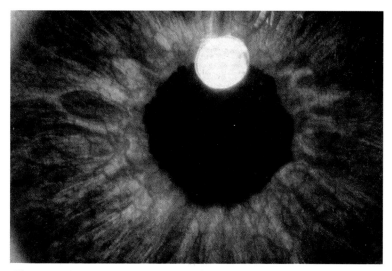

Fig. 23.1: Anterior segment neovascularisation secondary to Eales' disease.

adequately controlled with medical therapy. Further intervention is then contemplated. Trabeculectomy alone without antimetabolites has a poor chance of success. The use of mitomycin-C (MMC) greatly improves the chances of a successful outcome.[1-3] Trabeculectomy with MMC is most appropriate when the neovascular process has been controlled and the remaining angle is still closed or compromised. Conjunctiva should not be markedly inflamed or vascular. An additional surgical consideration is the presence of large new vessels on the iris (Fig. 23.1). These vessels make iridectomy at time of surgery hazardous and are likely to cause intraoperative bleeding that can be very difficult to control. Aqueous tube shunt devices offer an attractive surgical alternative.[4-6] The internal tube ostomy is less prone to fibrovascular occlusion. Conjunctival inflammation and vascularization are less of a problem. Additionally, no iridectomy is performed so that the chances of hyphema are minimized. The choice of implant can be individualized to the patient. A third option for eyes with poor visual potential is a cyclodestructive procedure such as neodymium:yttrium-aluminium-garnet (Nd:YAG) or diode laser cyclophotocoagulation.[7-10] Cyclocryoablation is also an option, although these patients may be at higher risk for complications with this procedure.[11,12] If pars plana vitrectomy (PPV) is being performed in order to address posterior segment pathology, then transpupillary endolaser[13,14] of the ciliary processes may be a viable treatment modality. A typical patient may be a diabetic with NVG where PPV is indicated to clear vitreous hemorrhage and augment the PRP.

GLAUCOMA OCCURRING AFTER RETINAL DETACHMENT SURGERY

Glaucoma occurring after retinal detachment surgery presents special challenges to the glaucoma surgeon. The conjunctiva is usually disrupted often in the locations used for trabeculectomy procedures. The presence of scleral buckling hardware makes the implantation of tube shunt devices more difficult. Scleral buckling surgery can cause intractable glaucoma mainly by an angle-closure mechanism. Structural changes induced by the buckle in addition to the use of intraocular gas and transient uveal effusions caused by injury to the vortex veins may also result in compromise to the drainage angle. Early postoperative IOP elevations are common and are treated medically.[15] Postoperative steroid drops are important to help in limiting anterior synechia formation. Adjustment of intraocular gas is sometimes necessary after surgery. Uveal effusion drainage or scleral buckle modification may all be needed in the early postoperative period.[16] If there is a question of pupillary block contributing to the raised pressure, then a laser iridotomy should be performed. If early attempts to control IOP have failed and permanent synechia develops then the pressure may be difficult to control medically. Additionally, glaucoma can develop by other mechanisms related or unrelated to the retinal pathology, such as NVG or open angle glaucoma. Surgical glaucoma management is often difficult. Trabeculectomy with MMC may be contemplated if sufficient conjunctiva is present. This can be assessed by rolling a cotton swab over the conjunctiva to evaluate if there is underlying scarring from the previous procedures. Inflammation and vascularity of the conjunctiva must also be considered as they will limit the success of trabeculectomy. A tube shunt procedure is a logical alternative to trabeculectomy. However, placing the episcleral plate over the preexisting hardware can be difficult. A technique has been described where a silicone tube connects the anterior chamber with the preexisting fibrous capsule around the buckle.[17] An ultimate success rate of 85% is reported by the authors with a mean follow-up time of 21.7 months. Surgical revisions to unblock the proximal or distal tube opening were required in 27% of patients in this small series. A related technique is to modify existing tube shunt devices. Fran et al. report a 72% chance of successful IOP control at 2 years using both modified long Denver–Krupin tubes and modified Baerveldt implants.[18] Finally, cycloablative procedures may be considered in eyes with limited visual potential as discussed below.

GLAUCOMA OCCURRING AFTER PENETRATING KERATOPLASTY

Penetrating keratoplasty may induce chronic glaucoma by a variety of mechanisms.[19] Commonly, chronic angle closure may result from the anatomic distortion of the drainage angle induced by the graft. Chronic pressure elevations have been reported in 18 per cent of penetrating keratoplasty patients.[20] High IOP in these patients is hazardous not only to the health of the optic nerve, but also to the corneal graft. When medical therapy fails to control the problem, surgical intervention is contemplated. Trabeculectomy with antimetabolites can be considered if sufficient conjunctiva exists. Extra care should be taken

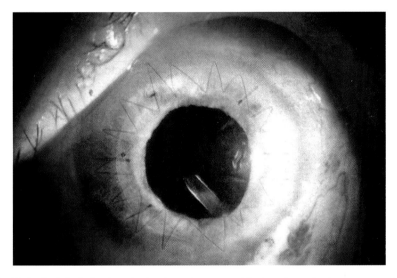

Fig. 23.2: An inferiorly placed tube shunt in an eye with chronic angle closure secondary to penetrating keratoplasty.

to avoid hypotony in the early postoperative period as compromise to the graft can take place in the presence of a flat chamber. Sutures may be tied more tightly than usual or placed in greater numbers with early postoperative suture lysis performed to control pressure elevations. Ayyala et al. reported a 17 mmHg average pressure decrease in 17 patients who underwent a trabeculectomy with MMC after PKP with two of the 17 grafts failing postoperative.[21] Tube shunts (Fig. 23.2) offer an alternative to trabeculectomy but also must be used with caution in these patients. Tube corneal touch will cause a graft to fail. Early postoperative hypotony must also be avoided. The valved implants like the Ahmed may have an advantage in this regard as they may allow early postoperative pressure control with less risk of hypotony.[22] Alternatively, placing the tube into the posterior segment through a PPV site could be beneficial if an aphakic or pseudophakic patient was undergoing PPV at the same time. Good success rates for control of IOP with tube shunts after PKP have been reported[23,24]; however, graft failure rates in these studies were quite high at 42% and 44% respectively. Cyclodestructive procedures may be considered in eyes with limited visual potential. Nd:YAG laser has been used successfully but often requires retreatment to be effective. A small series of patients undergoing this technique were studied and graft failure resulted in 6 of 14 patients, (43%), all of whom needed repeat treatments.[25] Cyclocryotherapy has also been used to treat postpenetrating keratoplasty glaucoma with reasonable success.[26]

UVEITIC GLAUCOMA

Glaucoma may result from uveitis for a variety of reasons. Anterior segment sequelae of the inflammation, such as posterior synechia, may result in iris bomb'e and subsequent angle closure. Chronic inflammation can also lead

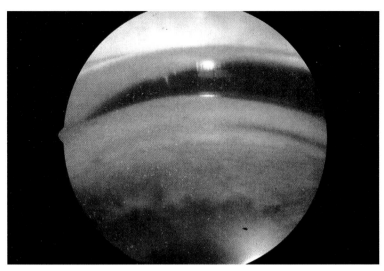

Fig. 23.3: Gonioscopic view of a partially open angle with peripheral anterior synechia in a patient with uveitic glaucoma.

to synechial closure of the angle in the absence of iris bomb'e. Open-angle glaucoma may also result, presumably from structural changes in the trabecular meshwork, from the inflammatory process (Fig. 23.3). In all cases, except for Fuchs' heterochromic iridocyclitis, control of the inflammatory process is the major concern. This along with antiglaucoma medications may control the IOP. When these measures fail, the usual surgical options are available. Trabeculectomy with antimetabolites has been shown to have good success rates.[27-29] The inflammatory process should be as quiet as possible since postoperative inflammation could compromise the outcome of filtration surgery. Additionally, a flat anterior chamber in the presence of active inflammation would cause further synechial closure of the angle. Steps should be taken to avoid this complication (see section on 'Glaucoma and Penetrating Keratoplasty'). Cataract progression may occur more often in the uveitic patient post trabeculectomy. Patitsas et al. noted cataract progression in nine out of 10 of their patients, of which seven required cataract extraction.[28]

Tube shunt devices are also an option especially in the presence of active inflammation. One to two years success rates of 79% were reported with Molteno implants.[29] Again, postoperative flat chambers are to be avoided, and the valve devices may be advantageous in this regard. Active inflammation should be controlled as much as possible because an inflamed conjunctiva could make the more posteriorly placed filtration area of the tube shunt device fail. For all surgical procedures control of perioperative inflammation is of utmost importance. Frequent topical steroids should be given pre- and postoperatively along with cycloplegic agents. Additionally, the use of periocular steroid injections (away from the intended filtration site) and the use of systemic steroids should be considered in the perioperative period. If a large amount of postoperative fibrin formation is encountered in the anterior chamber, intra-cameral tissue plasminogen activator (TPA) may be helpful in doses of 6–12.5 μg.[30] Hyphema may occur after injection and this drug should be used with caution in individuals prone to bleeding such as those with active neovascularization. Cycloablative procedures are, as usual, used as a last resort. Extra caution may be warranted in these patients because of the possibility of exacerbating the inflammatory process. Hypotony and phthisis bulbi are definite risks with these procedures. Nevertheless, cycloablative procedures such as diode and transcleral Nd:YAG lasers have been performed on patients with inflammatory glaucoma without unusually high complication rates, but the number of these patients in those studies was very small.[7,9,13]

MALIGNANT GLAUCOMA

Malignant glaucoma, also referred to as aqueous misdirection syndrome, is an uncommon condition that is classically described following incisional surgery for angle closure glaucoma.[31] The suspected pathogenesis involves aqueous being diverted posteriorly into the vitreous, leading to a forward movement of the lens–iris diaphragm and progressive shallowing of the anterior chamber with closure of the drainage angle in the presence of a patent iridectomy. Central chamber shallowing is an important feature of this syndrome and may help to distinguish it from other types of angle closure such as pupillary block. Usually associated with high IOP, this condition may start with normal or even low IOP in the setting of overfiltration or wound leak. Management is at first conservative with cycloplegic agents, typically atropine, in addition to ocular hypotensive therapy including oral hyperosmotics. This may be expected to break an attack in up to one-half of cases within 5 days. Cycloplegic therapy should then be continued indefinitely.[32]

If the attack is not broken medically, and in some cases concurrent with medical therapy, laser treatment can be attempted. The argon laser has been used to disrupt the ciliary processes if they are visible through the surgical iridotomy.[33] The Nd:YAG laser has been used to disrupt the anterior hyaloid face.[34,35] Should more conservative measures fail, surgical intervention is aimed at disrupting the vitreous. Chandler's technique involves inserting a needle through the pars plana in order to disrupt the anterior hyaloid face and remove some of the vitreous.[36,37] At the same time the anterior chamber is reformed with balanced salt solution (BSS). Pars plana anterior vitrectomy,[38] alone or in combination with lensectomy,[32] may also be used successfully to treat an attack of malignant glaucoma.

ANGLE-CLOSURE GLAUCOMA NOT RESPONSIVE TO LASER IRIDOTOMY

Primary angle closure or pupillary block glaucoma is normally treated with laser peripheral iridotomy. Oral or intravenous hyperosmotics are used to lower the IOP acutely along with topical medications which include 1% or 2% pilocarpine. Oral carbonic anhydrase inhibitors are also useful. Topical glycerine may be used to clear the cornea in order to facilitate a peripheral laser iridotomy, which is usually curative. If angle closure is due to posterior segment pathology pushing forward such as a uveal effusion, or when the patient has been in an attack of primary angle closure for more than several hours, the attack may be more difficult to break by the conventional means described above. In this sense, although not typically referred to as a refractory glaucoma, angle-closure glaucoma can be classified as refractory. We have found the technique of peripheral iridoplasty as described by Ritch et al.[39] to be very useful in these situations (see procedures section). This technique has even been used successfully as a primary treatment for angle closure prior to iridotomy.[40] It does not, however, take the place of laser iridotomy, which is necessary in both the affected and fellow eye. Should all measures fail, incisional surgery is sometimes necessary in primary acute angle closure. Attempts should be made to lower the IOP preoperatively as much as possible with ocular hypotensive agents. Trabeculectomy can be performed by the standard technique and the use of antimetabolites would be individualized to the patient's risk factors. If the lens was thought to play a major role in the angle-closure attack, consideration may be given to removing it, with subsequent placement of an intraocular lens. A technique of goniosynechiolysis has been described whereby peripheral anterior synechia (present less than 6–12 months) are swept from the angle with viscoelastic and a blunt instrument.[41] This may be helpful if done at the time of trabeculectomy.

PROCEDURES

Trabeculectomy

Trabeculectomy remains the most common surgical intervention for control of many forms of refractory glaucoma. With the introduction of antimetabolite agents such as mitomycin C (MMC) and 5-fluorouracil (5-FU), some patients who would formerly have had a poor prognosis with this procedure now enjoy improved success rates.[1-3,42-44] Patients who are particularly likely to benefit from the use of an antimetabolite are shown in Table 23.1.

Table 23.1: Indications of antimetabolites agents.

1. Prior failed trabeculectomy
2. Black race
3. Neovascular glaucoma
4. Inflammatory glaucoma
5. Aphakia or pseudophakia
6. Young patients (<40 years)

The site of trabeculectomy is normally superior, superotemporal or super-onasal. Inferior filtration blebs are associated with a higher risk of endoph-thalmitis and are best avoided.[45] The choice of site will partially depend on surgeon preference and on what conjunctiva is still mobile in the case of a previously operated eye. In an eye without prior trabeculectomy surgery, it is best to use either the superonasal or superotemporal quadrant. If an initial superonasal trabeculectomy failed, then conjunctiva would still be available superotemporally and possibly superiorly if a third trabeculectomy were ever needed. The conjunctival opening can be either limbal- or fornix-based.

Limbus-Based Flap

Constructing a limbus-based flap has the advantages of placing the incision line well under the lid and away from the site of antimetabolite application (if used). Wound leaks are less likely to be a problem given the posterior loca-tion. Disadvantages include the need for a traction suture in order to get ade-quate exposure, access to the limbus is more difficult, and closure time is often greater than with a comparable fornix-based flap. Despite its difficulties, the authors prefer the limbus-based flap. After the usual sterile preparation and draping, a large blade eyelid speculum is inserted. It is wise to mark the 12 o'clock limbus with a single dot of a fine surgical marking pen. This keeps one oriented when the eye is retracted inferiorly and helps to identify the expected location of the superior rectus muscle. A corneal traction suture is placed in the peripheral clear cornea approximately 1.5 mm from the limbus on the corneal side (Fig. 23.4). A superior rectus stay suture could also be used but has the disadvantage of potentially causing a subconjunctival hemorrhage. The authors feel exposure is best with the corneal suture and using 6-0 Dexon

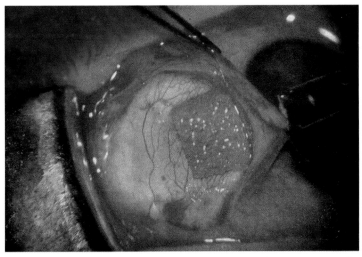

Fig. 23.4: Antimetabolite sponge in place—limbus-based flap. Note corneal traction suture.

on a DO-1 needle. Marking the conjunctiva along the intended incision line with the surgical marking pen can assist in identifying the conjunctival edges during closure. The incision should be placed 10 mm posterior and concentric to the limbus. Conjunctiva and Tenon's are opened separately with a Westcott scissors and this also facilitates accurate closure of the layers. Care must be taken to avoid the recti muscles as the incision line is well behind their insertion. Elevating the tissues off the globe before cutting helps to avoid damaging the muscles. An anteriorly placed incision is a potential cause of bleb failure. Contractional healing forces can cause the suture line to move anteriorly and this can critically limit the bleb if the original incision is not posterior enough. Dissection is carried forward to the limbus with sharp dissection under Tenon's capsule with the blunt Westcott's scissors, visualizing their tips through the conjunctiva. If necessary, remaining Tenon's insertions at the limbus can be lysed with the Gill knife. Enough limbal area needs to be exposed to create the scleral flap and also leave room for the sutures. Care is taken to control subconjunctival bleeding with light cautery. All bleeding vessels should be closed but excessive cautery should be avoided. It can cause shrinkage of the tissues and distortion of the subsequent scleral flap.

Fornix-Based Flap

Fornix-based flaps have the advantage of easier access to the surgical limbus in addition to faster closure time. They are especially useful when a cataract extraction procedure is being performed at the same time. Although some studies indicate similar success and complication rates as limbus-based flaps when antimetabolites are used in combined cataract and trabeculectomy surgery,[46] we feel that wound leaks and subsequent bleb failure is more likely, especially in the hands of a surgeon not thoroughly accustomed to this technique. When wound leaks do occur they are more difficult to eradicate without surgical intervention. The conjunctiva is disinserted from the limbus with a Westcott scissors or a number 69 blade. Relaxing radial incisions may be made on one or both sides of the conjunctival flap. The conjunctiva is undermined posteriorly with the Westcott scissors. All bleeding is controlled using light cautery.

Antimetabolites

The risk of significant complications is higher when antimetabolites are used. Hypotony and subsequent maculopathy[47] as well and bleb leaks[48] and late onset endophthalmitis[49] are all well-known side effects of trabeculectomy and occur more commonly with antimetabolite use. Therefore, many do not advocate the use of these agents in certain individuals, such as primary trabeculectomies or high myopes, unless they satisfy high-risk characteristics (Table 23.1). The choice of antimetabolites is essentially confined to intraoperative or postoperative 5-FU, or intraoperative MMC. For individuals with high-risk characteristics, MMC is the treatment of choice. It is typically applied on a soaked methylcellulose sponge cut to approximately twice the size of the filtration site (Fig. 23.4). The optimum exposure time and concentration of MMC is unknown. Typically, concentrations between 0.2 and 0.5 mg/ml of MMC are used with exposure times varying between 1 and 5 min. In general, the longer exposure times and higher concentrations are associated with a greater likelihood of complications.[50] Exposure time is adjusted relative to the patient's risk factor for failure. The sponge is usually applied on the sclera prior to dissection of the flap. Some surgeons prefer to partially dissect the scleral flap and place the sponge underneath.[51] If this method is chosen, care must be taken to ensure that the anterior chamber has not been inadvertently entered, as MMC inside the eye can have serious consequences. The conjunctival edges are carefully held away from the MMC sponge during the exposure. At the end of the exposure, the sponge is removed and the area is copiously irrigated with 30 ml of BSS. For individuals at lower surgical risk, an attractive alternative to MMC is intraoperative 5-FU. It is applied in a similar fashion to MMC. The concentration is 25–35 mg/ml and the exposure time is 5 min.[52,53] This technique gives the advantage of inhibiting fibrosis without the long-term impact of MMC. The trade-off is less antifibrosis effect, and is therefore only appropriate for moderate to lower risk patients.

The Scleral Flap

The scleral flap is then fashioned to approximately one-half corneal thickness. Square, trapezoidal or triangular flaps can all be used with success. The thinner the flap, the greater the filtration. Approximate dimensions are 3–4 mm along the limbus by 2–3 mm radially. Dissection of the flap should be carried forward into the clear cornea (Fig. 23.5). Failure to carry the dissection for enough anterior is a common cause of filtration failure and also makes the iridectomy difficult and prone to bleed if the iris root and ciliary body are incised. A paracentesis port is fashioned next, at a site that is readily accessible if the anterior chamber needed to be reformed postoperatively. We typically will use a temporal location. The anterior chamber is entered through the anterior extent of the scleral flap using a number 75 blade or similar knife. A Kelly Descemet's punch is used to fashion the ostomy, which should be punched from clear cornea and trabecular meshwork. A knife or Vannas scissors could also be used. The size and location of the ostomy also determines the filtration. In general, the ostomy should occupy the middle third of the scleral bed. Offsetting the ostomy to one side can increase filtration to that side. Increasing or decreasing the size of the ostomy will also increase or decrease the amount of filtration respectively. In addition, the closer the ostomy is to the posterior edge of the flap, the greater the filtration. A surgical iridectomy is performed next. The iris is grasped with toothed forceps and pulled through the ostomy. An iris scissors is used to make a single cut with care being taken to engage enough tissue in the scissors so that a full-thick-

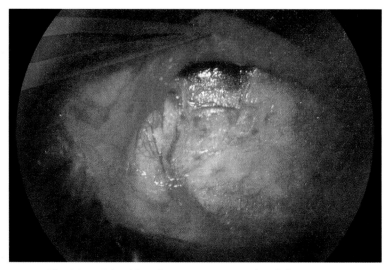

Fig. 23.5: Scleral flap dissection into peripheral clear cornea.

ness iridectomy is produced. The iridectomy should be just large enough to prevent the iris from plugging the filtration site. If vitreous is present in the anterior chamber or if it is likely to be there, as with surgical aphakia, then an anterior vitrectomy should be performed. This will prevent vitreous from obstructing the internal ostomy. The flap is repositioned using interrupted 10-0 nylon sutures. The more anterior the sutures in the sides of the flap, the more tightening effect they have. We place four to five sutures, two on the sides, two in the posterior corners and one in the back of the flap if necessary. The knots are buried so the ends will not perforate the conjunctiva at a late date. Filtration is assessed by irrigating BSS via the paracentesis port through a 30-gauge cannula. The sutured flap is dried first with a surgical sponge and then flow is assessed. A small amount of flow should be seen. Sutures are added as required. Some surgeons prefer the flap watertight and cut sutures soon after the surgery if the IOP is too high. This approach may be especially appropriate when large doses of antimetabolites are used. An alternative to buried interrupted sutures is the releasable suture. These techniques are well described elsewhere,[54] and remove the need for an argon or dye laser to perform the suture lysis.

Conjunctival Closure: Limbus Based

In the limbus-based technique, the closure is performed in one or two layers. We use 9-0 Vicryl on a cutting needle (TG 140) for the Tenon's capsule, which is closed in a running fashion. Conjunctiva is closed next using a monofilament 9-0 Vicryl on a vascular needle (BV 100), also in a running fashion. The conjunctiva is handled with nontoothed forceps to help avoid buttonholes. The closure can be performed in a single layer but we feel it is safer to close as described. This will help avoid wound leaks, especially when antimetabolites are used. Nonabsorbable sutures such as 10-0 nylon can also be used for the conjunctiva.

Conjunctival Closure: Fornix Based

The limbal corneal epithelium is denuded using a number 69 blade or cautery. The flap is then repositioned using two interrupted 9-0 Vicryl sutures on a spatulated needle. Alternatively, 10-0 nylon can be used. The limbal edge of the flap must be taut and this usually results in the edge of the conjunctiva being advanced 1–2 mm onto the cornea. If this edge is not watertight then additional 10-0 nylon sutures can be placed in a horizontal mattress or running fashion. The knots should be buried into the cornea. The radial relaxing incision(s) made in the conjunctiva may also require closure. If so, a 9-0 Vicryl on a cutting needle placed in a horizontal mattress fashion can be very useful.

Postoperative Care

Postoperatively, the eye is dressed with atropine ointment and an antibiotic. Atropine helps reduce the risk of an aqueous misdirection syndrome as well as aiding in postoperative comfort. Steroid eyedrops are mandatory after glaucoma filtration surgery. Prednisolone acetate or equivalent is used every 2 h while awake for 2–4 weeks and tapered slowly over the following months. An antibiotic-steroid combination ointment is used at night for the first month. Atropine is used two to four times daily for 1 month and then discontinued. Antibiotic drops are used for 2 weeks. Digital massage can aid in establishing flow through the filtration site in the immediate postoperative period.[50] Filtration is adjusted by suture lysis either with argon or dye laser or via releasable suture removal. If MMC has been used, suture lysis can be performed with good effect for up to 2 months. If no antimetabolites are used, then removing sutures after 2 weeks is unlikely to have much effect.

Postoperative Antimetabolites

Postoperative injections of 5-FU are also a method of delivering antimetabolite to the filtration site in patients at high risk for trabeculectomy failure.[42-44] The original protocol[42] called for two injections daily of 5 mg of 5-FU during the first postoperative week and then one injection of 5 mg daily for an additional week. The main disadvantage of this route is the need for daily postoperative follow-up and the discomfort associated with the injections. Injections are given with a 30-gauge needle, typically 90° to 180° away from the filtration site. The main toxicity is to the corneal epithelium, which can start to show punctate erosions that can progress to large corneal defects. Some surgeons will discontinue the injections once the epithelial toxicity occurs, others will continue. Another useful role of 5-FU is to augment the antimetabolite effect if the conjunctiva appears very inflamed or vascular in the early postoperative period. The authors often use this drug in the manner described above for four to eight injections, even if the patient has received intraoperative antimetabolites.

TUBE SHUNTS

Aqueous tube shunts represent an alternative to trabeculectomy under specific conditions where a trabeculectomy is likely to fail. These devices have significant complications associated with their use, which include corneal decompensation, cataract formation, tube extrusion with risk of infection, postoperative hypotony and diplopia.[55] For these reasons, tube shunts are reserved for these specific indications and should only be inserted by the eye surgeon familiar with their use (Table 23.2).

There are several different types of tube shunts currently in use. They can be broadly separated into restrictive (valved) and nonrestrictive (Table 23.3 and Figs. 23.6 and 23.7). These devices consist of a silastic tube attached to a plate, which is inserted posterior to the equator. They shunt aqueous through the tube to a reservoir formed by encapsulation of the plate. The restrictive implants limit flow through the tube until a specified level of IOP is reached. This is to help minimize postoperative hypotony. In reality, the Ahmed implant works better than the Krupin in this regard.[56] The nonvalved implants require specific surgical maneuvers (discussed later) in order to avoid postoperative hypotony. The choice of implant depends on several factors. It has been shown that the surface area of the plate is a major determining factor of postoperative pressure control.[57,58] For this reason, the double

Table 23.2: Indications of aqueous tube shunts.

1. Prior failed trabeculectomy with antimetabolite
2. Active neovascular glaucoma
3. Active uveitic glaucoma
4. Insufficient conjunctiva for a trabeculectomy

Table 23.3: Types of aqueous tube shunts.

Restrictive tube shunts (surface area in mm^2)
1. Ahmed (184)
2. Krupin disk (180)
Nonrestrictive tube shunts (surface area in mm^2)
1. Molteno, single and double plate (135,270)
2. Baerveldt (250,350,425)
3. Shockett (300)

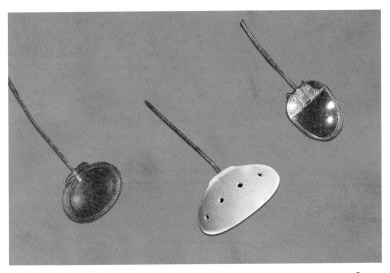

Fig. 23.6: Tube shunts—from left to right, Krupin disc, Baerveldt (350 mm²), Ahmed valve.

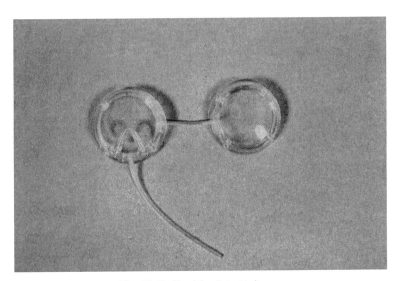

Fig. 23.7: Double plate Molteno.

plate Molteno implant and the Baerveldt implant are popular and have been shown to be comparable with respect to IOP control.[4] The double plate Molteno requires a two-quadrant dissection, and the Baerveldt only one, which may lead some to favor the Baerveldt. The Shockett implant consists of a tube connected to an encircling band. The surface area is comparable to the Molteno and Baerveldt, but this device is more complicated to insert, requiring a four-quadrant dissection and is therefore seldom used. The restrictive devices are single plates and therefore have smaller surface areas than the nonvalved implants. Nonetheless, their ease of insertion and the fact that special operative maneuvers to avoid hypotony are not required make them (especially the Ahmed) very popular. The plates are sutured near the extraocular muscles; therefore, postoperative diplopia is a concern. The size of the plate determines the size of the filtration bleb, which can affect ocular alignment. The Baerveldt implant is placed underneath the muscles and, therefore, incorporates the muscles into the fibrous capsule and postoperative diplopia has been a disadvantage.[58] Modifications in this implant, which consist of holes in the plate, are designed to limit bleb size and therefore reduce this complication. The Molteno implant has an interplate tube (Fig. 23.7), which is passed above or below the muscle and makes diplopia less of a concern. Krupin disk implantation may also be associated with intractable diplopia in some patients.[59,60] The quadrant in which the implant is placed can influence the occurrence of diplopia. In general, the superotemporal quadrant is the largest and usually employed for the Baerveldt and other single-plate devices. The inferonasal quadrant would be expected to cause the biggest problem with diplopia as the eye infraducts and converges for reading. Small misalignments in this location could be symptomatic. Concerns for closure of the conjunctiva as well as preexisting implant devices in superior quadrants may lead the surgeon to the inferior quadrants. In this situation, the authors will typically use a double plate Molteno with the tube insertion nasally. It has been suggested that Ahmed tube insertion should be avoided superonasally as the plate may damage the optic nerve if inserted too far posteriorly.[61]

The use of antimetabolites with glaucoma implant devices remains controversial. Some authors suggest it has no benefit when used over the intended plate site.[62] Others have found it to be beneficial at least during intermediate term follow-up of 2–3 years.[63,64]

Conjunctival Opening: All Devices

For the single-plate devices, a corneal traction suture is placed in a fashion described in the trabeculectomy section. The conjunctiva may be opened fornix based or limbus based, 4–6 mm from the limbus. The incision is smaller when the fornix-based opening is made. The conjunctival opening should be slightly more than 90° for the single-plate devices and approximately 220° for the double-plate Molteno. Radial relaxing incisions can aid exposure. The conjunctiva and Tenon's capsule are separated from the episcleral tissue using sharp dissection with the Westcott scissors. These scissors are then buried deep into the quadrant with their curve following that of the globe and the blades spread once and removed. Care should be taken to avoid damage to extraocular muscles and optic nerve. The extraocular muscles can be isolated with a muscle hook and 4-0 silk, and this also aids exposure especially with the two-plate device. Episcleral bleeding is controlled with light cautery. Exposure should be sufficient to allow placement of the plates at least 10 mm from the limbus.

Antimetabolites

If MMC is employed, 0.5 mg/ml is used at the site of plate attachment for 5 min. A cut surgical sponge with the handle attached is used for this purpose and the pledget is placed deep in the quadrant(s). Care is taken to avoid contact with the conjunctival edges. At the end of the exposure time the quadrant(s) is/are irrigated with 30 ml of BSS. Prior to insertion, all devices should be irrigated to assess patency. A 27-gauge cannula and BSS are used for this purpose. A full 1 ml of BSS should be irrigated through the device.

Plate Placement: Single-Plate Devices

The plate is sutured to the sclera 10–12 mm posterior to the limbus with a permanent suture such as 8-0 silk.

Plate Placement: Two-Plate Molteno

In order to avoid postoperative hypotony, we place a 4-0 Prolene suture through the anterior chamber tube and out the back of the proximal plate (the plate attached to the anterior chamber tube). Several centimeters are left extending out the back of the plate. This suture will be fed under the vertical rectus muscle and anchored to the sclera in a convenient location to facilitate later removal. This is referred to as the ripcord technique. The tube of the two-plate Molteno is usually inserted nasally. The proximal plate is passed from the temporal side either under or over the superior or inferior rectus muscle. If MMC is used, it is applied to both quadrants as described above. The plates are then sutured to the sclera as described for single plate devices.

Tube Insertion into the Anterior Chamber: All Devices

The tube insertion into the anterior chamber is a critical step and if done improperly can lead to tube-cornea touch, tube-lens touch or postoperative leaking around the tube and hypotony. The silastic tube is measured for size. Approximately, 2 mm should be visible inside the anterior chamber, and this is estimated by draping the tube over the cornea and estimating the correct length. The tube is then stretched and cut with a Vannas scissors creating a bevel toward the cornea. A 3 mm by 3 mm half-thickness scleral flap is raised at the intended entry site if the sclera is sufficiently thick. If not, this step can be omitted. The authors prefer to raise a flap as it can help prevent tube erosion at the limbus. A 23-gauge needle is used on a viscoelastic syringe. The anterior chamber is entered approximately 1 mm posterior to the limbus with the needle oriented in the plane of the iris. The needle should go straight in with care being taken to avoid side-to-side motion, which can enlarge the

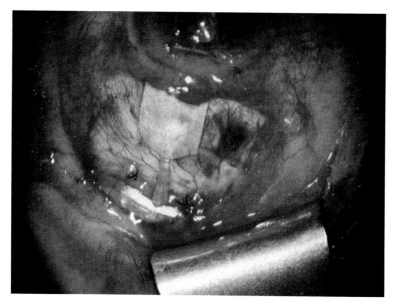

Fig. 23.8: Ahmed valve inserted superotemporally. Insertion site is covered with a scleral patch graft.

opening and cause leakage around the tube. As the needle is withdrawn, a small amount of viscoelastic is injected in order to lubricate the track. A tube forceps is then used to grasp the tube and insert it into the anterior chamber. If the tube position is not proper then it is removed and another pass of the needle can be made anterior or posterior to the original track, adjusting the angle of the needle appropriately. The tube is then anchored to the sclera with an 8-0 or 9-0 nylon suture in a horizontal mattress fashion and tied loosely. The scleral flap is repositioned with interrupted 10-0 nylon sutures with minimal tension being placed on the flap in order to avoid erosion. A scleral patch graft of (approximate dimension 4 mm by 6 mm) is then sutured over the anterior portion of the tube (Fig. 23.8).

Modification for Double-Plate Molteno: Occlusion of the Tube and Ventilation Slits

Prior to inserting the tube into the anterior chamber, the tube is occluded. A 9-0 nylon suture is tied in a clove hitch fashion near the tube–proximal plate junction, thus occluding the tube around the 4-0 Prolene suture (placed previously). A 27-gauge cannula is then inserted through the proximal end of the tube and BSS is irrigated into the lumen, ensuring that it is occluded. Anterior to this (closer to the cornea), the side of the tube is cut with a number 75 blade and a slit is made 2 lumen diameters long. This ventilation slit will allow aqueous to flow through it while encapsulation of the plate is occurring. Eventually, these slits close off as fibrosis occurs around the tube. The tube is then inserted and anchored as described above.

Conjunctival Closure: All Devices

Meticulous conjunctival closure is important with all devices. If a limbus-based flap was made then a single layer running closure with 9-0 Vicryl on a TG-140 needle is adequate. If a fornix-based opening was used then the conjunctiva should be reapproximated to the limbus with the same suture. A horizontal mattress suture to anchor the conjunctiva in front of the scleral graft is particularly important to avoid exposure of the graft. At the conclusion of the case antibiotics and a short-acting steroid are normally given as a subconjunctival injection.

POSTOPERATIVE CARE

Steroid eyedrops along with cycloplegics and antibiotics are given as described for trabeculectomy surgery. Careful evaluation of the tube position is important with early reoperation for tube-cornea or tube-lens touch. The ripcord is kept in place for 2–3 weeks if no antimetabolites have been used and for 6–8 weeks if they have been used. Removal of the ripcord is usually possible with a small incision under topical anesthesia.

CYCLODESTRUCTIVE PROCEDURES

Cyclodestructive procedures decrease IOP by destroying portions of the ciliary processes and the nonpigmented ciliary body epithelium, which produces the aqueous fluid. Advantages to the noninvasive forms of cyclodestruction include simplicity of the procedure and follow-up, generally lower cost and good success rates. Disadvantages include visual loss, postoperative inflammation and pain, transient IOP elevation, as well as phthisis bulbi. Rare reports of sympathetic ophthalmia have been described with the use of transscleral cyclophotocoagulation.[65] Because of the potential for serious complications, especially loss of vision, these procedures are typically reserved for eyes with visual acuity of 20/200 or less, or that are otherwise poor surgical candidates where the risk of elevated pressure outweighs the risks of the procedure.

CYCLOPHOTOCOAGULATION

Laser energy can be delivered to the ciliary body via a trans-scleral route or by direct visualization of the ciliary processes.

Trans-scleral

Both contact and noncontact methods are available to treat the ciliary processes. The Nd:YAG laser and newer semiconductor diode lasers are available for this purpose. Both lasers give good success rates for controlling

IOP although the various studies are hard to compare directly due to different follow-up times and success parameters. Hampton et al.[7] reported up to 95% success or qualified success rate after noncontact Nd:YAG laser when patients that needed retreatment were included (minimum 6 months follow-up). However, they also noted a 45% loss of vision in their patients, approximately half of which was due to the treatment. Schuman et al.[8] noted that contact Nd:YAG laser treatment reduced IOP below 25 mm Hg in 71% of eyes at 6 months follow-up. They reported only 7% of their patients lost two or more lines of Snellen acuity. The Diode Laser Ciliary Body Ablation Group[9] found that 72% of patients at 1 year and 52% of patients at 2 years had greater than 20% reduction in IOP or an IOP less than 23 mm Hg. Visual loss of more than five lines of acuity occurred in 19% of eyes in this study. Retrobulbar anesthesia is required for all forms of cycloablative procedures.[1] Noncontact Nd:YAG laser: The laser in the free-running thermal mode is used. For the Microruptor II (LASAG, Thun, Switzerland), maximum offset (position 9) of the aiming beam is used. Pulse duration is 20 ms and power is between 4 and 8 J. The patient is seated behind the slit lamp and the laser is aimed 1.5 mm posterior to the limbus superiorly and inferiorly, and 1 mm medially and temporally. Thirty to forty spots are applied over 360° avoiding the 3 and 9 o'clock positions where the ciliary nerves are located.[7] A special lens has been described to assist in placement of the YAG laser spots.[10] Energy settings vary with the type of machine.[2] Contact Nd:YAG laser: A sapphire-tipped probe is used for the Nd:YAG laser (Surgical Laser Technologies, PA, USA), which is used in continuous wave mode. Typical power settings are 7 W for 0.7 s. The probe is oriented 90° to the sclera and is centered 1.5 mm from the limbus by placing the anterior edge of the probe 0.5–1 mm from the limbus. The number of spots varies between 32 and 40 over 360°, avoiding the 3 and 9 o'clock positions. Contact diode laser: a similar probe is used with the solid state lasers and is referred to as G probe (Iris Medical, CA, USA). This handpiece is designed to place the tip of the probe 1.25 mm posterior to the limbus parallel to the visual axis. Typical laser settings for the Oculight system (Iris Medical) would be 1.5–2 W of power for 2–2.5 s duration.[9] Initially three quadrants are treated with six burns each for a total of 18 burns. Power is adjusted down if audible 'pops' are heard, which are caused by disruption of the ciliary process.

Transpupillary Endolaser during Pars Plana Vitrectomy

The ciliary processes can be treated at the time of pars plana vitrectomy via the argon endolaser probe used through the vitrectomy ports. Success rates of 76% and 78% have been reported.[13,14] A typical patient may be the one undergoing vitrectomy with endolaser for neovascular glaucoma. This technique is performed by vitreoretinal surgeons. After pars plana vitrectomy, the argon laser endoprobe is used at power settings of 500–700 mW with 0.5–1 s duration burns. Blue green argon laser light is used. The entire length of the ciliary process is coagulated with the endpoint being a visible whitening and central pit formation.[13] The amount of treatment is tailored to the patient, but typically 240° are treated.

Endoscopic Endolaser

A probe has been developed that combines a light source with an endoscope and an endolaser visualization with a diode laser. The ciliary processes are visualized directly via a television monitor and are precisely ablated. This can be accomplished by a pars plana approach,[66] or through a limbal incision.[67,68] Chen et al.[68] have reported a 90% success rate (average follow-up 12.9 months) for obtaining an IOP of less than 21 mm Hg. Visual loss of greater than two lines was observed in 6% of patients, with no cases of hypotony or phthisis. However, the expense of the instrumentation as well as the need for intraocular surgery may limit the widespread use of this technique.

Postoperative Care

A subconjunctival injection of a short-acting corticosteroid can help in reducing the postoperative inflammation. Frequent topical steroids approximately every 2 h while awake are used after the procedure and reduced as the inflammatory response subsides. Topical atropine is instilled into the eye and continued until the eye is comfortable, typically 2–4 weeks. If performed in conjunction with intraocular surgery, then topical antibiotics are also given for 2 weeks. The intraocular pressure can rise as a result of the procedure and should be checked on postoperative day 1. Commonly an immediate decrease of the IOP is noted.[7] Our experience suggests that this early response is often short-lived. Decisions on retreatment are delayed for 4–6 weeks at which point additional treatments are given for inadequate pressure response. Not infrequently, two or more treatments are needed to gain control of the IOP.

CYCLOCRYOTHERAPY

Cyclocryotherapy has the highest complication rate of all the cyclodestructive procedures and, therefore, is typically used only as a last resort. Approximately 60% of people will suffer visual loss,[11] and the phthisis rate ranges from 12–34% with the highest risk occurring in individuals with neovascular glaucoma.[11,12] A recent review of this treatment for refractory pediatric glaucoma has shown a 50% phthisis rate in a small group of patients with aniridia.[69] Overtreatment can be associated with anterior segment ischemia and hypotony. Success rates have been reported as high as 92% with aphakic glaucoma,[70] but much less with neovascular glaucoma.[12] Retrobulbar anesthetic is used. A nitrous oxide cryounit is normally used. A 2.5-mm probe is typical, but a 1.5–4 mm cryoprobe can be used. For the 2.5-mm probe, the anterior edge of the probe is placed 1.5 mm posterior to the limbus superiorly and 1 mm in the other quadrants. The cryotip temperature is –80°C, and the application lasts 60 s, with the iceball extending 1–2 mm into the peripheral clear cornea. Moderate pressure on the probe facilitates penetration of the iceball to the tips of the ciliary processes. The probe tip is allowed to thaw for 60 s and then be irrigated with BSS to help prevent tearing the conjunctiva. One spot should be placed per clock hour for 180° and this should be the maximum per session. If retreatment is necessary, the same area can be treated again. Not treating more than 270° in total may help to prevent anterior segment ischemia.[71] At the conclusion of the procedure a subconjunctival injection of steroid is advisable in order to treat postoperative inflammation. Topical atropine should be instilled into the eye. Postoperative care intraocular pressure elevations are frequent. The patient's IOP should be monitored the next day. All preoperative pressure medications should be continued and topical steroid drops should be given every 2 h initially and slowly tapered as the inflammatory response subsides. Retreatment can be considered in 4–6 weeks based on pressure response.

PERIPHERAL IRIDOPLASTY

The technique of argon laser peripheral iridoplasty is useful in the management of acute angle closure attacks that are not responsive to laser iridotomy and also when laser iridotomy is not immediately obtainable.[39,40]

Technique

Topical anesthetic is applied to the eye. An Abraham iridotomy lens or a Goldmann three-mirror lens (the central portion) can be used. The authors prefer the latter as the angle that is being treated can be viewed through the gonio mirror immediately after the treatment to assess the effect. The argon laser is used on the green wavelength. Red wavelengths are also very useful when corneal edema is present. A 500-μm spot size is used with powers of 200–400 mW and a 0.5 s duration burn. The spots should be placed at the extreme periphery of the cornea, ignoring any arcus senilis that may be present. Power should be titrated to visible contraction of the iris stroma, but avoiding charring of the stroma and gas bubble formation. Getting the patient to look toward the quadrant being treated may be helpful. Approximately 24 burns are placed around 360°. The patient's IOP is monitored postoperatively. Frequent topical steroids are used six to eight times daily following the procedure until the anterior chamber reaction has settled. As mentioned earlier, this technique is not a substitute for laser iridotomy, which should be performed as soon as possible in both the affected and fellow eye.

REFERENCES

1. Palmer SS. Mitomycin as adjunct chemotherapy with trabeculectomy. Ophthalmology. 1991;98(3):317-21.
2. Skuta GL, Beeson CC, Higginbotham EJ, et al. Intraoperative mitomycin versus postoperative 5-fluorouracil in high risk glaucoma filtering surgery. Ophthalmology. 1992;99(3):438-44.
3. Katz GJ, Higginbotham EJ, Lichter PR, et al. Intraoperative mitomycin versus postoperative 5-fluorouracil in high risk glaucoma filtering surgery—extended follow-up. Ophthalmology. 1995:102:1263-9.
4. Smith MF, Doyle JW, Sherwood MB. Comparison of the Baerveldt implant with the double plate Molteno drainage implant. Arch Ophthalmol. 1995;113(4): 444-7.
5. Lloyd MA, Baerveldt G, Heuer DK, et al. Initial clinical experience with the Baerveldt implant in complicated glaucomas. Ophthalmology. 1994;101(4):640-50.
6. The Krupin Eye Valve Filtering Surgery Study Group. Krupin eye valve with disk for filtration surgery. Ophthalmology. 1994;101(4):651-8.
7. Hampton C, Shields MB, Miller KN et al. Evaluation of a protocol for transscleral neodymium: YAG cyclophotocoagulation in one hundred eyes. Ophthalmology. 1990;97(7):910-7.
8. Schuman JS, Puliafito CA, Allingham RR, et al. Contact transscleral continuous wave neodymium:YAG laser cyclophotocoagulation. Ophthalmology. 1990;97:571-80.
9. Kosoko O, Gaasterland DE, Pollack IP, et al. Long-term outcome of initial ciliary body ablation with contact diode laser transscleral cyclophotocoagulation for severe glaucoma. Ophthalmology. 1996;103:1294-302.
10. Simmons RB, Shields MB, Blasini M et al. Transscleral Nd:YAG laser cyclophotocoagulation with a contact lens. Am J Ophthalmol. 1991; 112: 671-7.
11. Brindley G, Shields MB. Value and limitations of cyclocryotherapy. Graefes Arch Clin Exp Ophthalmol. 1986;224(6):545-8.
12. Krupin T, Mitchell KB, Becker B. Cyclocryotherapy in neovascular glaucoma. Am J Ophthalmol. 1978;86:24-6.
13. Zarbin MA, Michels RG, de Bustros S, et al. Endolaser treatment of the ciliary body for severe glaucoma. Ophthalmology. 1988; 95(12):1639-48.
14. Patel A, Thompson JT, Michels RG, et al. Endolaser treatment of the ciliary body for uncontrolled glaucoma. Ophthalmology. 1986;93(6):825-30.
15. Sebestyen JG, Schepens CL, Rosenthal ML. Retinal detachment and glaucoma. I—tonometric and gonioscopic study of 160 cases. Arch Ophthalmol. 1962;67(6):736.
16. Williams GA, Aaberg TM Sr. Techniques of scleral buckling. In Tasman W, Jaeger EA, (Eds): Duane's Clinical Ophthalmology, revised edition. Philadelphia, PA: Lippincott Raven; 1995. Vol. 59, p. 28.
17. Sidoti PA, Minckler DS, Baerveldt G, et al. Aqueous tube shunt to a pre-existing episcleral encircling element in the treatment of complicated glaucomas. Ophthalmology. 1994;101(6):1036-43.

18. Smith MF, Doyle JW, Fanous MM. Modified aqueous drainage implants in the treatment of complicated glaucomas in eyes with pre-existing episcleral bands. Ophthalmology. 1998;105(12):2237-42.
19. Shields MB. Glaucoma following ocular surgery. In: Darlene Barela Cook (Ed). Textbook of Glaucoma, 4th edition. Baltimore, MD: Williams and Wilkins; 1998. p. 359.
20. Foulks GN. Glaucoma associated with penetrating keratoplasty. Ophthalmology. 1987;94(7):871-4.
21. Ayyala RS, Pieroth L, Vinals AF, et al. Comparison of mitomycin C trabeculectomy, glaucoma drainage device implantation, and laser neodymium:YAG cyclophotocoagulation in the management of intractable glaucoma after penetrating keratoplasty. Ophthalmology. 1998;105(8):1550-6.
22. WuDunn D, Alfonso E, Palmberg PF. Combined penetrating keratoplasty and trabeculectomy with mitomycin C. Ophthalmology. 1999;106(2):3 96-400.
23. McDonell PJ, Robin JB, Schanzlin DJ, et al. Molteno implant for control of glaucoma in eyes after penetrating keratoplasty. Ophthalmology. 1988;95(3):364-9.
24. Rapuano CJ, Schmidt CM, Cohen EJ et al. Results of alloplastic tube shunt procedures before, during or after penetrating keratoplasty. Cornea. 1995;14(1): 26-32.
25. Cohen EJ, Schwartz LW, Luskind RD, et al. Neodymium:YAG laser transscleral cyclophotocoagulation for glaucoma after penetrating keratoplasty. Ophthalmic Surg. 1989;20(10):713-6.
26. Binder PS, Abel R Jr, Kaufman HE. Cyclocryotherapy for glaucoma after penetrating keratoplasty. Am J Ophthalmol. 1975;79(3):489-92.
27. Prata JA, Neves RA, Minckler DS, et al. Trabeculectomy with mitomycin C in glaucomas associated with uveitis. Ophthalmic Surg. 1994;25(9): 616-20.
28. Patitsas CJ, Rockwood EJ, Meisler DM, et al. Glaucoma filtering surgery with postoperative 5-fluorouracil in patients with intraocular inflammatory disease. Ophthalmology. 1993;99(4):594-9.
29. Hill RA, Nguyen QH, Baerveldt G, et al. Trabeculectomy and Molteno implantation for glaucomas associated with uveitis. Ophthalmology. 1993;100(6): 903-8.
30. Lundy DC, Sidoti P, Winarko, T et al. Intracameral tissue plasminogen activator after glaucoma surgery—indications, effectiveness and complications. Ophthalmology. 1996;103(2):274-82.
31. Yakub MK, Simmons RB, Simmons RJ. Malignant glaucoma. In El Sayyad F, Spaeth GL, Shields MB, et al. Editors. The Refractory Glaucomas. New York: Igaku-Shoin; 1995. pp. 107-42.
32. Shields MB. Glaucoma following ocular surgery. In Cook DB (Ed). Textbook of Glaucoma, 4th edition. Baltimore, MD: Williams and Wilkins; 1998. pp. 345-68.
33. Herschler J. Laser shrinkage of the ciliary processes—a treatment for malignant (ciliary block) glaucoma. Ophthalmology. 1980;87(11):1155-9.

34. Epstein DL, Steinert RF, Puliafito CA. Neodymium-YAG laser therapy to the anterior hyaloid face in aphakic malignant (ciliovitreal block) glaucoma. Am J Ophthalmol. 1984;98(2):137-43.

35. Melamed S, Ashkenazi I, Blumenthal M. Nd-YAG laser hyaloidotomy for malignant glaucoma following one-piece 7 mm intraocular lens implantation. Br J Ophthalmol. 1991;75(8):501-3.

36. Chandler PA, Simmons RJ, Grant WM. Malignant glaucoma—medical and surgical treatment. Am J Ophthalmol. 1968;66(3):495-502.

37. Shaffer RN, Hoskins HD Jr. Ciliary block (malignant) glaucoma. Ophthalmology. 1978;85(3):215-21.

38. Byrnes GA, Leen MM, Wong TP, et al. Vitrectomy for ciliary block (malignant) glaucoma. Ophthalmology. 1995;102(9):1308-11.

39. Ritch R, Liebmann JM. Argon laser peripheral iridoplasty. Ophthal Surg Lasers. 1996;27(4):289-300.

40. Lam DS, Lai JS, Tham CC. Immediate argon laser peripheral iridoplasty as treatment for acute angle closure attack of primary angle-closure glaucoma— a preliminary report. Ophthalmology. 1998;105(12):2231-6.

41. Shingleton BJ, Chang MA, Bellows AR et al. Surgical goniosynechialysis for angle closure glaucoma. Ophthalmology. 1990; 97(5):551-6.

42. The Fluorouracil Filtering Surgery Study Group. Fluorouracil Filtering Surgery Study one-year follow-up. Am J Ophthalmol. 1989;108(6):625-35.

43. The Fluorouracil Filtering Surgery Study Group. Three-year follow-up of fluorouracil filtering surgery study. Am J Ophthalmol. 1993;115(1):82-92.

44. The Fluorouracil Filtering Surgery Study Group. Five-year follow-up of the fluorouracil filtering study group. Am J Ophthalmol. 1996;121(4): 349-66.

45. Higginbotham EJ, Steven RK, Musch DC, et al. Bleb related endophthalmitis after trabeculectomy with mitomycin C. Ophthalmology. 1996;103(4): 650-6.

46. Bereska JS, Brown SV. Limbus versus fornix-based conjunctival flaps in combined phacoemulsification and mitomycin C trabeculectomy surgery. Ophthalmology. 1997;104(2):187-96.

47. Stamper RL, McMenemy MM Lieberman MF et al. Hypotonous maculopathy after trabeculectomy with subconjunctival 5-fluorouracil. Am J Ophthalmol. 1992;114(5):544-53.

48. Greenfield DS, Liebmann JM, Jee J, et al. Late-onset bleb leaks after glaucoma filtering surgery. Arch Ophthalmol. 1998;116(4):443-7.

49. Greenfield DS, Suner IJ, Miller MP, et al. Endophthalmitis after filtering surgery with mitomycin. Arch Ophthalmol. 1996;114(8):943-9.

50. Katz JL, Costa VP, Spaeth GL. Filtration surgery. In Ritch R, Shields MB, Krupin T (Eds). The Glaucomas, 2nd edition. St Louis, MO: Mosby-Year Book; 1996. Vol. 2, pp. 1684-5.

51. Beatty S, Potamitis T, Kheterpal S et al. Trabeculectomy augmented with mitomycin C application under the scleral flap. Br J Ophthalmol. 1998;82(4): 397-403.

52. Smith MF, Sherwood MB, Doyle JW, et al. Results of intraoperative 5fluorouracil supplementation on trabeculectomy for open-angle glaucoma. Am J Ophthalmol. 1992:114(6):737-41.

53. Lanigan L, Sturmer J, Baez K, et al. Single intraoperative application of 5fluorouracil during filtration surgery—early results. Br J Ophthalmol. 1994;78(1): 33-7.

54. Spaeth GL, Katz LJ, Terebuh AK. Glaucoma surgery. In Tasman W, Jaeger EA (Eds). Duane's Clinical Ophthalmology, revised edition. Philadelphia, PA: Lippincott-Raven; 1995. Vol. 5, p. 37.

55. Rosenberg LF, Krupin T. Implants in glaucoma surgery. In Ritch R, Shields MB, Krupin T (Eds). The Glaucomas, 2nd edition. St. Louis, MO: Mosby Year Book; 1996. Vol. 3, pp. 1783-1807.

56. Francis BA, Cortes A, Chen J et al. Characteristics of glaucoma drainage implants during dynamic and steady-state flow conditions. Ophthalmology. 1998;105(9):1708-15.

57. Heuer DK, Lloyd MA, Abrams DA et al. Which is better? One or two? A randomized clinical trial of single versus double-plate Molteno implantation for glaucomas in aphakia and pseudophakia. Ophthalmology. 1992;99(10):1512-9.

58. Lloyd MA, Baerveldt G, Fellenbaum PS, et al. Intermediate-term results of a randomized clinical trial of the 350 versus the 500 mm2 Baerveldt implant. Ophthalmology. 1994;101(8):1456-64.

59. Frank JW, Perkins TW, Kushner BJ. Ocular motility defects in patients with the Krupin valve. Ophthalmic Surg. 1995;26(3):228-32.

60. Cardakli UF, Perkins TW. Recalcitrant diplopia after implantation of a Krupin valve with disk. Ophthalmic Surg. 1994;25(4):256-8.

61. Leen MM, Witkop GS, George DP. Anatomic considerations in the implantation of the Ahmed glaucoma valve. Arch Ophthalmol. 1996;114(2): 223-4.

62. Lee D, Shin DH, Birt CM et al. The effect of adjunctive mitomycin C in Molteno implant surgery. Ophthalmology. 1997;104(12):2126-35.

63. Perkins TW, Cardakli UF, Eisele JR et al. Adjunctive mitomycin C in Molteno implant surgery. Ophthalmology. 1995;102(1):91-7.

64. Perkins TW, Gangnon R, Ladd W et al. Molteno implant with mitomycin C—intermediate-term results. J Glaucoma. 1998;7(2):86-92.

65. Lam S, Tessler HH, Lam BL et al. High incidence of sympathetic ophthalmia after contact and non-contact neodymium:YAG cyclotherapy. Ophthalmology. 1992;99:1818-9.

66. Uram M. Ophthalmic laser endomicroscope ciliary process ablation in the management of neovascular glaucoma. Ophthalmology. 1992;99(12): 1823-8.

67. Uram M. Combined phacoemulsification, endoscopic ciliary process ablation, and intraocular lens implantation in glaucoma management. Ophthalmol Surg. 1995;26:3346-52.

68. Chen J, Cohn RA, Shan CL et al. Endoscopic photocoagulation of the ciliary body for the treatment of refractory glaucomas. Am J Ophthalmol. 1997;124(6): 787-96.

69. Wagle NS, Freedman SF, Buckley EG et al. Long term outcome of cyclocryotherapy for refractory pediatric glaucoma. Ophthalmology. 1998;105:1921-7.
70. Bellows AR, Grant WM. Cyclocryotherapy of chronic open angle glaucoma in aphakic eyes. Am J Ophthalmol. 1978;85(5 Pt 1):615-21.
71. Stewart WC, Brindley GO, Shields MB. Cyclodestructive procedures. In Ritch R, Shields MB, Krupin T (Eds). The Glaucomas, 2nd edition. St Louis, MO: Mosby-Year Book Inc; 1996. Vol. 3, pp. 1605-20.

Index

Page numbers followed by *f* refer to figure and *t* refer to table.